THE ENGLISH–CHINESE ENCYCLOPEDIA OF PRACTICAL TRADITIONAL CHINESE MEDICINE

Chief Editor   Xu Xiangcai

Assistants   You Ke   Kang Kai

                 Bao Xuequan   Lu Yubin

英汉实用中医药大全

主　编　　徐象才

主编助理　尤　可　　康　凯

　　　　　鲍学全　　路玉滨

D1670499

Higher Education Press
高等教育出版社

20
护 理

	中文	英文	
主　编	辛守璞	寻建英	
副主编	于梅志	何筑丽	
编　者	杨　杰	张公平	丁瑞凤
	葛庆梅	张爱华	聂清浦
审　校		J·布莱克	

NURSING

	English	Chinese
Chief Editor	Xun Jianying	Xin Shoupu
Deputy Chief Editors	He Zhuli	Yu Meizhi
Editors	Zhang Gongping	Yang Jie
	Ding Ruifeng	Ge Qingmei
	Zhang Aihua	
	Nie Qingpu	
Reviser	John Black (New Zealand)	

(京) 112 号

The English-Chinese

Encyclopedia of Practical TCM

Chief Editor　Xu Xiangcai

20

NURSING

English Chief Editor　Xun Jianying

Chinese Chief Editor　Xin Shoupu

英汉实用中医药大全

主编　徐象才

20

护　理

中文主编　辛守璞

英文主编　寻建英

*

高等教育出版社出版

新华书店总店北京科技发行所发行

高等教育出版社激光照排技术部照排

高等教育出版社印刷厂印装

*

开本 850×1168　1/32　印张 17.25　字数 440 000

1992 年 12 月第 1 版　1992 年 12 月第 1 次印刷

印数 0 001—4 273

ISBN7—04—003880—3/R·18

定价　　　元

The Leading Commission of Compilation and Translation
编译领导委员会

The Commission of Compilation and Translation
编译委员会

Preface

I am delighted to learn that THE ENGLISH—CHINESE ENCYCLOPEDIA OF PRACTICAL TRADITIONAL CHINESE MEDICINE will soon come into the world.

TCM has experienced many vicissitudes of times but has remained evergreen. It has made great contributions not only to the power and prosperity of our Chinese nation but to the enrichment and improvement of world medicine. Unfortunately, differences in nations, states and languages have slowed down its spreading and flowing outside China. At present, however, an upsurge in learning, researching and applying Traditional Chinese Medicine (TCM) is unfolding. In order to maximize the effect of this upsurge and to lead TCM, one of the brilliant cultural heritages of the Chinese nation, to the world for it to expand and bring benefit to the people of all nations, Mr. Xu Xiangcai called intellectuals of noble aspirations and high intelligence together from Shandong and many other provinces in China and took charge of the work of both compilation and translation of THE ENGLISH—CHINESE ENCYCLOPEDIA OF PRACTICAL TRADITIONAL CHINESE MEDICINE. With great pleasure, the medical staff both at home and abroad will hail the appearance of this encyclopedia.

I believe that the day when the world's medicine is fully

developed will be the day when TCM has spread throughout the world.

I am pleased to give it my preface.

Prof. Dr. Hu Ximing

    Deputy Ministerof the Ministry of Public Health of the People's Republic of China,

    Director General of the State Administrative Bureau of Traditional Chinese Medicine and Pharmacology,

    President of the World Federation of Acupuncture—Moxibustion Societies,

    Member of China Association of Science & Technology,

    Deputy President of All—China Association of Traditional Chinese Medicine,

    President of China Acupuncture & Moxibustion Society.

December, 1989

Preface

The Chinese nation has been through a long, arduous course of struggling against diseases and has developed its own traditional medicine—Traditional Chinese Medicine and Pharmacology (TCMP). TCMP has a unique, comprehensive, scientific system including both theories and clinical practice. Some thousand years since its beginnings, not only has it been well preserved but also continuously developed. It has special advantages, such as remarkable curative effects and few side effects. Hence it is an effective means by which people prevent and treat diseases and keep themselves strong and healthy.

All achievements attained by any nation in the development of medicine are the public wealth of all mankind. They should not be confined within a single country. What is more, the need to set them free to flow throughout the world as quickly and precisely as possible is greater than that of any other kind of science. During my more than thirty years of being engaged in Traditional Chinese Medicine(TCM), I have been looking forward to the day when TCMP will have spread all over the world and made its contributions to the elimination of diseases of all mankind. However it is to be deeply regretted that the pace of TCMP in extending outside China has been unsatisfactory due to the major difficulties in expressing its concepts in foreign languages.

Mr. Xu Xiangcai, a teacher of Shandong College of TCM, has sponsored and taken charge of the work of compilation and translation of The English—Chinese Encyclopedia of Practical Traditional Chinese Medicine—an extensive series. This work is a great project, a large—scale scientific research, a courageous effort and a novel creation. I deeply esteem Mr. Xu Xiangcai and his compilers and translators, who have been working day and night for such a long time, for their hard labor and for their firm and indomitable will displayed in overcoming one difficulty after another, and for their great success achieved in this way. As a leader in the circles of TCM, I am duty—bound to do my best to support them.

I believe this encyclopedia will be certain to find its position both in the history of Chinese medicine and in the history of world science and technology.

Mr. Zhang Qiwen

Member of the Standing Committee of
All—China Association of TCM,
Deputy Head of the Health Department
of Shandong Province.

March, 1990

Publisher's Preface

Traditional Chinese Medicine(TCM) is one of China's great cultural heritages. Since the founding of the People's Republic of China in 1949, guided by the farsighted TCM policy of the Chinese Communist Party and the Chinese government, the treasure house of the theories of TCM has been continuously explored and the plentiful literature researched and compiled. As a result, great success has been achieved. Today there has appeared a world—wide upsurge in the studying and researching of TCM. To promote even more vigorous development of this trend in order that TCM may better serve all mankind, efforts are required to further it throughout the world. To bring this about, the language barriers must be overcome as soon as possible in order that TCM can be accurately expressed in foreign languages.

Thus the compilation and translation of a series of English—Chinese books of basic knowledge of TCM has become of great urgency to serve the needs of medical and educational circles both inside and outside China.

In recent years, at the request of the health departments, satisfactory achievements have been made in researching the expression of TCM in English. Based on the investigation into the history and current state of the research work mentioned above, the English—Chinese Encyclopedia of Practical TCM has been published to meet the needs of extending the knowledge of TCM around the world.

The encyclopedia consists of twenty—one volumes, each dealing with a particular branch of TCM. In the process of compilation, the distinguishing features of TCM have been given close attention and great efforts have been made to ensure that the content is scientific, practical, comprehensive and concise. The chief writers of the Chinese manuscripts include professors or associate professors with at least twenty years of practical clinical and / or teaching experience in TCM. The Chinese manuscript of each volume has been checked and approved by a specialist of the relevant branch of TCM. The team of the translators and revisers of the English versions consists of TCM specialists with a good command of English professional medical translators, and teachers of English from TCM colleges or universities. At a symposium to standardize the English versions, scholars from twenty—two colleges or universities, research institutes of TCM or other health institutes probed the question of how to express TCM in English more comprehensively, systematically and accurately, and discussed and deliberated in detail the English versions of some volumes in order to upgrade the English versions of the whole series. The English version of each volume has been re—examined and then given a final checking.

Obviously this encyclopedia will provide extensive reading material of TCM English for senior students in colleges of TCM in China and will also greatly benefit foreigners studying TCM.

The assiduous efforts of compiling and translating this encyclopedia have been supported by the responsible leaders of the State Education Commission of the People's Republic of China, the State Administrative Bureau of TCM and Pharmacy, and the Education Commission and Health Department of Shandong

Province. Under the direction of the Higher Education Department of the State Education Commission, the leading board of compilation and translation of this encyclopedia was set up. The leaders of many colleges of TCM and pharmaceutical factories of TCM have also given assistance.

We hope that this encyclopedia will bring about a good effect on enhancing the teaching of TCM English at the colleges of TCM in China, on cultivating skills in medical circles in exchanging ideas of TCM with patients in English, and on giving an impetus to the study of TCM outside China.

Higher Education Press

March, 1990

Foreword

The English—Chinese Encyclopedia of Practical Traditional Chinese Medicine is an extensive series of twenty—one volumes. Based on the fundamental theories of traditional Chinese medicine(TCM) and with emphasis on the clinical practice of TCM, it is a semi—advanced English—Chinese academic works which is quite comprehensive, systematic, concise, practical and easy to read. It caters mainly to the following readers: senior students of colleges of TCM, young and middle—aged teachers of colleges of TCM, young and middle—aged physicians of hospitals of TCM, personnel of scientific research institutions of TCM, teachers giving correspondence courses in TCM to foreigners, TCM personnel going abroad in the capacity of lecturers or physicians, those trained in Western medicine but wishing to study TCM, and foreigners coming to China to learn TCM or to take refresher courses in TCM.

Because Traditional Chinese Medicine and Pharmacology is unique to our Chinese nation, putting TCM into English has been the crux of the compilation and translation of this encyclopedia. Owing to the fact that no one can be proficient both in the theories of Traditional Chinese Medicine and Pharmacology and the clinical practice of every branch of TCM, as well as in English, to ensure that the English versions express accurately the inherent meanings of TCM, collective translation measures have been taken. That is, teachers of English familiar with TCM, professional medical translators, teachers or physicians of TCM and even teachers of palaeography with a strong command of English were all invited together to co—translate the Chinese manuscripts and, then, to co—deliberate and discuss the English versions. Finally English—speaking foreigners studying TCM or teaching English in China were asked to polish the English versions. In this way, the skills of the above translators and foreigners were merged to ensure the quality of the English versions. However, even using this method, the uncertainty that the English versions will be wholly accepted still remains. As for the Chinese manuscripts, they do reflect the essence, and give a general picture, of traditional Chinese medicine and pharmacology. It is not asserted, though, that they are perfect, I whole—heartedly look forward to any criticisms or opinions from readers in order to make improvements to future editions.

More than 200 people have taken part in the activities of compiling, translating and revising this encyclopedia. They come from twenty—eight institutions in all parts of China. Among these institutions, there are fifteen colleges of TCM:Shandong, Beijing, Shanghai, Tianjin, Nanjing, Zhejiang, Anhui, Henan, Hubei, Guangxi, Guiyang, Gansu, Chengdu, Shanxi and Changchun, and scientific research centers of TCM such as China Academy of TCM and Shandong Scientific Research Institute of TCM.

The Education Commission of Shandong province has included the compilation and translation of this encyclopedia in its scientific research projects and allocated funds accordingly. The Health Department of Shandong Province has also given financial aid together with a number of pharmaceutical factories of TCM. The subsidization from Jinan Pharmaceutical Factory of

TCM provided the impetus for the work of compilation and translation to get under way.

The success of compiling and translating this encyclopedia is not only the fruit of the collective labor of all the compilers, translators and revisers but also the result of the support of the responsible leaders of the relevant leading institutions. As the encyclopedia is going to be published, I express my heartfelt thanks to all the compilers. translators and revisers for their sincere cooperation, and to the specialists, professors, leaders at all levels and pharmaceutical factories of TCM for their warm support.

It is my most profound wish that the publication of this encyclopedia will take its role in cultivating talented persons of TCM having a very good command of TCM English and in extending, rapidly, comprehensive knowledge of TCM to all corners of the globe.

Chief Editor   Xu Xiangcai
Shandong College of TCM
March, 1990

Contents

Notes

NURSING is the twentith volume of THE ENGLISH—CHINESE ENCYCLOPEDIA OF PRACTICAL TRADITIONAL CHINESE MEDICINE.

The volume consists of six chapters. Chapter one deals with the introduction, characteristics of TCM nursing, psychological nursing, diet care and the administration of herbal medicines. Chapter two describes the routine procedures of TCM nursing in emergency cases, nursing implemented according to syndrome differentiation, and measures proposed for first—aid. The remaining four chapters highlight the actual nursing practice of the commonly—encountered diseases in the departments of internal medicine, surgery, gynecology and pediatrics. Each of these four chapters starts with a description of general nursing, which is then followed by differentiated nursing on the basis of disease types. This in fact manifests the TCM view that human body is an organic entity formed by the chanel system, internal organs, superficial body tissues and organs, etc. , and in affinity with the seasonal changes, local geography, environment, emotions and diet.

Guided by the theory of TCM syndrome differentiation, this volume is intended to combine the introduction to the knowledge of TCM nursing with the comprehensive therapeutic approaches of TCM such as those applied in acupuncture, massage and other external therapies, and to emphasize the significance of giving priority to disease prevention.

Deputy nurse director Gui Meifen, director of Nursing Department of Beijing TCM Hospital, deputy minister member in charge of Chinese Nursing Institute and nursing speciality in combination of TCM and Western Medicine has checked the Chinese manuscript, while Prof. Jiang Qi Yuan Ms. Lin Xiaoqi and Associate Prof. Wu Weitong helped go over the English manuscript at the symposiums held in Taian of Shandong Province for standardizing the English versions of The English—Chinese Encyclopedia of Practical Traditional Chinese Medicine. Here express our thanks to them.

The Editor

1 Introduction

1.1 A Brief History of the Development of Traditional Chinese Medicine (TCM) Nursing

TCM nursing has been developed alongside traditional Chinese medicine itself. Thus it has a long history and rich contents.

The ancient treatment and nursing were combined into one. As recorded *The Biogmphies of Bian Que and Cang Gone in Shiji*, Bian Que, who lived in about the fifth to fourth century B. C. , had a great command of medical knowledge in various clinical branches, he treated patients by needling, moxibustion, herbal decoction and hot compress. When he rescued a critically ill Prince Guo, he first used acupuncture and herbal decoction, then put hot medicinal compress on both hypochondriac regions to restore the body temperature. This demonstrates that diagnosis, treatment and nursing were all undertaken by the physician. Nursing was not a profession then, nor an independent branch of learning. But a great deal of nursing knowledge and experience were recorded in historical literature throughout the ages, forming an important constituent of TCM.

In the earliest records of Chinese culture, there are various references concerning wet fango compress, bandaging, bone setting, "acting for resisting cold" "remaining in the shade to prevent sunstroke", etc. . These indicate the beginning of nursing in traditional Chinese medicine.

Huangdi Nei Jing (The yellow Emperor's canon of Internal Medicine) , the earliest book on medicine written during the Warring States Period (770——221 B.C), not only summarizesa wealth of experience that ancient Chinese accumulated in fighting against diseases, but also makes a systematic exposition of body structure and function as well as the pathogenesis, etiology, diagnosis and treatment of disease. Meanwhile, it also deals with every aspect of TCM nursing including moral cultivation, life style, environmental sanitation, diet regulation, contraindication, herbal administration and the nursing thereafter. The book has laid a theoretical foundation for the development of TCM nursing.

Shang Han Lun (Treatise on Febrile Disease) and *Jin Gui Yao Lue* (Synopsis of Prescription of the Golden Chamber) written by Zhang Zhongjing during the Han Dynasty (D. C25——220) , contain concrete material concerning nursing according to differentiation of patient's herbal administration. Zhang Zhongjing also invented the pigs bile enema, which shows that enemas were used early in the Han Dynasty. Hua Tuo, another famous ancient physician, who was skilled in surgery, first created anesthesia that enriched the knowledge of surgical nursing. He laid great emphasis on the importance of physical exercises and devised five animal simulations, *Wu Qin Xi,* an exercise of imitating the motions of tiger. dear, monkey, bear and bird, affording a new method of building up health, preventing disease and recovery from chronic illness.

Zhouhou Jiucu Fang(Prescriptions for Emergencies) written by Ge Hong during the Jin Dynasty (365——420A. D) records surgical passive immunization therapy in which rabid dog brain was applied to the part bitten by rabid dog. *Jia Yi Jing* (Systematic Classic of Acupuncture and Moxibustion) compiled by Huangfu Mi carries forward the theory of acupuncture and moxibustion. Both books contribute greatly to the development of TCM nursing.

Chen Shiliang of the Tang Dynasty (618——907D. C) put forward in his book *Shixing Ben Cao* (A Dietetic Materia Medica) prescriptions for dietetic therapy and advice on the diet in the four seasons. It is also in this book that he elaborated important relationship between diet care and medical treatment. Sun Simiao (a person of the Tang Dynasty 618——907D. C) made the emphasis in his book *Qian Jin Yao Fang* (Valuable) Prescriptions that those who Practised medicine ought to have professional morals. They should treat patients equally, disregarding their nepotism, money status, age or appearance, and should have sympathy and responsibility. Such a fine tradition has been handed down to today with its resultant impact on clinical practice. Sun Simiao also emphasized health preservation. He was good at preserving his health and maintained that a good physician was one able to prevent potential disease before its onset. *Qian Jin Yao Fang* and *Qian Jin Yi Fang* (A Supplement to valuable Prescription) also contain much rich experience about massage, diet, dressing, infant nursing, etc. . Sun Simiao stressed that food should be cooked before eating, it is better to rinse out the mouth and take a walk after meals, and furthermore, compatible living may reduce the posibility of developing diseases. He was the first to apply Ahshi Points in acupuncture. It was also he who invented urethral catheterization by using a fine onion tube as the urinary catheter, demonstrating that this skill began to exist since the Tang Dynasty in China. *Wai Tai Mi Yao* (the Medical Secrets of an Official) by Wang Tao records various external therapies and nursing methods for neonates such as breast feeding, the way to wrap and bathe the neonates.

The book *Ben Cao Yan Yi* (Amplification on Materia Medica) written by Kou Zongshi in the Song Dynasty (960——1279) mentiones the relationship between table salt and diseases, pointing out that salt was contraindicated for patients with edema, viz, a low salt or salt—free diet is suggested in case of any disease with edema. In the book *Xiao Er Yao Zheng Zhi Jue*(Key to Therapeutices of Children's Disease) by Qian Zhongyang, it was advocated that a child with febrile condition may be treated with bathing, viz, lower the body temperature by washing and rubbing with lukewarm water which could be used as an assisting therapy. In *Xiao Er Fang Lun,* Yan Xiaozhong pointed out methods concerning how to feed babies of different months of age, such as feeding babies over six months old with rice juice, and babies more than ten months old with thin gruel and mashed food to support *Qi* of the middle—*Jiao* so as to boost immunity against disease. Raw, cold, oily, greasy or sweet food should be avoided. In addition, in *Fu Ren Da Quan Liang Fang* (The Complete Record of Effective Prescription for Women) by Chen Ziming, special chapters are devoted to contraindications, such as "Theory in Diet", "Nursing for Pregnant Women", "Postpartum Nursing", "Method of Puerperal Recuperation" which offered very valuable experiences for gynecological nursing in TCM.

The four famous physicians of Jin and Yuan Dynasties, Liu Wansu, Zhang Zihe, Li Dongyuan and Zhu Danxi all stressed the importance of nursing, although they held different academic viewpoints due to their different medical knowledge. Zhang Zihe dealt with many nursing problems in his book *Ru Men Shi Qin* (Prerequistite knowledge for Physicians) . It was he who invented sitz bath treating prolapse of rectum. He introduced his psychotherapy characterized by emotion conquering emotion, such as "feat and fright over joy, grief over anger and anger over worry, ···"Viewing that the spleen and stomach are the source for providing the acquired energy, Li Dong—Yuan stressed the importance of diet regulation of the acquired constitution and advocated that diet should be light, not rich or fatty, etc.

During the Ming and Qing Dynasties (1368——1840) , TCM nursing underwent new developments. Hu Zhengxin in the Ming Dynasty wrote"In a family with a patient suffering from infectious epidemic disease, the patient's clothes must be steamed in a cooking utensil, so that other members of the family will not be affected. "This explains that disinfection by use of steam was already in use to sterilize clothes or daily belongings touched by patients with infection. In the Qing Dynasty, Ye Tianshi carried out intensive studies in greater depth on the treatment and nursing of geriatric diseases, stressing that the elderly should learn how to maintain good health. He put forward that they should keep warm in cold, enjoy light diet by avoiding alcohol or greasy food, keep calm, cheerful and avoid anger. In addition, a person should take part in labour, exercise, go to bed and get up early, etc. . These methods of disease prevention and resistance to aging are elementary knowledge of keeping healthy as is practised in china.

Since traditional Chinese medicine regards medical treatment and nursing as complementary to each other and constituents of medical work, nursing work plays a very important role in the field of medicine. Constantly replenished and developed through the ages especially since the development and application of acupuncture, moxibustion, *Guasha* (a treatment for sunstroke by scraping the patient's neck, chest or back) , cupping, external therapy, massage, *Qigong* and *Taiji quan,* the contents of TCM nursing have been increasingly enriched.

Since the birth of new China, the Party's policies of TCM have created a favourable conditions for the development and improvement of the nursing cause. Vast medical workers and nursing staff in all parts of the country constantly sum up all their experiences concerning nursing of TCM through the combination of TCM with western medicine. Theories concerning the nursing science of the vast and rich contents of TCM have been explored and systematized and such books as "Nursing Science of TCM" are published continually. Nursing education has also been developed and paid attention. There are over ten training schools of TCM nursing in the whole country. There is a nursing department of TCM attached to some colleges of TCM. The nursing science of TCM has officially been formed as an independent subject. Particularly under the favourable situation in which traditional Chinese medicine is now being promoted in all parts of the country, the nursing staff of TCM is attempting to combine clinical practice based on the characteristics of TCM nursing and acquire new skills of modern nursing science to further develop and improve TCM nursing and enable it to serve the socialist construction better.

1. 2   The Characteristics of TCM Nursing

Following the theory of traditional Chinese medicine, TCM nursing has been developed the basic features of which may be summed up as four parts as follows.

1. The Wholistic Approach

Traditional Chinese Medicine perceives the human body as an organic entity with *Zang—Fu* (hollow organs and solid organs), channels and collaterals as the core. Man and everything in nature, including weather, physical and social environment, etc. , are all the unity of opposites and the relative balance between *Zang—Fu* organs in the body, between internal and external environment must be kept. Once imbalance appears, disorder will occur. Therefore when patients are cared for, a favorable external environment should be maintained. While observing the patient's condition, the nursing staff should pay attention not only to pathological changes but at the same time to the changes of interrelated *Zang— Fu* organs. For example, oral ulceration is caused by flaring—up of the heart—fire because the heart opens into the tongue. It may be accompanied by dark urine diffieulty and pricking pain in urination enused by exeessive heat in the small intestine, because the heart is externally—internally related to the small intestine and may transmit pathogenic heat to small intestine. In the case of the above symptoms, besides local treatment such as applying *Bingpeng, Xilei* or *Wugu* powder to the oral cavity, heart—fire should be purged with diuretics such as Herba Lophatheri and Rhizoma Imperatae which are decocted for frequent oral use. In addition, the patients should take more heat—clearing and fire—purging foods such as green gram soup, fruit, vegetables, while refraining from eating peppery and fried food. Traditonal Chinese medicine emphasizes the influence of seasonal changes, geographical environment and the patient's constitutions on disease, so the nursing staff must carefully consider factors of every aspect, make a concrete analysis of concrete conditions and adopt nursing method according to climate and seasonal conditions, geographical locations and the individual condition.

1) Climatic and seasonal conditions: In accordance with the characteristics of climate and seasons, appropriate therapeutic and nursing method are used. For example, a common cold contracted in summer is most likely to be a wind—heat type as the climate is burming hot resulting in dispersing of *Yang* and the pores remaining open. When taking medicine to relieve exterior syndrome, patients should be guided to prevent excessive sweating so as to avoid exhaustion of *Yin*—fluids. A cold contracted in winter tends to be a wind—cold type as the climate is cold and the pathogenic cold can easily cause the pores to stay closed. When taking medicine for relieving exterior syndrome, patients should drink hot and thin gruel or hot boiled water and be covered with a thick quilt to keep warm for sweating so as to remove pathogenic factors with sweating.

2) Geographical Locations: The appropriate therapeutic and nursing methods should be determined according to different geographical locations and climatic condition. Therefore, therapeutic and nursing methods should be different. For example, the climate in the south is hot and damp, while in the north, dry with less rainfall, therefore even the same illness requires dif-

ferent nursing therapy.

3) Individual conditions: Since there are differences in sex, age and constitution, the symptoms of the same disease may also differ, so different nursing methods should be adopted accordingly.

As the human body is an organic entity, whether the emotion is normal is closely related to the health. Normal emotion assists in normalizing the body to adapt to the surrounding environment and seasonal changes as well as in providing defense from exopathic invasion. Otherwise if the emotion is abnormal and internally injured, abnormal descending and ascending of *Qi* and the circulation of the qi and blood will be disrupted in addition to disturbance of *Wuzang* (five *Zang*) organs, thus causing various kinds of diseases. For example, an excess of joy injures the heart, manifested as palpitation, insomnia, mental confusion, and in severe cases, mania may occur. Anger injures the liver, resulting in stagnation of liver—*Qi* and poor appetite, and in severe cases, pale complexion, shivering of the limbs and even syncope may occur. Worry injures the spleen and affects the transporting and transforming function of the spleen, causing abdominal distention, loose stools, dizziness, insomnia, frequent dreaming, poor memory, etc. . Fear and fright injure the kidney causing incontinence of urination, etc. . Therefore, nursing staff should know the patient's emotional condition, be aware of his emotional changes and give him patient and careful advise to reassure him. The patient will then be at ease and in stable mood when he is treated.

In addition to the treatment of maintaining use of medicinal herbs, traditional Chinese medicine places much importance on diet as dietcare is a major aspect in TCM nursing . The rule of traditional dietetic therapy is to take the theory of traditional Chinese medicine as the basis. In the light of the four natures of foods (cold, hot, warm and cool), five kinds of flavor (sour, bitter, sweet, pungent and salty) and their channel tropism, differential analysis is given to the causative factors, location of pathological changes, nature of the disease and main clinical manifestations obtained by applying the four diagnostic methods (inspection, auscultation and olfaction, interrogation, pulse feeling and palpation), then food may be chosen to make up prescription of dietetic therapy. Taking opigastralgia as an example, all primary cases, whether due to excess syndrome or pathogenic factors invading the stomach, should be treated with the prescription of dietetic therapy for promoting circulation of Qi and blood as main means to expel pathogenic evils. All prolonged diseases, deficiency syndromes or irregular functioning of $Zang$— Fu should be treated mainly with the prescription of dietetic therapy for tonification to regulate the function of $Zang$—Fu.

2. Nursing According to Syndrome Differentiation

Differentiation of syndromes forms an important basis for the nursing of TCM. Diagnosis and an effective treatment are based on a comprehensive analysis of a patient's signs and symptoms obtained by applying the four diagnosic methods and the eight principles according to the basic theories of TCM. The theory also guides the practice of the nursing work. Taking fever as an example, the nursing principles for different patients with fever are also different because of the different pathogenesis, mechanism, signs and symptoms. If fever accompanied by chills, anhidrosis. white tongue coating and absence of thirst. it is due to the pathogenic factors on the exterior of the body. The principle of the treatment should be to relieve the exterior syndrome and the nursing principle is to avoid wind cold so as to prevent the body from invasion of exogenous pathogenic factors. The body should be kept warm and hot or sweet—ginger water should be drunk in order to promote sweating. If the fever is very high, accompanied by extreme thirst, profuse perspiration and yellow tongue coating, it is due to pathogenic factors going deep into the interior of the body and turning into heat. In nursing, the room should be well ventilated and light beverage should be mostly drunk; if the fever is caused by Qi deficiency accompanied by spontaneous perspiration, intolerance of cold, etc. warmth should be maintained and sweating should be avoided. Since the developing stages of a disease are different, the nursing should be changed accordingly. Taking a case due to damp—heat as an example, since it is manifested as serious damp and light heat at the initial stage, the patient's room should not be too cool, the clothes should not be too thin, and raw and cold food is contraindicated. It is manifested as damp retention and heat flaring at the later stage, so the temperature of the room should be low and appropriate amount of cold beverage should be drunk, etc.. In addition, when treating diseases, traditional Chinese medicine strictly adheres to the mechanism, that is, in differentiation of syndromes, focusing on the developments and changes of a disease. So in the course of nursing, the nursing staff should be completely aware of the developing patterns of various diseases so as to know the developing tendency of a disease.

3. Traditional Therapies

The contents of traditional therapies of Chinese medicine are wide, rich and varied and the therapies such as acupuncture, moxibustion, massage, cupping, *Guasna,* external therapies, including adhesive plaster, hot compress, pericompress, fumigation and washing, etc. , medicinal therapy, dietetic therapy and others all constitute valuable heritage of TCM. These therapies are not only important media of TCM in treating a disease, but also essential methods in the nursing of TCM. As these therapies have rapid remarkable therapeutic effects and few side effects, and they are safe and reliable and easy to learn and use, in recent years, they have been applied in a large scale in clinics, have broken through the range of traditional treatment and have developed and improved still further. For example, after operation on the abdomen, acupuncture is used to improve intestinal peristalsis to reduce abdominal distention; massage is applied to relieve the retention of urine occuring after operation; ear needing can prevent complications resulting from venous transfusion and blood transfusion. Senna leaf is taken after being infused in hot water instead of cleaning enemas; hot bran compress (an external therapy of applying heated bran wrapped in a cloth to an affected part) can assist healing of pleuritic intestine—cohesion which may occur soon after gastrointestinal operation, etc. .

4. Preventive Treatment of Disease

" Disease prevention prior to its treatment" is said in "Huangdi Nei Jing (Huangdi's Internal Classic) . It includes two aspects, namely, prevention before the attack of a disease and prevention from deterioration after occurrence of a disease. Traditional Chinese medicine advocates health preservation, requiring that man be moderate in diet, regular in life style and avoid overstrain in daily life. Physical exercises should be attended to in order to regulate the emotion to keep the body in vigorous vital—*Qi* and balance of *Yin* and *Yang*, which may reduce the attack of a disease. Therefore the sick person should be guided to keep good living habits, stable emotion and do strengthening exercises such as walking after meals, *Qi—Gong*, *Tai — Ji Quan* and others. Importance is attached to early diagnosis and treatment of a disease for fear of its negative development. Therefore the nursing staff is required to observe the patient's condition to know the premonitory of occurrence and development of a disease so as to take appropriate measures to control it.

1.3　Psychological Nursing

Psychological nursing has great clinical significance because traditional Chinese medicine realizes that the human body is an organic entity. Whether the emotion is normal is closely related to the health. When the emotion is normal, *Yin* and *Yang* are in balance, Vital— *Qi* is kept in the interior and the body in normal condition adapts to surrounding circumstances and seasonal changes so as to prevent invasion of exogenous pathogenic factors. Otherwise, when the emotion surpasses the limits of its normality, the mind will be injured in the interior, causing abnormal descending or ascending of *Qi*, disorder of the *Qi* and blood circulation and failure of the function of the *Wuzang* (five solid organs), easily resulting in various disorders.

Different emotional changes will result in different pathological changes of *Zang—Fu* such as violentrage damaging the liver, excessive joy injuring the heart, deep worry—the spleen, excessive grief—the lung, great fear and fright—the kidney, etc. , which are all actually significant in clinical analysis. For example, violent rage will cause hyperactivity of the liver— *Yang,* manifested as headache, dizziness, dry mouth and tongue, dryness of eyes, insomnia, poor memory, etc. , excessive worry will injure the spleen bringing about dysfunction of the spleen in transportation, manifested as poor appetite, distension and fullness sensation in the epigastric region after meal, lassitude, etc. .

In addition, according to five— element theory, "fear and fright over joy", "grief over anger", "anger over worry", "excessive joy over melancholy" and "worry over fear", that is to say, one mood is taken to calm down another mood that has exceeded reasonable limits. This is the psychotherapy characterized by emotion conquering emotion.

Special importance is attached to psychological nursing in TCM and the nursing personnel are required to be fully conversant with patient's psychological and ideological condition to bring his positive factors into play. At first, the patients should be made aware of effects of their emotional condition on their illness to bring their internal cause into play. For example, those with liver trouble should avoid anger, those with heart trouble should avoid excitement , and those with lung trouble should keep the mind optimistic, while for dangerous and serious cases, it is necessary to calm their spirit, try to eliminate bad emotional stimuli such as nervousness, fear, anxiety worry, giving them advices and confidence to defeat their disease and have them coordinate better with treatment to reduce their suffering and recover earlier, In order to do psyckological nursing well, on one hand, the nursing personnel should strengthen their self —cultivation, cultivating good medical morality and quality and have a steady, firm, careful and responsible approach to work and treat every patient equally disregarding nepotism, money status, age or appearance. On the other hand, they should master certain knowledge of basic theory of TCM, applying it clinically to do effective psycological nursing with a definite object in view taking into consideration both the patients illness and ideological condition.

1.4 Diet Care

Food is an important material assisting in treating disease and recovering the health. It is written in the book "Nei Jing" that "the treatment of diseases with medicine should be supplemented by proper diet. ". While doctors of TCM treat a disease with herbal medicine, they also place importance on the function of dietetic regulation and nourishing. Dietetic regulation and nourishing is also one of the important contents of TCM Nursing, so the nursing personnel should master the principles of nursing so as to improve the nursing quality.

1. Selection of Food

(1) The relationship between food and disease: A disease may be distinguished between *Yin* and *Yang*, cold and heat , deficiency and excess, exterior and interior types, and food has cold, heat, warm, and cool nature, as well as pungent, sweet, sour, bitter and salty taste so the nature and taste of food must be coordinated with the characteristics of a disease, otherwise it may bring about the opposite effect to that required, thus interfering with treatment rather than supporting it. When patient's food intake is guided, it is necessary to choose food with particular nature and function according to the characteristic of a disease, so as to achieve the goal, "illness of deficiency type being treated by

tonifying", "excess syndromes being treated with the method of purgation and reduction", "treating the cold—syndrome with hot natured foods", "heat syndrome being treated with foods of cold or cool in nature". For example, a person with a heat—syndrome should eat cool—natured food and refrain from eating heat—natured food such as peppery and fried food, and drinking alcohol; a person with a cold—syndrome should eat warm—natured food and refrain from eating cool—natured food like raw or cold fruits; a person with *Yang*—deficiency should eat warm—natured and tonifying food and avoid cold or cool—natured food; a person with *Yin* deficiency should eat tonifying, light, thin and moist food and avoid warm and heat—natured food; a person suffering from nail—like boil and carbuncle due to the fire—pathogenic factors should not eat oily or greasy food, meat or fish so as to prevent supporting fire and producing phlegm to aggravate the condition; a person suffering from skin trouble should generally avoid such fresh food as fish and shrimp, etc. which may induce a recurrence of the disease, to prevent escalating itchiness due to production of wind and skin eruption. A person suffering from hemorrhoids should refrain from eating irritative food like peppery one to prevent constipation causing hemafecia and pains after passing stool.

(2) Relationship between foods and herbs: Foods and herbs originate from same source, namely plants and animals. The nature, taste, channel tropism and properties of herbs have parallels in foods. Thus the nature and energy of herbs and foods may have the function of coordinating with and controlling each other, and the coordination may increase curative effects. For example, Radix Angelicae Sinensis taken with mutton and raw gin-

ger can increase the function of warming and recuperating to promote generation of blood; carp stewed in water with red bean can strengthen the effect of diuresis. Radix Astragali seu Hedysari plus Tob's tears seed can boost the effect of alleviating water retention by excreting dampness. If the nature and energy of foods taken is contrary to those of the prescribed herbs, the foods may reduce the efficacy and even cause side effects. For example, radish taken with *shen lei* herbs (Radix Ginseng, Radix Sophorae Flavescentis, Radix Scrophulariae, Radix Codonopsis Pilosulae, etc.) and Radix Rehmanniae can promote digestion and consume *Qi* resulting in *shenlei* herbs and Radix Rehmanniae to lose their function of tonifying *Qi*. In addition, Herba Schizonepetae should not be taken with fish and crab nor should Rhizoma Atractylodis Macrocephalae be taken with peach and plum; honey with onion; Radix Glycyr hizae with silver carp; Ferrum Pulveratum with tea—leaves; Rhizoma Coptidis, Radix Platycodi and Fructus Mume with pork, etc.

(3) Relationship Between Foods

The nature and function of each food are different, while there are differences of mutual reinforcement, mutual assistance, mutual restraint and incompatibility between two foods when mixed. For examples, mutton and fresh ginger both are warm in nature and may be coordinated to play a role to strengthen their warming— tonifying function and treat abdominal pain due to cold of insufficiency type; crab and fresh ginger may be taken together bacause one is cold and the other is warm in nature, and cold can be relieved with foods warm in nature. But crab and persimmon should not be taken together because both are of cold nature and after taking, they may bring about cold syndrome of the stomach. Only by being fully conversant with the nature, function and selection of foods, can you mix foods rationally to strengthen the coordinated function of food and raise the curative effects.

(4) Relationship Between Cooking of Food and Diseases

There are many methods to cook and process food. The same food may be indicated or contraindicated for a disease according to different cooking methods, hence food should be cooked in a way suitable for the needs of the patient. health condition, For example, meat and poultry such as chicken and duck thoroughly cooked on low heat can promote digestion and absorption of the food and is indicated for gastrointestinal troubles or both *Qi* and blood deficiency due to prolonged disease. This kind of food, stir—fried, deep—fried, roasted or smoked is apt to cause internal heat syndrome by impairing the stomach—*Yin* due to its increased dryness and heat; eggs steamed, egg—soup boiled or poached are generally not contraindicated; but fried and stir—fired eggs can damage the stomach and are not easily digested. Therefore, to cook food rationally is significant in coordination of treatment.

2. Basic Requirements for Dietetic Nursing

(1) Implementation Based on Differentiation of Syndrome on Guiding Diet in the Light of Theory of Traditional Chinses Medicine;

Food suitable for the health and healing a disease should be chosen according to the patient's health condition and the different syndromes. The nature of a food must be suited to the property of a disease. For example, for a cold syndrome, foods warm in nature are indicated and food cold and cool in nature are contraindicated; for heat syndrome, foods cold and cool in nature are indicated but those warm and hot in nature are contraindicated. If these guidelines are neglected, the disease may be worsened. Clinical practice has proved that occurrence of some diseases, their sudden changes, prolonged period of recovery and their recurrence, etc. are mostly related to laxness of diet. Therefore, dietetic nursing is a key link in the clinical nursing chain.

(2) The Regulation of Diet;

The four—seasonal regulation of diet should be attended to , appetite controlled, time and quantity of meal fixed and neither excessive hunger nor fullness is permitted. The coldness and heat of diet should be suitable, the hardness and softness should be moderate to assure the normal function of food digestion and transportation of the spleen and stomach benefiting recovery of a disease. Conversely, improper diet will damage the function of the spleen and stomach resulting in disharmony between *Ying* and blood making the disease more severe.

(3) Attention to Dietetic Hygiene;

Food should be clean and fresh, the hands washed before meals and the mouth rinsed after eating to prevent pathogens from entering the body through the mouth. Diet should be regular and food should be eaten until hunger is felt. Excessive fill, partiality for particular kind of food, greed for eating and much eating in the evening should be avoided. A walk should be taken after meal and lying immediately after fill should be avoided. In addition, ease of mind should be kept before meals and anger before or after eating be avoided in order that the stomach and spleen will benefit from the food and maintain their normal functions of food digestion and fluid transportation promoting a quick recovery.

3. Classification of Food

The variety of food is too large to mention individually. According to the conventional classification of traditional Chinese medicine, foods are summarized in such categories as grain, vegetable, fruit and meat. In the light of difference of their nature, taste and function, they are classified as follows.

(1) Pungent categories; Ginger, onion, garlic, pepper, alcohol and other foods warm in nature and promoting fire are included. They are indicated for cold — syndrome and are contraindicated for heat—syndrome.

(2) Uncooked and cold categories; Melon and fruit, shredded raw and cool vegetable, cold food and drink, and those which are cool in nature cool—prepared food, are included. They are indicated for heat—syndrome but should be used little or with caution for patients ill with insufficiency of spleen—stomach—*Yang*.

(3) Fatty meat and fine grain or rich food: Such categories as poultry, eggs, meat, milk, and fried, stir—fired, deep—fired, roasted or quickly fried food should not be used for heat—syndrome because they are dry and hot in nature and easily damage stomach—*Yin*.

(4) Tonifying categories: Various foods have certain tonifying functions which are generally classified as even, clearing and warming reinforcing, etc. because of their differences in nature and taste. Food should be used flexibly according to the requirements of the patient's condition, bodily health and four—seasonal changes of weather.

4. Nature of food

This generally refers to the four natures, that is, cold, hot, warm and cool. Slightly cold nature is generally included as being cool, largely warm nature as being hot and moderate nature is called neutral, so they are clinically classified as three kinds—— warm and hot, cold and cool, and neutral.

(1) Food of Warm and Hot Nature

a. Meat: dog meat, beef, chicken, turtle, mutton, sparrow, shrimp, long—noded pit viper, black— tail snake and others.

b. Vegetables: soybean, broad bean, sword bean, mussel, carrot, onion, garlic, fragrant— flowered garlic, leaf mustard, rape, coriander, pepper, hot pepper, etc. .

c. Others: brown sugar, wheat flour, goat's milk, polished glutinous rice, etc. .

(2) Food of Cold and Cool Nature

a. Meat: duck meat, goose, rabbit, soft—shelled turtle, oyster, crab and so on.

b. Vegetables: spinach, Chinese cabbage, celery, three—coloured amaranth, bamboo shoots, cucumber, balsam pear, eggplant, wax gourd, laver, etc. .

c. Fruits: pear, watermelon. mandarin orange, orange, shaddock, etc. .

d. Others: barley, mung bean, white sugar, uncooked honey, and so on.

(3) Neutral Food

a. Meat: pork, carp, cuttlefish, etc. .

b. Vegetables: red bean, black bean, cowpea, kidney bean, towel gourd, jew's earfungus, lily bulb, lotus seed, Chinese date, potato, day lily, etc. .

c. **Others**: duck egg, Chinese yam, apricot kernal, grape, peach, fig, etc.

5. The Main Effects of Food Noted as Follows

(1) Relieving exterior syndromes: This may be done with food pungent in flavor and warm in nature, such as fresh ginger, scallion stalk coriander, etc. ; relieving the exterior syndrome with food pungent in flavor and cool in nature such as light—prepared soybean, tea—leaves and carambola, etc. .

(2) Clearing heat and expelling toxins: wax gourd, pumpkin, cucumber, watermelon, balsam pear, mung bean, hyacinth bean, spinach, river snail, duck's meat, pear, three— coloured amaranth, tomato, etc. .

(3) Clearing heat and relieving summer heat: mung bean, hyacinth bean, watermelon, muskmelon, tea—leaves, lemon, etc. .

(4) Removing intense heat from the throat: balsam pear, powder on the surface of dried persimmon, water chestnut, duck's eggs, cucumber, sweet potato, peppermint and others.

(5) Eliminating dampness and promoting diuresis: red bean, broad bean, kelp, laver, carp, snakeheaded fish, watermelon, wax gourd, Chinese cabbage, celery and so on.

(6) Relieving cough and dissolving the phlegm: radish, crystal sugar. pear, apricot kernel, gingko nut, orange and so on.

(7) Strengthening the spleen and replenishing the stomach: malt sugar, Chinese date, lotus seed, Chinese yam, peanut, fresh ginger, onion, garlic, hawthorn, Chinese prickly ash, fennel, etc. .

(8) Reinforcing: even reinforcing: pork, carp, snakeheaded fish, black carp, grape, eggs and so on; clearing; gingko, lily bulb, soft—shelled turtle, sea slug, etc. ; warming: mutton, dog

meat, chicken, sparrow's meat, etc. .

(9) Prevention against catching cold: fresh ginger, garlic. onion, vinegar, prepared soybean and others.

(10) Promoting eruption of rash: coriander, mushroom, water chestnut, yellow croaker, fresh carp, fresh shrimp and so on.

(11) Relieving toxin: fresh ginger, vinegar are used for relieving seafood poisoning: tealeaves, white hyacinth bean are used for relieving herbal poisoning; goat's blood and kongxincal are used for relieving meat poisoning; honey is used for various detoxification; garlic is used for antibacterial effects and detoxification.

(12) Moistening intestines and relaxing the bowels; mulberry, honey, banana, kernel of walnut, sesame oil, pine nut, kelp, and pork, etc. .

(13) Relieving diarrhea with astringents: lotus seed, fried Chinese yam and lotus root are indicated for diarrhea due to spleen— deficiency; garlic and portulaca are indicated for diarrhea due to heat; hawthorn, charred malt and rice aprouts are indicated for diarrhea due to improper diet, etc. .

(14) Expelling parasites: pomegranate, seed of pumpkin, quisqualis fruit, torreya seed, garlic, coconut, carrot, etc. .

(15) Stopping bleeding: day lily, lotus root starch, jew's ear fungus, cicai, dried persimmon, banana, lettuce, fragrant— flowered garlic and so on.

(16) Lowering the blood pressure and blood—fat and preventing arteriosclerosis: kelp, jelly fish, laver, jew's ear fungus, hawthorn, onion, mushroom, garlic, tea—leaves, celery, honey, bean products, and so on. .

(17) Lactogenesis: crucian carp, pig's foot, lettuce, carp and silver carp are used for shortness of milk due to *Qi* and blood deficiency and so on.

(18) Treating diabetes: polished glutinous rice, pork tripe, pork, mulberry, different kinds of bean, Chinese yam, onion, wild rice stem.

6. Examples of Dietetic Selection for Common Diseases

The respiratory disease includes acute and chronic tracheitis, asthma, lung abscess, pulmonary tuberculosis, pleurisy and others often marked by cough, phlegm, dyspnea, etc. . During the acute attack, it is most often caused by exterior pathogenic evils, so it is not suitable for the patient to take rich and greasy food too early. Conversely, the pathogenic factors are easily retained in the body. The patient should eat light food, plenty of fruits and fresh vegetables while avoiding pungent, peppery, oily, greasy and sweet food, smoking and alcohol. If there is cough with yellow phlegm due to the excessive lung—heat, the patient should eat radish, orange, pear, loquat, etc. or gruel made of polished round — grained nonglutinous rice so as to clear heat and eliminate phlegm; if there is phlegm with blood, pieces and juice of lotus root should be eaten to clear heat and relieve blood; if there is *Yin*— deficiency of the lung due to prolonged disease after the pathogen has been removed, lily bulb, tremella and soft—shelled turtle, etc. should be eaten to nourish *Yin* and supplement the lungs.

The hepatic and biliary diseases include cirrhosis, acute and chronic hepatitis, infection of biliary tract and cholelithiasis. The patient should eat light food with plenty of vegetables, lean meat, chicken, fish and so on while avoiding pungent and peppery products, smoking and alcohol, and eat little animal fat. During an acute attack, the patient should follow a mainly vegetarian diet, eating a small amount of meat during the recovery. If there is hepatosplenomegaly, the patient may eat some soft—shelled turtle and mussel, etc. . To relieve ascites, he / she may eat crucian carp, red bean soup or astragalus root, gruel made of Chinese date and polished round—grained nonglutinous rice, animal liver and have a little or no salt in the diet. Day lily, Chinese date, raisins, river snail, etc. may be eaten to relieve jaundice.

1.5 Nursing in Administration of Herbal Medicine

There are many forms of prepared Chinese drugs, decoctions, extracts, pellets, pills, powders, tinctura, etc, which are often used clinically. Their effect is varied. With the constant reform and development of forms of Chinese drugs, and in order to overcome difficulties of administering decoction and for convenience of storage and portability, mixtures, powder preparations, tablets, injections, etc. are prepared. Nursing staff should thoroughly understand herbal properties, and master methods of using each form of prepared Chinese drugs and nursing well in administration, which will increase efficacy and promote early recovery.

1. Commonly Used Forms of Prepared Drugs

(1) Decoction: Medicinal solution is obtained by boiling herbs with an appropriate amount of water for a period of time, then the dregs removed. It is characterized by flexibility of prescription, modification with symptoms and signs, immediate effi-

cacy and indicated for both acute and chronic disease, complex syndrome and external application, decoction is not only taken orally but also applied externally, being mostly used for fumigation and washing.

(2) Pill: A Pharmaceutical preparation as a globular mass is made of medicinal powder mixed with honey (or water), with the characteristics of slower absorpation but lasting effect and portability, it is indicated for chronic diseases.

(3) Soft extract: for oral administration usually made by concentrating a decoction to syrupy consistency with addition of sugar or honey, such as *Yimucaogao* (soft extract of motherwort) *Lutaigao* (soft extract of deer fetus), ointment or plaster for external use.

(4) Powder: a preparation of drugs ground into powder for oral administration or external application.

(5) Tinctura: a pharmaceutial preparation made by immersion of medicines in alcohol for a period of time, making their effective composition dissolve in alcohol and then the dregs being filtered.

(6) Danji: a kind of sublimated crystalline preparations of minerals with various colours such as red and white. It is made from minerals such as salt, vitriol, nitre and silver by healing, mostly for external use and more costly pills with especial curative effect are known as *Dan* such as *Zixuedan, Zhibaodan* and *Piwendan,* usually for oral use.

(7) Soluble granule preparations: a granular preparation made of the extract of drugs, which is dissolved in boiling water for oral use, e. g. *Ganmaochongji,* (A Pharmaceutical Preparation for Common Cold), *Jiangyachongji* (A Pharmacentical

Preparation for High Blood Pressure) .

(8) Tablets: a medicinal formulae made up of a kind or various kinds of herbs. The herbs are ground into fine powder, to which suitable assisting material is added and the mixture is pressed and prepared into tablets. e. g. *Xilingjiedu Pian, Niuhuangjiedu Pian.*

2. The Preparation of Decoction

Decoction is a form of prepared Chinese medicine, often used clinically, the method of decocting herbs being significantly related to curative effect.

(1) Containers for decocting herbs: Casserol and earthenware are suitable, enamelware and aluminiumware are also used but ironware must be avoided so as to prevent chemical reactions with herbs which decrease the curative effect.

(2) Preparation before decocting herbs: Before being decocted, the herbs are soaked in water for an hour or so , which benefits the dissolution of the active components from the herbs. The amount of water used may vary depending on the nature of herbs. Those with powdery property and large amounts of starch must be well diluted because such herbs have a high affinity for water; shell and mineral types require little water; reinforcing herbs must be well diluted because they must be decocted for a long time; the herbs for relieving pathogenic factors from the exterior require little water because they must be decocted only for a short time.

(3) The decocting time and fire — temperature control: These depend upon herbal property, e. g. the diaphoretic herbs must be decocted with a strong fire for a short time (about five minutes after boiling) and tonifying herbs must be decocted with

soft fire for a long time (about 30—60 minutes after boiling) .

（4）During the process of decocting herbs, appropriate measures should be taken to ensure the curative effects of the herbs based on their particular characteristics.

a. To be decocted first: Certain kinds of shell, mineral, fruit, root and stem herbs must be decocted for 15—30 minutes prior to other drugs (e. g Magnetitum, ochra Os Draconis Fossilia Ossis Mastodi, Concha Ostreae, Plastrum Testudinis, Concha Arcae, Concha Haliotidis, Os Sepiella seu Sepiae) . Some toxic herbs must be decocted first for several hours so as to decrease their toxin, such as Rhizoma Pinelliae (raw) , Radix Aconiti, Radix Aconiti Kusnezoffii and others.

b. To be decocted later: Some fragrant and pungent herbs such as Herba Menthae, Herba Agastachis, Ramulus Uncariae cum Uncis, Radix et Rhizoma Rhei, etc. must be added when the other herbs are semi—decocted so as to preserve their effective components, being decocted for only about 3—5 minutes.

c. Decoction of a wrapped drug: Some drugs such as Flos Inulae, semen Plantaginis, Indigo Naturalis, Halloysitum Rubrum should be wrapped in a piece of cloth before they are decocted with other drugs.

d. Dissolution by heat: Certain medicine such as Colla Corii Asini, Colla Cornus Cervi, Saccharum Cranorum and others should be melted by heat in the decoction or water, taken after they have dissolved.

e. To be taken after being infused in hot water or decoction: Certain medicines are only soaked in boiling water and taken as tea, such as Folium Cassiae Semen Sterculiae Seuphigerae, Flos Chrysanthemi, Radix Glycyrhizae, etc.

f. Decocting costly medicines: Certain costly herbs such as Radix Ginseng, Radix Panacis Quinguefolii, Cornu Saigae Tataricae, etc. should be decocted singly and then taken after being mixed with the decoction.

3. Methods of Administration

There are different requirements for administration according to the mildness, seriousness, acuteness or chronicness, the location and properties of a disease, and different herbal nature and function.

(1) Depending on how serious a disease: a dose of decoction is generally taken twice a day, at intervals of 4——6 hours; a patient in serious condition may take two doses of herbs daily and once every two hours: a dangerously ill patient may be fed little and frequently: a patient who is unconscious or can't take medicine orally for some reason can be given decoction by nasal feeding: a patient who vomits readily may frequently take little of the concentrated decoction.

(2) Based on the position of a disease: A patient ill in the lower warmer should take decoction before a meal, ill in upper warmer or suffering from common diseases should all take decoction after a meal.

(3) Based on the herbal function; Tonifying herbs are suitable for taking on an empty stomach; herbs stimulating the gastrointinal tract should be taken after a meal; herbs tranquilizing the spirit and loosing the bowel to relieve constipation should be taken before sleeping; herbs preventing and curing malaria should be taken two hours prior to the attack; decoction expelling parasites should be taken before sleeping and also on an empty stomach early in the morning; decoction regulating

menstruation begins to be taken several days prior to menstruation.

(4) According to the characteristics of a disease; A decoction for a common disease should be taken warm, for cold — syndrome, should be taken hot, and for heat— syndrome, should be taken cold; heat syndrome with pseudo— cold syndrome or cold syndrome with pseudo—heat symptoms must be treated by using corrigent, that is , herbs cold in nature must be taken hot or herbs hot in nature must be taken cold; decoction used to induce sweating and dispel exopathogens must be taken hot so as to promote sweating.

(5) Other forms of prepared Chinese drugs; Powder should be taken following its infusion with hot decoction or after mixing with honey or may be taken in capsule form. Pills such as water—paste pills can be directly taken with boiled water, a honeyed pill can be swallowed after being divided into small pills or taken after dissolution in warm water. Soft extract should be taken following its infusion with boiling water.

4. Watching and Nursing during Administration

It is very important to observe patients carefully and nurse them seriously after administration since the herbal funcion, nadture, taste and features are all different.

(1) When decoction promoting sweating is taken, the correct amount must be administered and the patient should drink hot thin gruel or hot water after administering, and lie in a bed well covered to support the effect of the medicine, causing the whole body to sweat slightly. However, over sweating resulting in exhaustion of body fluids must be guarded against. The patient should not be given raw or cold fruits.

(2) When a patient takes purgative herbs, the patient should be asked to take note of the times of bowel movements as well as the color and amount of stool. If the curative goal is achieved, administration of purgatives should be stopped at once.

(3) After herbs for expelling parasites are taken, the patient must be watched for if there is toxic reaction of the herbs and parasites are removed through the examination of the bowels.

(4) When herbs for discharging stones are taken, the patient should be watched for to see if abdominal pain occurs. Examination of bowels and urine should be carried out to check for discharged stones.

(5) Administering of tinctura should be based on a patient's capacity for liquor. Over drinking must be avoied to protect the patient from harmful reactions such as dizziness, vomiting, palpitation, etc. .

(6) A patient ill with vomiting must rest for a while after vomiting so as to bring about decending of the stomach—Qi, then take several drops of ginger juice or be needled at the point "Neiguan" (P6) to relieve vomiting before taking medicine.

(7) When a patient takes downward discharging herbs or drastic purgatives, harmful reactions likely to follow should be explained to the patient so that the patient will not be shocked by sudden reactions such as diarrhea so as to avoid worry and nervousness. After the medicine is taken, the patient's reaction must be closely watched for, and if abnormal phenomena is found, it must be dealt with promptly.

2　Nursing In Critical Cases

2.1　High Fever Nursing

Fever is one of the common clinical symptoms and occurs in many diseases. It is usually caused by exopathogen or internal injury. Fever caused by internal injury is usually manifested by gradual onset, long duration, absence of aversion to cold, or aversion to cold that will be relieved by additional clothing or bedclothing, intermittent fever, or sometimes regular fever, feverish sensation of the palms and soles with dizziness, lassitude, spontaneous perspiration and night sweating, week pulse and feeling of weekness, etc. Fever caused by exopathogen is manifested by sudden onset, short duration, aversion to cold that is not relieved by putting on more clothes and bedclothes, headache, stuffy nose, and floating pulse, etc. .

1. A patient with high fever should have bed rest.

2. Ward temperature and humidity should be suitable, and the light should not be too strong. The air should be fresh and the ward should be ventilated, but wind should not be directed straight at the patients.

3. The fever may be aggravated by unease of mind, disorder of the liver—Qi and fire—syndrome due to stagnation of Qi. So the patients need good emotional care, especially those with fever caused by internal injury, as the course of their disease is longer

and the condition is more complex. The patients should be encouraged to reduce their mental burden and boost their spirits in order to recover more quickly.

4. Diet should be light and fresh, nutritious and easily digested. Patients should be put on liquid or semi—liquid diet according to their feverish condition. Meat or fish, greasy and peppery food is contraindicated. Meanwhile their specific diet depends on the differentiation of signs and symptoms.

5. Fever mostly consumes body fluids, clinically manifested by thirst and scanty, dark coloured urine. Patients should be encouraged to drink plenty of water and liquid made with ophiopogon root, lophatherum, rush pith, etc. taken as tea. Patients with exopathogenic wind— heat syndrome should have plenty of cool drinks, such as lukewarm boiled water, water—melon or other fruit juice. Those with exopathogenic wind—cold syndrome should have more hot drinks, such as hot porridge, hot ginger liquid, etc. and avoid cold and uncooked food.

6. Intensify oral care. Because patients with fever have shortness of breath and sweat, and their body fluids are wasted, the patients have dry mouths and tongues, and they are subject to stomatitis. The mouth should be rinsed out with decoction of Flos Lonicerae, Fructus Forsythiae (forsythia fruit), Rhizoma Coptidis (coptis root) , Dandelion Taraxacum. Garlic injection or injection of Flavescent Sophora root is applied in the patients with fungous infection. *Bingpeng San, Xilei San, Shishuang* (persimmon frost) , *Wuku San* (Galla Chinensis 36 g plus white sugar 3 g parched into yellowish colour by moderate heating and then dried alum 25 g added are together and ground into fine powder, then stored in a bottle for use) may be applied in those

who suffer from mouth ulcers. Oil may be applied in those who have dry mouths with cracked lips.

7. The skin should be kept clean and dried with towel after sweating. Sweaty and damp clothes and bedclothes should be changed promptly to prevent the patients from catching cold. Skin nursing should be given to the patients who are in bed for a long time to prevent bedsores.

8. Changes of body temperature should be observed carefully. The temperature should be taken and recorded every four hours, and any other time it is deemed necessary. Suitable measures should be taken to lower the temperature of patients with high fever according to their conditions, but the careful observation of feverish pattern should not be affected lest diagnosis should be delayed or collapse should be caused. Therefore, the cause of fever should be ascertained first. If heat is in the surface of the body, physical cooling should be avoided to prevent closure of sweat glands, which are then unable to relieve the heat because of accumulation of heat in the interior. The method of relieving exterior syndrome by means of diaphoresis should be used to transmit pathogenic heat outward. Physical cooling may be given for interior heat syndrome marked by high fever, thirst, etc.. Patients with constipation due to high fever should be given *Daihuang* Powder 3 g (rhubarb powder 3 g) or *Daihuang* tablet 5 (rhubarb tablets) for oral use.

9. Acupuncture cooling:

Quchi(LI11) , Dazhui(DU14) , Fengchi(GB20) , should be selected combining Yintang (EX−HN3) , Taiyang (EX−HN5) , Hegu(LI4) or double Taiyang, Yintang, Shixuan (EX−UE11) and Chize(LU5) should be pricked with three edged—needles for bloodletting in small amounts. Auricular points, Shenmen (HT7), *subcortex, sympathetic* should be applied with moderate stimulation, with retention of needles for 30 minutes after the needles are twirled for five minutes.

10. Patients with high fever, restlessness, coma, delirium and even convulsion due to heat pathogen in the pericardium should take 1. 5—3 g of *Zixue Dan* or one pill of *Angong Niuhuang Wan* (Bezoar Bolus for Resurrection) at once and the doctor should be reported to take measures.

11. If prostration syndrome, manifested as sudden cooling, sweating and cold limbs, pale complexion, dim expressness, thready and rapid pulse or extremely abnormal weak pulse, appears, the doctor should be assisted promptly to give emergency treatment.

12. The doctor should be reported to immediately to give emergency treatment if there appear hematemesis, epistaxis, eruption of the skin, hematuria and hemafecia due to heat acting on *Ying* system and blood.

13. Observe such changes as cold, fever, perspiration, thirst, drinking, tongue coating, pulse condition, emotion, breathing, complexion, urine and feces. Any abnormal conditions found should be treated promptly.

14. Patients with fever due to exopathogen should take hot decoction and plenty of hot drink, and additional clothes and bedclothes should be put on; while those with fever due to interior injury should take warm decoction. The condition of perspiration should be observed after decoction is taken, such as duration, location, nature and odor of perspiration. If sweating is excessive, the doctor should be reported to and herbal administra-

tion should be stopped.

2.2　Coma Nursing

The main clinical manifestations of coma are loss of conciousness, metal confusion and loss of normal reaction to various stimuli. There are many causes causing coma, such as craniocerebral diseases, poisoning caused by medicine or chemicals, etc. regardless of the cause, coma patients are always regarded as critical cases.

1. The location and environment of wards for the critical cases should be quiet, with suitable light and fresh air. Articles and medicines for emergency treatment should be conveniently located and ready for use.

2. Arrange special nursing and prepare and nursing plan. Establish a special record. Observe and record the changes of temperature, pulse condition, breathing, blood pressure and the pupils carefully. Abnormal changes should be reported to the docctor promptly in order that necessary treatment may be given.

3. Observe the change of condition closely:

1) Observe changes in degree of coma. Gradually increasing consciousness indicates improvement of patient's condition. Deepening of coma indicates exacerbation of their condition. Under this condition, the doctor should be assisted to give emergency treatment.

2) If patients have pale complexion, an open mouth, relaxed hands, low and weak breath, cold limbs, cold sticky sweat, fall of blood pressure, thready weak pulse, which show that crisis of *Bi* syndrome developing into prostration syndrome is occuring, the

doctor must be coordinated with to give emergency treatment effectively.

3) The patients with coma whose cause has not been determined should be observed carefully. If any accompanying symptoms appear, such as high fever, stiffness of nape, headache, convulsion, hemiparalysis, vomiting, jaundice, etc. , the doctor must be reported to immediately in order to assist diagnosis and treatment.

4. Keep the respiratory tract unobstructed. Sputum and vomit should be removed promptly. Generally, the patient should be in the supine position, the head inclined to one side, dentures removed and the glossocoma pulled lest the tract should be obstructed. If there are manifestations of rapid breath, cyanotic complexion and limb convulsion in patients, oxygen should be given. In severe cases, a tracheotomy may be necessary.

5. Intensify oral care to prevent complications. Apply a pad at the tooth occlusal surface of the patients with convulsion to prevent injury to the mouth and tongue. Black plum may be used to rub the teeth, or needles inserted into Xiaguan (ST7) , Jiache (ST6) (mandible) Hegu (LI4) etc. , in the case of patients with gnathospasmus. For those who breathe with open mouth, a layer of wet gauze may be placed to cover on their lips to keep mucosa moist.

6. The eyes should be protected carefully. Eye drop may be used regularly or the eyes covered by wet gauze with normal saline as the patient with coma often have dysraphism of the eyelids. So corneal ulcer and inflammation due to exrosis corneae may be prevented.

7. Intensify skin care. In the patients with urine and stool

incontinence, proper method should be taken lest the skin be irritated and the buttocks should be cleaned promptly. Nurse well the limbs of the patients with paralysis or hemiparalysis.

8. Prevent urinary infection. Note the quantities of urine passed. If there is no urine for more than six hours, uroschesis, oliguria, or anuresis should be distinguished out in order to give appropriate treatment.

9. Keep the bowels open. Give caccagogue or enema to the patients who haven't defecated for 3 days.

10. The patients in initial stages of coma should fast for 2—3 days. Their nutritional requirement is supplied intravenously. Those who remain unconscious after two or three days should be put on nasal feeding of liquid diet. In principle, light diet is desirable in primary period, while in its later stage, sufficient nutrition must be guaranteed and enough moisture content provided. When the patient's condition improves and they regain their ability to swallow, nasal feeding should be stopped and replaced by oral intake.

11. Patients with excess syndrome of stoke and those with prostration syndrome are treated separately according to doctor's orders.

1) *Bi* syndrome (excess syndrome of stroke): Give nasal feeding of *Angong Niuhuang Wan, Zhibao Dan* (Treasured Bolus) , *Zixue Dan* or injection of *Qingkailing* by intravenous drip to the patients with heatblockage; or puncture Shuigou (DU26), Shixuan (EX—UE11), Baihui(DU20), Hegu(LI4) , Yongquan(KI1) , or bloodlet at Shixuan; Give nasal feeding of *Suhexiang Wan* to the patients with turbid—blockage; Give nasal feeding of bamboo solution and ginger juice to those with

mental disorder due to stagnation of phlegm or puncture the acupoints of Tiantu (RN22), Fenglong (ST40) , Neiguan (PC6) etc..

2) Prostration syndrome: *Shenfu Tang* should be given to the patients with *Yang* depletion. Moxibustion may be applied over such points as Qihai(RN6), Guanyuan(RN4), Baihui(DU20), Danzhong(RW17), Shenque (RN8) (moxibustion over the salt on the point) ; or needles may be inserted into Shuigou(DU26), Hegu, Zusanli(ST36) ; Patients with *Yin* depletion should take *Shengmai San* (pulse— activating Powder) or *Yixin Koufu Yie*(Oral Juice For Reinforcing Heart) .

2.3 Syncope Nursing

Syncope is mainly manifested as sudden fainting, unconsciousness, pale complexion and cold limbs. Generally, the time for fainting spell is short, there is no sequel of hemiparalysis and aphasia, and deviating mouths and eyes, etc. after regaining consciousness. Shock, fainting spells, heat—stroke, coma due to hypoglycemia and psycological diseases, etc. are all within the range of syncope in modern medicine. Because the causes resulting in it are different, clinically, it is also divided into syncope resulting from disorder of *Qi*, syncope due to excessive bleeding, phlegm syncope, syncope due to summer heat and crapulent syncope.

1. Keep the patients in the supine position or with the head lowered. The head of the patients with vomiting and sputum should be towards one side, the clothes and button being loosened and opened. Take care to keep the patients warm.

2. Keep the ward environment quiet; light in the ward

should be dimmed; keep the patients well rested.

3. Give the patients sugar solution or boiled water when they have cold limbs. After wakening, they should be put on light liquid or semiliquid diet.

4. Observe and note carefully any changes of consciousness, pupil, comlexion, body temperature, breath, pulse condition, blood pressure, urine and stool. If abnormality is found, the doctor should be reported to immediately to take measures.

5. Take care to ask medical history and predisposing factors. Observe the patient's general condition and make a complete examination, distinguish excess from deficiency and give treatment and nursing of primary disease in accordance with the cause of the disease.

6. If Syncope is caused by an allergic reaction due to medicine, one ml of 0. 1% of adrenalin hydrochloride should be immediately injected subcutaneously, oxygen inhalation should be given and the doctor should be told at once in order to give emergency treatment.

7. Excess syndrome can be treated with acupuncture and moxibustion therapy. Needles may be inserted into shugou (DU26) , Chengjiang(RN24) , Shixuan(EX−UE11) , Yongquan (KI1) with strong stimulation and the needles are manipulated every 3—5 minutes. Deficiency syndrome can be treated with acupuncture combined with moxibustion which is applied to Baihui(DU20) , Qihai(RN6) , until the patient return to normal.

8. Syncope resulting from disorder of *Qi* is often induced by emotional irritability. So psychological nursing should be especially emphasized. The patients and their relatives should be ad-

vised to relieve their mental stress and phobic psychology and avoid negative stimulation.

9. Take blood pressure promptly in patients with syncope due to excessive bleeding. Observe any changes in blood pressure and get ready to give blood transfusion. The patients with deficiency syndrome may take *Dushen Tang,* and should be given treatment for primary disease and nursing according to their medical history. They should be advised to give priority to recuperation and avoid overfatigue, take care of regimen in order to build up their health.

10. The lateral recumbent position should be assumed by patients with phlegm syncope. When expectoration of sputum is difficult, their backs may be patted. If necessary, sputum may be aspirated with a sputum aspirator, or 30 ml. of bamboo juice is taken to eliminate sputamentum and keep the respiratary tract unobstructed.

11. The room of patients with syncope due to summer heat should be ventilated and cool. Physical cooling should be given without delay. Medicine for removing heat from the heart in order to restore to consciousness should be taken at once, such as one pill of *Niuhuang Qingxin Wan* taken after it is infused in cold boiled water, or *Shi Di Shui* (ten drops) and *Ren Dan,* etc. The patients should take plenty of cooling drink, such as cool boiled water, soup of mung bean, and watermelon juice.

12. Patients with crapulent syncope should fast temporarily. Gastric content may be removed by inducing vomiting or using emetic agent of Chinese herbs, and they may take medicine, such as *Baohe Wan* (lentive pill) , *Sixiao Tang* (sugar of promoting digestin) to normalize the function of the stomach and spleen,

clear food retention, and promote digestion. Patients with abdominal distention and constipation may take caccagogue, such as *Daihuang Pian* (rhubarb tablets) , *Fanxieye* (Senna leaf) in hot water taken as tea.

13. Patients with coma resulting from syncope for a prolonged period should be taken care of in the light of coma nursing.

14. It is still necessary to keep watch for changes of the condition after remission of syncope syndrome in order to prevent relapse.

2.4　Palpitation Nursing

Palpitation refers to unduly rapid beating of the heart which is felt by the patient himself and accompanied by uncomfortable sensation in the precardium. In traditional Chinese medicine, palpitation is divided into two types: palpitation due to fright and severe palpitation. The former often results from exopathogenic factors. Its symptoms are milder and of short duration. But it may develop into severe palpitation with prolonged onset. The latter mainly results from endopathic factors. Its symptoms are more severe, and its attack is frequent. Occurance of palpitation is related to mental factor, insufficiency of heart blood, failure of the heart—*Yang,* and retention of excessive fluids in the body, obstruction of blood stasis in the channels and collaterals, etc. .

1. The ward environment should be quiet and noise should be avoided lest stimulation of fright result in attack of palpitation.

2. Attack of palpitation is often related to excessive mental

stress, excitement or worry. So psychological nursing should be directed towards boosting morale in order to give patients ease of mind and help them to adopt a positive attitude towards disease and actively cooperate with the doctor during the treatment.

3. Severe cases or patients having an attack of palpitation should stay in bed. When they are companied with dyspnea, semirecumbent position should be taken and oxygen inhalation should be given, The mild cases may have a moderate exercise. The level of activities should be increased gradually so as not to aggravate the symptom. The patients should avoid fatigue and strenuous exercise.

4. A tonic or nourishing food should be supplied, such as the Chinese yam (Rhzoma Pioscoreae) , Chinese date, lotus seed (Semen Nelumbinis) , longan, soft—shelled turtle, pig heart, sea cucumber, etc. Patients should have small frequent meals, avoiding overeating, smoking, alcohol, pungent and irritative food. The patients with copious sputum should be prohibited from eating fat, sweet or greasy food. Intake of sodium salt should be controlled in the patients acompanied with edema.

5. Keep a close watch for changes of condition:

(1) Pay attention to the condition of palpitation attack (whether it is frequent or paroxysmal) and its relationship to activities, spirit and food—intake in order to assist diagnosis.

(2) Observe symptoms by which palpitation is accompanied. It is heart failure if palpitation is accompanied by cough, chest pain, oppressed feeling in the chest, dyspnea, oliguria and edema. If palpitation is accompanied by chest pain, cold sweating and lowed blood pressure, it is suggestive of myocardial infarction. If palpitation is accompanied by high fever and severe toxic symptoms in general body, the possibility of toxic myocarditis should be considered. If the above conditions are found, the doctor should be informed so as to treat promptly.

(3) Observe the features, duration and regularity of palpitation attack.

(4) Keep watch over changes of blood pressure, heart rate and rhythm of the heart. If abnormality is found, the doctor should be informed so as to treat promptly.

(5) Pay attention to changes of complexion, appearance of the tongue and pulse condition. Dry hot face, flushed texture of tongue and thready and rapid pulse are usually indicative of hyperativity of fire due to *Yin* deficiency; Pale complexion, pale tongue and weak and small pulse indicate insufficiency of *Yang*— *Qi*; rough complexion, dark red tongue and weak, thready and uneven pulse, or knotted and intermittent pulse indicate stagnation of heart— blood; and swelling face, sticky tongue coating, slow and slippery pulse suggest phlegm— dampness or coldness.

6. With the onset of palpitation, Xinshu(BL15) , Neiguan (PC6) , Shenmen(HT7) , Danzhong(RN17) may be punctured.

7. To keep the bowels open, the patients with constipation should be given light diaphoretic prescription, such as *Qingning* pill 3 g, taking twice a day.

8. If the patient's heart stops beating suddenly, emergency measures should be taken immediately, such as closed cardic massage, artificial respiration, endocardial injection, etc.

9. Before use of digitalis patient's pulse should be felt, their heart rate should be taken for one minute. In case of less than sixty beats per minute, stopping medicine should be considered and

possible poisoning reaction to digitalis should be checked for. In the case of any such reaction, the doctor should be informed at once in order to take measures.

3 Nursing for Commonly Encountered Medical Diseases

3.1 Common Cold

Common Cold is a common exogenous ailment, characterized by stuffy nose, nasal discharge, headache, cough, fever, aversion to cold, etc. . The mild type is known as invasion by wind. The severe type is known in TCM as severe invasion by wind. If there is an epidemic manifested with similar symptoms and signs, it is known as influenza or epidemic influenza.

General Nursing

1. The air in the room should be fresh and well ventilated but the patients should not be in any draught which may worsen the cold. The patient's body should be kept warm and the patient's garments and bed clothes should be increased according to weather changes.

2. Cases of epidemic influenza should be isolated as per the isolation method of respiratory infectious disease. The air in the ward may be sterilized by steaming vinegar, 1—2 parts water to 1 part vinegar, 5—10 ml of vinegar is diluted with water for each cubic metre of room. The sterilization is given once a day or every other day.

3. A mild case does not require rest. But a severe or feverish case must rest in bed, getting up only after the fever has subsided and returning to work only after the symptoms and signs have disappeared, striking a proper balance between work and rest.

4. The patient's food should be nourishing, light and easy to digest, while oily, greasy or sweet food is contraindicated. A patient ill with common cold may eat semifluid food but one with influenza should drink vegetarian fluid diet and plenty of water.

5. Take note of any changes of fever, aversion to cold, sweating, as well as the tongue and pulse condition.

6. Decoction must be decocted for only a short time, not over boiled. A Dose of decoction is generally separated into two parts to be taken at different times. But if after the first part of the decoction has been taken, the fever greatly reduces, the doctor should be notified immediately and the other part is then contraindicated. Sweating, in order to expel pathogenic factors, must not be excessive; light sweating all over the body should be allowed as the normal. After sweating, the patient should avoid wind and keep the body warm to avoid any relapse. If the patient does not perspire after taking medicine and the fever continuously rises, a doctor should be informed.

7. The patients should take exercise to build up their disease—resistant ability.

Nursing According to Syndrome Differentiation

1. Wind—cold Syndrome
Clinical Manifestations
Chills, low fever, anhidrosis, headache, pantalgia, stuffy

running nose, cough, asthma due to phlegm, no thirst or preference for hot drinks, thin and white tongue coating, superficial and tense pulse.

Nursing

(1) The ward temperature should be a little on the high side.

(2) Raw and cold food is contraindicated but plenty of hot drinks of water are suitable.

(3) Herbs pungent in taste and warm in nature, for relieving the exterior syndrome and venilating the lung and expelling cold should be administered. The selected prescription is *Jingfang Baidu San* with modification (Modified Antiphlogistic powder of Schizonepeta and Ledebouriella), the decoction being administered hot. After administration, the patient should be warmly covered and meanwhile, be given more hot water gruel or rice soup to drink so as to support the herbal effect.

(4) High fever should not be lowered by physiotherapy in order to prevent sweat pores from closing up and thus maintaining pathogenic evils.

(5) Acupuncture is used with the purpose of expelling wind and cold, relieving exterior syndromes and ventilating the lung. Lieque (LU7), Yingxiang (LI20), Fengchi (GB20), Hegu (LI4), are selected. Yintang (EX−HN3), and Taiyang (EX−HN5) are added for headache.

(6) Fresh Ginger 3 pieces, onion 5 pieces and Prepared Soybean 9 g are decocted in water for oral use, or *Xiling Jiedu Pian* is taken three times a day.

2. Wind——heat Syndrome

Clinical Manifestations

High fever, slight aversion to wind and cold, non—smooth

perspiration, headache, red eyes, yellow and thick nasal discharge, cough with mucous or yellow sputum, swelling and sore throat, thirst, white tongue coating, superficial and rapid pulse.

Nursing

(1) Keep the ward cool and well ventilated.

(2) Plenty of fruits such as water—melon, peach, should be eaten. Much drink which is cool in nature such as mung bean soup, should be taken.

(3) Herbs pungent in flavor and cool in nature should be taken to relieve the exterior syndrome, ventilate the lung and clear away heat; the prescription is *Yingqiao San* with modification (powder of Lonicera and Forsythia). The decoction should be taken warm, and the patient should be kept warm with dry clothes so as to avoid any relapse.

(4) Needling is given to Chize(LU5) , Yuji(LU10) , Quchi(LI11) , Dazhui(DU14) , Waiguan(SJ5) to dispel wind heat and clear lung— *Qi*. Shaoshang(LU11) is added for sore throat and pricked with three— edged needles for bleeding, or *Houzhen Wan* and *Liu Shen Wan* can be taken.

(5) Lophatherum 12 g, Herba Menthae 3 g, Semen Armeniacae Amarum 3 g and Fructus Forsythiae 3 g are decocted with water for oral use. A sack of Sangju Ganmao Chongji can also be taken orally, three times a day.

3. Summer—heat Wetness Syndrome

Clinical Manifestations

General fever, slight aversion to wind, little perspiration, heavy head, heavy and sore limbs, cough with mucous, thick nasal discharge, restlessness, thirst but little inclination to drink, feeling of fullness and oppression over the chest, abdominal distention due to severe vomiting, loose stool, thick and greasy or yellow and greasy tongue coating, soggy or soggy rapid pulse.

Nursing

(1) Light and fluid diet is suitable for the cases with obvious symptoms of gastrointestinal tract.

(2) Herbs should be taken to eliminate summer heat from superficies of the body by diaphoresis and eliminate dampness with aromatics. The prescription is *Xinjia Xiangru Yin* with modification (Modified Decoiction of Elsholtzia with Supplements), the decoction of which should be taken warm. The case with obvious symptoms of gastrointestinal tract should take the decoction frequently but a little each time and may also take it with fresh ginger juice.

(3) Acupuncture and moxibustion is used to eliminate summer—heat and dampness, and disperse the evils from the superficies and regulate the interior. Zhongwan (RN12), Hegu (LI4), Zusanli (ST36), can be used. Dazhui (DU14) and Quchi (LI11) are included for high fever and Yinlingquan (SP9) is added for serious wetness.

(4) *Liuyi San* (Six to one Powder)12 g and Herba Menthae 6 g are taken after being infused in boiling water, or *Huoxiang Zhengqi Wan* 1~ 2 pills (Pills of Agastachis for Restoring Health) are taken twice a day.

3.2 Dysentery

Dysentery is an intestinal infectious disease commonly encountered in summer and autumn, marked by abdominal pain, diarrhea, tenesmus and frequent stools containing blood and mucus.

General Nursing

1. Protection of the digestive canal is necessary to prevent cross infection. The excreta, eating utersile, chamberware and anything touched by the patient ill with dysentery must be thoroughly sterilized. After three consecutive tests show that stool culture is negative, the isolation may be relaxed.

2. The air in the ward should be fresh and the temperature must be suitable. Emergency cases must take bed rest and chronic cases should do proper physical exercises to build up their health.

3. Note abdominal pain, bowel movement times and colour, and the general body condition and inform a doctor immediately to take emergency measures if critical conditions appear such as high fever, coma and convulsion due to invasion of the heart—*Ying* by pathogen.

4. After bowel movement, the anus should be rubbed with soft paper and washed clean with warm water. If necessary, talcum powder or little oil may be applied.

Nursing According to Syndrome Differentiation

1. Damp—heat Dysentery
Clinical Manifestations
Fever, aversion to cold, abdominal pain, diarrhea, bloody or mucous stools, burning, sensation of the anus, tenesmus, dry mouth and preference for cold, yellow sticky tongue coating, slippery and rapid pulse.

Nursing

(1) Liquid or semiliquid and light diet is suitable. Patients are encouraged to drink plenty of warmly boiled water or light salt solution so as to replenish fluid and avoid damage of body fluids.

(2) Herbs should be administered for eliminating dampness and heat, and promoting flow of Qi and blood circulation, the selected prescriptions being *Shaoyao Tang* (Peony Decoction), *Gegen Qin Lian Tang* with modification (Modified Decoction of Pueraria, Scutellaria and Coptis), their decoction being taken warm.

(3) Needling is given to Tianshu(ST25), Dachangshu (BL25) Geshu(BL17), Zusanli(ST36), Xuehai(SP10).

2. Fulminant Dysentery

Clinical Manifestations

Sudden onset, frequent stools containing blood and mucus, intense abdominal pain, tenesmus, high fever, flushed face, thirst, irritability, delirium in a severe case, coma and convulsion, red and crimson tongue with yellowish coating, flooding and rapid pulse.

Nursing

(1) A severe case may temporarily fast for 6—8 hours. After the patient's condition stabilizes, he should have fluid diet and plenty of water to maintain water—electrolytic balance and gradually return to the normal diet during the period of his recovery. Greasy, fried and not easily digested food is contraindicated.

(2) Take care to watch for any changes in body temperature; a case with high fever should be reported to a doctor for appropriate treatment. (refer to 2. 1 Nursing of High Fe-

ver) .

(3) Watch the patient's condition, and inform the doctor to take treatment measures when the patient shows unconsciousness, delirium, clonus or convulsion, restlessness, pale complexion, thin and weak pulse, etc. (refer to 2. 3 Syncope Nursing) . If there is appearance of irregular depth and rhythm of respiration or sighing known as crisis of respiratory failure, a doctor should be informed immediately in order to take emergency measures.

(4) Heat—clearing and detoxifying herbs should be taken, the selected prescription being *Baitouweng Tang* with modification (Modified Pulsatilla Decoction) .

(5) Needling is given to Dazhui(DU14), Neiguan(PC6), Tianshu(ST25), Sifeng(EX−UE10), Shixuan(EX−UE11).

3. Deficiency—Cold Dysentery

Clinical Manifestations

Frequent loose stools with purple and dark colour with mucosity, prolonged dysentery, abdominal pain, tenesmus, chills and cold limbs, lassitude, loss of appetite, thin and pale tongue coating, deep and thin pulse.

Nursing

(1) The patient's abdomen should be kept warm. When abdominal pains occur, hot compress is given with hot—water bag or heated table salt or Fructurs Foenicuii wrapped in cloth.

(2) The patient should be given nourishing and easily digested food, some hot in nature such as garlic, onion, ginger, while fatty, rough, greasy, raw and cold food should be limited.

(3) Herbs should be administered for warming and tonifying the spleen and kidney, and relieving diarrhea. The prescrip-

tion is based on *Yangzang Tang* (Decoction Tonifying Zang Organs) and *Sishen Wan* (Pill of Four Miraculous Drugs) with modification, the decoction being taken hot.

(4) Moxibustion is applied to the points, Zusanli(ST36), Tianshu(ST25), Shenque(RN8), Dachangshu(BL25).

4. Recurrent Dysentery

Clinical Manifestations

Dysentery occurring on and off, difficult to cure, abdominal pain in dysentery, tenesmus, stool with mucosity or little blood and pus, thin and pale tongue coating, thin and weak pulse.

Nursing

(1) Diet should be regulated carefully. Nourishment should be stressed for delicated patients. Herbs should be taken frequently for strengthening the spleen, replenishing *Qi* and removing the stagnation of food to restore normal function of the stomach, the selected prescription being *Liu Junzi Tang* with modification (Modified Decoction of Six Ingrendients), and *Xianglian Wan* (Aucklandia and Coptis Pill) is added when the disease attacks, the decoction should be taken warm.

(2) Acupuncture and moxibustion treatment is given to Zusanli(ST36) Zhongwan (RN12) Pishu(UL20).

3.3 Bronchitis

Bronchitis falls into two kinds; acute and chronic, belonging to cough range of TCM. Acute bronchitis is cough generally due to invasion by the exogenous pathogenic factors; chronic bronchitis is cough generally caused by internal injury. The disease occurs mostly in the changeable seasons, spring and winter, mostly in those persons, the elderly and weak. It is mainly characerized by cough, expectoration and dyspnea.

General Nursing

1. Keep room clean with air circulating and at suitable temperature and humidity to avoid dryness and prevent accumulation and circulation of dust, smoking and particular smells that may induce cough or make it more severe.

2. A case with fever should rest in bed , the elderly and weak may prolong the rest period.

3. A suitable diet for such patients is one of high calorie, light and easily digested food. Plenty of water should be drunk. Peppery and irritative food, smoking and alcohol are contraindicated.

4. Observe carefully any changes of fever, cough, sputum property, coating and pulse condition.

Nursing According to Syndrome Differentiation

1. Impairment of Dispersing and Descending Function of the Lung Due to Attack of the Lung by Exogenous Pathogenic Wind —cold (Wind—cold type)

Clinical Manifestations

Cough with thin and white sputum, aversion to cold with slight fever, nasal obstruction and discharge, itching of the throat and hoarse voice, thin white tongue coating and superficial pulse.

Nursing

(1) Ensure that body is kept warm. The room temperature should be on the warm side and weather changes are taken into

account. When going outside, the patient should wear a gauze mask to prevent secondary attack of exopathogen which may make the patient's condition more severe.

(2) Raw and cold fruits are contraindicated.

(3) Herbs are taken to disperse wind and cold, release inhibited Lung—energy and relieve cough. The prescription is *Xing Su San* with modification (Modified Apricot—kernel and Perilla Powder), which is taken hot, the result after administration being observed.

(4) *Tong Xuan Li Fei Wan* (1—2 pills Releasing Inhibited Lung—energy) can be taken twice a day.

(5) Acupuncture and moxibustion treatment is given to the points; Lieque(LU7), Hegu(LI4), Feishu(BL13), Waiguan(SJ5).

2. Dysfunction of the Lung due to Wind—heat Attacking the Superficies of the Body (Wind—heat Type)

Clinical Manifestations

Cough with thick sputum, choking cough, thirst, sore throat, fever, yellow tongue coating, superficial and rapid pulse.

Nursing

(1) Keep the room air fresh and cool but prevent draught from blowing directly on to patients.

(2) Let patients eat food that will clear heat and resolve phlegm, such as orange, shaddock, radish, beef, and have plenty of cool drink.

(3) Herbs should be taken to disperse wind, clear heat, ventilate the lung and stop cough, the selected prescription being *Sengju Yin* with modification (Modified Decoction of Mulberry Leaf and Chrysanthemum), the decoction being taken warm.

(4) The patient with choking cough due to thick phlegm should sit upright or in a semireclining position, the back being gently tapped or Flos Lonicerae 3 g, Radix Platycodi 3 g and Radix Polygalae 3 g are decocted for spray inhalation so as to dilute phlegm and ease its removal.

(5) Take the temperature of a feverish patient promptly and inform the doctor of the result. (refer to 2. 1 Pyrexia Nursing)

(6) Both acupuncture and moxibustion are given to the points: Chize(LU5), Feishu(BL13), Quchi(LI11), Dazhui (DU14) .

(7) *Sangju Pian* 3 tablets (Tablet of Mulberry Leaf and Chrysanthemum) are taken three times a day or Folium Mori 9 g, Semen Armeniacae Amarum 9 g, Gypsum Fibrosum (raw) 30 g, Radix Glycyrrhizae 1 g are decocted with water for oral use.

(8) The patient's mouth should be kept clean. *Yinqin Tang* (Flos Lonicerae 9 g, Herba Taraxaci 9 g, Rhizoma Coptidis 9 g, Radix Scutellariae 9 g are decocted with water leaving 500 ml of decoction) is used to rinse the mouth.

3. Accumulation of Phlegm—dampness in the Lung due to Dysfunction of the Spleen

Clinical Manifestations

Cough with profuse, white and mucous or thin sputum, stuffiness and depression in the chest, white, sticky tongue coating, soggy and slippery pulse.

Nursing

(1) Diet should be light. Smoking, alcohol, fat and meat are contraindicated so as to prevent restoration of dampness and production of phlegm.

(2) Herbs should be taken to strengthen the spleen, elimi-

nate dampness, resolve phlegm and regulate the function of the lung, the selected prescription being *Erchen Tang* with modification (Modified Two Old Drugs Decoction). The result after taking the medicine must be noted carefully.

(3) Both acupuncture and moxibustion are given to the points: Zhongwan(RN12), Fenglong(ST40), Feishu (BL13) .

(4) *Juhong Wan*1— 2 pills (Red Tangerine Peel Pill) is taken twice a day, or Rhizoma Pinelliae 9 g, Poria 12 g, Pericarpium Citri Reticulatae 3 g, Radix Glycyrrhizae 3 g are decocted with water for oral use.

4. Fire Acting on the Lung due to Stagnation of the Liver— *Qi*

Clinical Manifestations

Cough due to reversed flow of *Qi*, redish complexion, dry throat, purulent and thick sputum, vexation, thirst, thin and yellow tongue coating with little body fluids, wiry and rapid pulse.

Nursing

(1) Take care of the patient's emotion, preventing excitement in order to ease patient's mind.

(2) Herbs are administered to calm the liver in order to purge intense heat, remove heat from the lung, and lower the adverse flow of *Qi*. A modified prescription treating hemoptysis is selected.

(3) Both acupuncture and moxibustion are given to the points: Feishu(BL13) , Ganshu(BL18) , Jingqu(LU8) , Taichong(LR3) .

(4) Cortex Mori Radicis 9 g, Radix Scutellariae 9 g, *Dai Ge San* 9 g (powder of Indigo and Clam Shell) are decocted with water for oral use.

3.4 Bronchial Asthma

Asthma is a common disease characterized by repeated attacks of paroxysmal dyspnea with wheezing, breath shortness and difficulty. The severe case opens his mouth, raises his shoulder, nares flaring and can not lie on his back, which are called asthma, The first attack is usually symptomatic of excess syndrome, but repeated attacks form excess into deficiency syndrome.

General Nursing

1. Facilities in the room should be kept simple and the room maintains cleanliness and tidiness, quietness and ventilation. Plants or other things with stimulating smells are not placed in the room.

2. When asthma attacks, the patient should have bed rest, sitting in semireclining position or upright and be given oxygen promptly.

3. Counsel the patient with a smoking habit to give up smoking.

4. Diet should be light, and food inducing attacks of asthma such as eggs, milk, fish, shrimp, etc. are avoided. Raw, cold, excessive salty or sweet food is contraindicated.

5. Take care of the phychological nursing, easing the patient's mind to prevent relapse due to mental factors. When the asthma attacks, the patient should be given comfort to ease his nervous emotion.

6. Patients should be advised to avoid smog, dust and irritative smells as far as possible, so as to avoid relapses of asthma.

7. Watch for sign of an impending asthma attack, such as oppressed feeling in the chest, dyspnea, itching feeling in nose and throat, sneezing, nose running, etc. which should be treated as early as possible.

8. Pay close attention to the time of asthma attack, degree of mildness or severity, duration of attack, accompanying symptoms, the condition of expectoration, the changes of body temperature, tongue and pulse condition.

9. Investigate the patient's living environment, dietetic habits and family allergy history, etc. to search for inducing factors which should be avoided to get in touch with.

10. Patients with difficult expectoration may be given herbal decoction for spray inhalation or gently patting the back.

11. Encourage the patients to take physical exercises, such as *Qigong*, breathing exercises, *Taiji quan,* etc. to build up their health.

Nursing According to Syndrome Differentiation

1. Excess Syndrome
(1) Retention of cold in the Lung
Clinical Manifestations
Shortness of breath, wheezing in the throat, thin, whitish or frothy sputum, stuffiness sensation in the chest and epigastric region, gloomy complexion, absence of thirst or thirst with preference for hot drink, headache, fever, chills, anhidrosis, etc. , white and slippery tongue coating, superficial and tight pulse.
Nursing
(a) Patients should keep the body warm to avoid cooling

and wear a gauze mask outside.

(b) Herbs can be taken to warm the lungs and dispel cold, eliminate phlegm for resuscitation and anti— asthma, The selected prescription is *Sheganmahuang Tang* with modification (Modified Decoction of Belamcanda and Ephedra), which is taken warm. Plenty of hot drink should be taken, raw and cold diet being contraindicated.

(c) Acupuncture and moxibustion are given to the points: Lieque (LU7), Chize(LU5), Fengmen(BL12), Feishu(BL13).

(d) *Xiaochuan Wan* 3 pills (Asthma pills) are taken before sleep each evening. Datura leaves are prepared into a cigarette type which is lit and inhaled in an attack, in order to relieve the syndrome.

(2) Accumulation of Phlegm and Heat in the Lung

Clinical Manifestations

Cough, dyspnea, thick and yellow sputum, reddish complexion with fever, perspiration, thirst, restlessness, chest pain due to cough, yellow and sticky tongue coating, slippery and rapid pulse.

Nursing

(a) Attention should be paid to mouth nursing. *Yinqin Tang* (Decoction of Honeysuckle Flower and Scutellaria Root) may be given to rinse the mouth.

(b) Watch feverish patients for changes of the body tamperature.

(c) Herbs should be taken to clear heat and promote the dispersing function of the lungs, resolve phlegm and lower the adverse flow of *Qi*. The selected prescription is *Maxingshigan Tang* with modification (Modified Decoction of Ephedra, Apricot Rernel Seed, Cypsum and Licorice) , which is taken warm, the effects being noted after administration.

(d) Both acupuncture and moxibustion are applied to Hegu (LI4), Dazhui(DU14), Fenglong(ST40), Danzhong (RN17) Fire cupping is done on the added points Feishu (BL13) and Yunmen(LU2) for severe dyspnea.

(e) 1 bottle of *Shedanchuanbei San* (Powder of Snake Gall and Sichuan Fritillary Bulb) is taken three times daily.

2. Asthma due to Deficiency Syndrome

Clinical Manifestations

Slow attack, longstanding asthma, shortness of breath, feeble voice, spontaneous perspiration, aversion to wind, dyspnea on exertion, blue lips and nails, cold limbs, dark purple tongue, thin and rapid pulse.

Nursing

(1) Tiredness and emotional irritation should be prevented so as to avoid inducing asthma.

(2) As weather changes, the patients should be careful to keep warm and seriously prevent catching cold.

(3) Herbs should be taken to tonify the lung and benefit the kidney, lower the adverse flow of *Qi* and resolve phlegm. The selected prescription is *Pingchuanguben Tang* with modification (Modified Decoction for Relieving Asthma and Consolidating Root), which is taken hot.

(4) A case with deficiency of lung *Qi* should be given *Huangqin Gao* 15 g (Soft Extract of Scutellaria Root) which is taken three times a day.

(5) Acupuncture and moxibustion are given to the points, Dingchuan(EXB1), Gaohuang(BL43), Feishu(BL13), Taiyuan (LU9).

3.5 Pulmonary Abscess

Pulmonary abscess known in TCM is a disease due to retention of wind and virulent heat in the lung leading to blood stasis and the formation of pus, characterized by fever, chest pain, cough with discharge of foul purulent sputum or even bloody pus. According to each chronological stage in the course of disease, clinically the period of the disease is divided into inital days, abscess stage, stadium suppurationis and recovery stage.

General Nursing

1. The ward should be kept clean and well ventilated with fresh air.

2. Take care to regulate the room temperature, preventing cold and maintaining warmth well so as to prevent superinfection and exacerbation of the disease.

3. During the acute stage, as the patients run a fever, expectorate purulent sputum and hemoptysis occur, they should remain in bed and be permitted to move about only after they are on the way to recovery, which may improve discharge of purulent sputum.

4. Diet should be light with plenty of vegetables but not excessively salty. Peppery or greasy food, some seafood which can cause relapse of the disease, such as yellow croaker, shrimp, crab should be contraindicated and plenty of water should be taken.

5. Smoking and drinking are forbidden.

6. Observe the changes of patient's body temperature, breath, tongue coating and pulse, taking careful notes.

7. Observe the condition of expectoration and its changes

such as color, quality, quantity and smell.

Nursing According to Sydrome Differentiation

1. The Inital Stage
Clinical Manifestations
Chills, fever, cough, white and sticky foamy sputum, the quantity of which varies from little to much, dyspnea, dry mouth and nose, thin and yellow or thin and white tongue coating, superficial rapid and slippery pulse.

Nursing
(1) Observe the changes of cough, chest pain and sputum quantity.

(2) Herbs to clear away the lung— heat and dispel pathogens from the body exterior should be taken. The selected prescription is *Yinqiao San* with modification (Modified powder of Lonicera and Forsythia) . The decoction should not be boiled for too long, and be taken warm but the effects after administration should be observed, formed abscess being prevented.

2. Formed Abscess Stage
Clinical Manifestations
Fever with perspiration, chills, oppressed feelings and pains in the chest, cough with short breath, expectoration of purulent sputum with stinking smell as of rotten fish, restlessness, yellow and sticky coating, slippery and rapid pulse.

Nursing
(1) Observe the changes of fever, chest pain, sputum quantity, colour and smell. High fever, chills, oppressed feelings in the chest, dull pain of dragging chest in cough and sputum with stink-

ing smell as of rotten fish indicate that pulmonary abscess has developed.

(2) Herbs Should be taken to remove heat from the lung and dispel stasis to relieve boils, the selected prescripton being *Weijing Tang* with modification (Modified Reed Stem Decoction) .

(3) Patients with constipation may be prescribed mild laxatives to keep the bowels open.

3. Stadium Suppurationis

Clinical Manifestations

Expectoration of a great quantity of purulent and bloody sputum with horrible stinking smell as of rotten fish, restlessness, fullness and pain in the chest, inability to lie down due to asthma, fever with reddish complexion, morbid thirst and desire for drink, red or dark red tongue with yellow and sticky coating, slippery and rapid pulse.

Nursing

(1) Patients with fever should be given semifluid diet and eat mostly fruits such as orange, pear, loquat, radish so as to nourish the lung and resolve phlegm, They can eat job's tears gruel so as to improve the expectoration of phlegm, and have more cold drink and boiled water of fresh reed rhizome taken as tea.

(2) Care of mouth cavity should be emphasized. *Yin qiao Tang* (Decoction of Lonicera and Forsythia) or light salt water is given to gargle.

(3) Ensure the sterilization of spittoon, in which disinfectant liquid should be put.

(4) Medicinal herbs for evacuating pus and relieving toxin

should be taken, the selected prescription being *Jiaweijiegeng Tang* with modification (Modified Decoction of Platycodon Root) .

(5) The patients with thick sputum difficult to be expectorated should be given herbal decoction in the form of spray inhalation to clear heat and resolve phlegm so as to promote discharge of sputum.

(6) Proper arrangement of body position is made for benefiting the release of phlegm by postural drainage.

(7) Watch patient's condition carefully. If a great quantity of blood is expectorated, the nurse should watch out for appearance of blood clot obstructing air passage, or crisis of exhaustion of *Qi* resulting from hemorrhea. Once the crisis appeares, the doctor must be immediately reported to for emergency treatment.

(8) Proper amount of Radix Coicis (fresh) is pounded into pieces from which juice is drawn and boiled, then taken hot three times a day to improve discharge of sputum, or a suitable amount of lotus leaf is decocted to thick juice to which white honey is added for oral use.

4. Recovery Stage

Clinical Manifestations

The symptoms such as fever, cough and expectoration of purulent and bloody sputum become milder gradually, or are manifested by dull pain in the chest and hypochondrium, shortness of breath, spontaneous perspiration, night sweat, low fever, tidal fever, pale complexion, emaciation, red or light—red tongue, thin, rapid and weak pulse.

Nursing

(1) Encourage the patients to walk about but not over exert

themselves.

(2) Give the patients high calorie and high—proten diet. The amount of food should be gradually increased but not be excessive so as to avoid damaging the stomach and spleen.

(3) Since the period of disease is long and patient's mental burden is heavy, psycholigical nursing should be stressed to ease the patient's mind so as to benefit the recovery.

3.6 Hypertension Disease

Hypertension is included in the range of ailments known as "headache" or "dizziness" in traditional Chinese medicine, characterized by intermittent headache and dizziness, or heavy sensation in the head and unsteady walk, and a rise in blood pressure.

General Nursing

1. Ward light should not be strong, the environment should be quiet and comfortable, and sleeping time should be assured.

2. The patient with initial hypertension may take part in work, but must not be overtired, and should regularly do exercises such as *Taiji quan, Qigong,* etc.

3. Diet should be low calorie, light, plenty of vegetables, fruits, high in vitamins and with a little salt. Peppery, sweat, fat and greasy food is contraindicated and drinking must be abstained from completely.

4. Watch for changes of blood pressure, if the blood pressure is in obvious undulation, the doctor should be informed in order to take measures.

Nursing According to Syndrome Differentiation

1. Fire—syndrome due to Stagnation of the Liver—*Qi* and Hyperactivity of the Liver *Yang*.

Clinical Manifestations

Dizziness, flushed complexion, red eyes, irritability, bitter taste in the mouth, dry throat, scanty and dark urination, reddish tongue, wiry, rapid and forceful pulse.

Nursing

(1) Understand the patient's psychology, give the patient psychological nursing to assist him to free his mind of anxiety and anger, keep ease of mind and optimistic attitude.

(2) Herbs should be taken to clear and purge liver—heat and assist in nourishing *Yin*. The selected prescription is *Longdan Xiegan Tang* with modification (Modified Decoction of Gentiana for Purging the Liver—fire) .

(3) Acupuncture and moxibustion are given to the points, Xingjian(LR 2) , Shuiquan(KI5) , Yintang(EX–HN3) ; ear seeds implanting is applied to Shenmen(HT7) and Jiangyagou (ear acupoint, indication: hypertension) .

(4) Flos Chrysanthemi 60g is boiled for oral use instead of tea. *Longdan Xiegan Wan* (Pill to Purge the Liver Fire with Gentiana) 9 g is taken each time, twice a day.

2. Hyperactivity of the Liver—*Yang* due to Both Deficiency of the Liver—*Yin* and Kideny—*Yin*.

Clinical Manifestations

Dizziness, tinnitus, insomnia, frequent dreaming, irritability, difficult and dark urine, lumbago and lassitude in legs, numbness of limbs in the severe case, wiry and thin pulse and dark red tongue.

Nursing

(1) Watch carefully for changes of patient's condition, in the case of symptoms and signs of apoplexy such as numbness of lips and tongue, numbness of extremities, deviation of the eye and mouth, the patient must take immediate bed rest and the doctor should be notified promptly to give treatment.

(2) Since every attack of the disease is due to tiredness or anger, rest and emotional care are essential.

(3) Acupuncture and moxibustion are given to Ganshu(BL18), Shenshu(BL23), Sanyinjiao(SP6) Zusanli(ST36).

(4) *Naoliqing* 10—20 pills is taken each time, twice a day.

(5) Herbs should be taken to nourish liver— *Yin* and kidney — *Yin,* tranquilize and subdue hyperactive liver— *Yang*. The selected prescription is *Zhengan Xifeng Tang* with modification (Modified Tranquilizing the Liver— wind Decoction). The decoction should be taken warm.

3. Upward Invasion of *Yang* due to Deficiency of Both *Yin* and *Yang*

Clinical Manifestations

Headache, dizziness, blurred vision, tinnitus, light red face, dry mouth, spontaneous— perspiration, insomnia, frequent dreaming, soreness of the loins, cold limbs, muscular twiching and cramp, short breath on exertion, dark red tongue with scanty coating, wiry and thin pulse.

Nursing

(1) Diet should be supervised strictly, Chinese date, sesame seed, Chinese yam, walnut, etc. should be mostly eaten.

(2) Herbs should be taken for nourishing the kidney— *Yin,* warming the kidney— *Yang*. The selected prescription is *Shenqiwan* with modification (Modified Bolus for Tonifying the

Kidney—*Qi*).

(3) Acupuncture and moxibustion treatment is given to Qihai(RN6), Sanyinjiao(SP6), Zusanli(ST36), Pishu (BL20).

(4) *Guifudihuang Wan* (Pills of Chinnamon Twig, Prepared Aconite Root and Rehmannia Root) 1 pill is taken each time, twice daily.

3.7 Cerebrovascular Disease

The diseases are known as wind stroke in TCM, character-ized by falling down in a fit with loss of consciousness accom-panied by deviation of the eyes and mouth, hemiplegia, slurred speech, or only by deviated mouth and hemiplegia without unconsciousness. Wind stroke caused by invasion of exogenous evils is known as apoplexy from exogenous wind. In mild cases there are only symptoms showing dysfunction of the channels and collaterals, while in severe cases both dysfunction of *Zang—Fu* organs and that of the channels and collaterals are manifested. Therefore it is clinically divided into two major kinds: attack on the meridians, the symptoms of which are mild and generally without emotional changes; attack on the *Zang—Fu* organs the symptoms of which are severe and commonly accompanied with unconsciousness.

General Nursing

1. A coma case is nursed according to coma nursing (refer to 2. 2, coma nursing).

2. The ward environment should be quiet and clean and the

air should be fresh.

3. During the acute period, the patient must take complete bed rest and avoid movement.

4. According to the patient's condition, light semifuid or fl. id diet and a plenty of water should be given, but nasal feeding is given to the unconscious case. Smoking, drinking, fat, sweet and irritant food must be forbidden.

5. Closely observe the changes of patient's condition such as emotions, pupils, blood pressure, appearance of the tongue, pulse, body's temperature, breathing, urination and defecation, speech, limb and body condition and take careful note.

6. Since emotional hurt and overacting of the five emotions is one of the important factors of the disease attack, phychological nursing should be done well to ease the patient's mind, keep their minds on their health and make them cooperate actively with the doctor's treatment.

Nursing According to Syndrome Differentiation

1. Attack on the Channels and Collaterals

Clinical Manifestations

Headache, dizziness, sudden deviation of the eyes and mouth, excessive flow of saliva, slurring of speech, numbness of the limbs, chills, fever, subjective sensation of contraction of the body, soreness and pain of joints, hemiplegia in a severe case, thin and whitish tongue coating, superficial and rapid pulse.

Nursing

(1) In the primary attack, sick persons should have complete bed rest, their heads and body being on the same level. As

the illness eases, they may gradually restore movement.

(2) Herbs should be administered for calming the liver to stop the wind and resolving phlegm to remove obstruction in the channels. The selected prescription is based on *Qianzheng San* and *Daotan Tang* with modification (Modified Decoction based on Powder for Treating Wry—mouth and Decoction for Expelling Phlegm).

(3) Watch carefully for the patient's condition dealing with any deterioration promptly so as to avoid repeated attacks causing aggravation of the patient's condition with appearance of syndromes involving *Zang—Fu* organs.

(4) After the patient's condition stabilizes, treatments such as pressing and rubbling, massage, acupuncture, moxibustion, etc. should be given as well as guidance in practising *Qigong*, *Taiji Quan* so as to facilitate recovery of the body's function.

(5) Hemostatis are contraindicated so as to avoid blood stasis affecting curative effects.

2. Attack on the *Zang—Fu* Organs

(1) *Bi* (Tense) Syndrome

Clinical Manifestations

Falling down in a fit with loss of consciousness, trismus, red face and flushed eyes, deviation of the eyes and mouth, hemiplegia or with subjective sensation of contraction of the body, inability in urination and defecation, red tongue with yellow coating, rolling and rapid pulse.

Nursing

a. The patient must lie in bed on one side, the head being higher than the body, avoiding movement as far as possible so as to prevent deterioration of the disease.

b. Keep the mouth cavity clean and in good condition.

c. Keep the respiratory tract unobstructed and give sputum aspiration if necessary.

d. The patient with excess—syndrome of coma accompanied by heat syndrome may be fed orally or nasally; the prescription, composite *Zhibao Dan* (Composite Treasured Bolus) or *Angong Niuhuang Wan* (Bezoar Bolus for Resurrection) being used. The patient with excess—syndrome of coma accompanied with cold manifestations may be given *Suhexiang Wan* (Storax Pill) dissolved in warm water for oral or nasal feeding.

e. Herbs should be taken for calming the endopathic wind and removing fire, eliminating phlegm for resuscitation, the selected prescription being *Lingyang Gouteng Tang* with modification (Modified Decoction of Antelope's Horn and Uncaria Stem) .

f. A case of incompletely closed eyes can be given gauze steeped in saline solution to cover the eyes so as to protect the cornea from dryness causing damage, if necessary, eye drops of chloramphenicol may be given.

g. Watch for changes of the body temperature. The sick person with over 39℃ may be given an ice bag placed on his head, or sponge bath with alcohol and in summer an electric fan can be used in the room.

h. closely watch for the patient's changes in emotion, pupilla, breathing, blood pressure and so on. In the case of abnormal condition, a doctor must be informed timely to proceed with emergency treatment.

i. Bowel and bladder movements are kept free. A case with constipation may take laxatives, e. g. *Shengdaihuang Fen* 5 g

(Powder of Raw Rhubarb) or Senna leaf steeped in boiling water for drinking instead of tea. *Kaisailu* may also be used. A case with uroschesis or retention of urine may be given massage on Jimen (SP11) point or needling Zhongji (RN3) and Sanyinjiao (SP6) . If necessary, urethral catheterization and enema may be performed.

j. Acupuncture and moxibustion treatment is given to Shuigou (DU26) Shierjing, (twelve jin points) Taichong (LR3) , Fenglong (ST40), Laogong (PC8) to calm the liver to stop the wind, and eliminate phlegm for resusciation. Dicang (ST4) and Jiache (ST6) are added for trismus. Zhaohai (KI6) and Tiantu (RN22) are added for dysphagia.

(2) Prostration Syndrome

Clinical Manifestations

Coma with eyes closed and mouth agape, flaccid paralysis of limbs, incontinence of urine, snoring but feeble breathing, cold limbs, thin, weak or minute pulse.

Nursing

a. Herbs for emergency treatment to rescue the patient from perishing of *Yin* and *Yang* should be administered. The selected prescription is based on *Shenfu Tang* (Decoction of Ginseng and Prepared Aconite) and *Shengmai San* Pulse–activating powder) with modification. The effect after administration should be noted.

b. Watch for the changes of breathing, perspiration, limb temperature, blood pressure, etc. . Cold oily sweat, flushed face, small and indistinct pulse or floating and big pulse without root belong to critical signs and should be reported to the doctor immediately for emergency treatment.

c. Moxibustion is applied to Guanyuan(RN4) and Shenque (RN8) so as to restore *Yang* from collapse.

(3) Sequelae

Clinical Manifestations

Hemiplegia, deviation of the eyes and mouth, slurring of speech, etc. .

Nursing

a. Take good care of the patient's emotion, avoid emotional stimuli and keep the patient's mind at ease.

b. Daily life should be normal to prevent invasion of any of the six climatic conditions in excess as pathogenic factors from aggravating the patient's condition.

c. Diet should be regular, light and easily digestible. Fat, sweet and irritative food should be avoided.

d. After the patient's condition stabilizes, the patient should be guided in dirigibility of their limbs gradually, Therapies such as massage, *Taiji,* walking, may be used.

e. A case of hemiplegia should be given acupuncture and moxibustion, the selected points being Hegu(LI4), Shousanli (LI10) Quchi(LI11), Jianjing(GB21) Huantiao (GB30), Xuehai(SP10) , Yanglingquan(GB34) Zusanli(ST36) , Kunlun(BL60) · Shenmai(UB62) , Naohui(SI13) Wangu (SI4) , Hegu(LI4) , Xingjian(LR2) and Yanglingquan (GB34) are applicable to itching of hand and foot with inability to grasp things. Scalp acupuncture may also be used, motor area of foot—kinesthetic area and speech area of cerebrum being selected. Otopuncture is applied to relevant points of hemiplegia.

f. A case of dysphasia should be given speech training in the early stages, the method being taken from the simple to the complicated.

3.8 Coronary Arteriosclerotic Cardiopathy

The disease is characterized by paroxysmal or continuous, choking precordia pain radiating to the neck, arm or upper abdomen, shortness of breath, inability to lie flat due to dyspnea and sometimes accompanied with cold and cyanotic limbs, minute and thin pulse. It belongs to the TCM range of "angina pectoris" or obstruction of *Qi* in the chest.

General Nursing

1. A mild case can move about properly, a case with shortness of breath and inability to lie flat may take a semireclining position and a severe case should take complete bed rest.

2. The diet should be regular and light. Fruits, vegetables and small frequent meals should be mostly had. Excessive fat, sweet, raw and cold food must be avoided, and smoking and alcohol must be forbidden so as to avoid impairing the spleen and stomach, causing the recurrence due to dysfunction of the spleen and stomach in transportation and transformation, or the exacerbation of the disease.

3. Emotional disturbance is the major factor of the occurrence and the exacerbation of the disease, so emotional care should be done well to help patients free their minds of apprehesions, avoid nervousness and excitement, keep their minds stable and to make them actively cooperate with doctor's treatments.

4. Closely observe the patient's changes in the painful loca-

tion, feature, degree, duration and cause, tongue and pulse condition, breath, heart rate, heart rhythm, blood pressure and perspiration, etc. , which are treated promptly and noted carefully.

5. Bowel movements are kept free. The patient is made to cultivate the hebits of regular bowel movements and not to force a compulsive bowel movement by excessive increase of abdominal pressure so as to avoid any accident occurring. The case with constipation should eat mostly vegetables, fruits, honey, etc. to make bowels loose. If necessary, the patient may be given slow—acting purgative prescription such as *Daihung Pian* (Rhubarb Tablet), Folium Cassiae.

6. The case with sudden and more severe pain in the precordia must take a rest immediately, may take *Guanxin Suhexiang Wan* 1 pill *Xiaosuan gan you Pian* (Nitroglycerin Tablet) 0. 3—0. 6 mg is sucked under the tongue. Acupuncture and moxibustion treatment can be given to Danzhong (RN17) , Neiguan(PC6) , Zusanli (ST36) , Tongli(HT5) Quchi(LI11) Shenmen(HT7) , Jianshi(PC5) Ximen(PC4) .

7. The patient with oppressed feeling in the chest, shortness of breath and dyspnea should be given oxygen inhalation.

8. After the condition has stabilized, the patients are instructed to do suitable physical exercise such as *Taiji quan, Qigong,* but avoiding tiredness and strenuous exercise.

Nursing According to Syndrome Differentiation

1. Obstruction of Heart Vessels due to Hypofunction of Chest—*Yang*

Clinical Manifestations

Oppressed feeling in the chest, paroxysmal cardialgia, palpitation, shortness of breath, pale complexion, aversion to cold, cold limbs, spontaneous perspiration, insomnia, poor appetite, clear and profuse urination, loose stool, white moist or sticky tongue coating, sinking moderate or knotted and intermittant pulse.

Nursing

(1) The room temperature should be suitable, the patients should attend to keeping their body warm to prevent catching cold and the exacerbation of the disease.

(2) The patients should be given easily digested food, eating that which has the function of restoring *Yang* such as sword bean, prawn, and walnut kernel, and refrain from eating raw and cold food.

(3) The herbs warming and restoring heart— *Yang* and dredging the channels and collaterals should be taken, the selected prescription being *Gualou Xiebai Guizhi Tang* with modification (Modified Decoction of Trichosanthes, Allium and Cinnamom twig) , taken warm.

(4) Acupuncture and moxibustion treatment is given to Xinshu(UB15) , Jueyinshu(BL14) , Neiguan(PC6) , Tongli(HT5) , etc. . After acupuncture, moxibustion is added to restore *Yang* and disperse cold.

2. Obstruction of Heart Collaterals due to Stagnation of *Qi* and Blood

Clinical Manifestations

Paroxysmal, pricking pain in the chest, radiating to the shoulder and back, oppressed feeling in the chest, shortness of breath, dark tongue, sinking, choppy or knotted and intermittant pulse.

Nursing

(1) Watch carefully for the condition of chest pain and deal with it promptly.

(2) Herbs for promoting the circulation of *Qi* and blood, removing blood stasis and obstruction in the channels should be taken. The selected prescription is *Xuefu Zhuyu Tong* with modification (Modified Decoction for Removing Blood Stasis in the chest) .

(3) Acupuncture and moxibustion treatment is given to Danzhong(RN17) , Juque(RN14) , Geshu(BL17) , Xinshu (UB15) , which are needled with reducing method.

(4) Faeces Trogopterorum 30 g and Pollen Typhae 30 g are ground together into powder. 6 g of the powder is taken with millet wine each time.

3. Obstruction of Heart Collaterals Resulting from Phlegm Collection due to Spleen Deficiency

Clinical Manifestations

Body being mostly fat, somnolence, lassitude, cough with thin sputum, oppressed feeling and pain in the chest, tightly bound feeling over the head, palpitation, white or sticky tongue coating, slippery or wiry slippery pulse.

Nursing

(1) Patients should be moderate in eating and drinking and avoid excessive intake of food so as to lose their weight and lower the burden of the heart. Excessive sweet, fatty and fried food should be contraindicated to avoid restoring wetness, producing phlegm.

(2) Herbs for strengthening the spleen and resolving phlegm, and removing wetness and nourishing the heart should

be taken, the selected prescription is *Daotan Tang* with modification (Modified Decoction for Expelling Phlegm) .

(3) Acupuncture and moxibustion treatment is given to Juque(RN14) , Danzhong (RN17) , Ximen(PC4) , Taiyuan (LU9) , Fenglong (ST40) , etc. which are needled with reducing method to activate *Yang* and dispel turbidness.

4. Stagnation of Heart—blood due to *Yin* deficiency of the Liver and Kidney

Clinical Manifestations

Oppressed feeling in the chest, chest pain at nights, dizziness, tinnitus, dry mouth, margins of eyelids, poor sleeping, night perspiration, soreness and weakness of back and legs, etc. slightly red tongue, thin and rapid or thin and choppy pulse.

Nursing

(1) The case with insomnia may take 10g of Chinese date seed powder before sleeping, or is given auricular—plaster therapy to such points as heart, kidney, and Shenmen(HT7) .

(2) The patient with night perspiration should be given *Wubeizi* powder (Powder of Chinese Gall) applied externally to the acupoint, Shenque(RN8) after mixing with vinegar before sleeping each night.

(3) Angina cordis often attacks at nights, so an inspection tour at nights should be done routinely. If indication of onset appears, treatment should be given promptly.

(4) Herbs for nourishing the liver and kidney,. activating blood flow and eliminating blood stasis should be taken, the selected prescription is *Yangyin Tong Bi Tang* with modification (Modified Decoction Tonifying *Yin* and Removing Stagnation —syndrome of Blood and *Qi*) .

5. Deficiency of Both *Yin* and *Yang* and Insufficiency of *Qi* and Blood

Clinical Manifestations

Oppressed feelings in the chest, epigastric pain, sometimes being woken up due to the oppressed feeling at nights, palpitation, shortness of breath, dizziness tinnitus, loss of appetite, lassitude, aversion to wind, cold limbs, or feverish sensation in the palms, purplish, dark tongue with pale coating, short of fluids, thin, frail, knotted and intermittant pulse.

Nursing

(1) If there appears continued epigastric pain, or a fit of cold limbs with cyanosis, minute and thin pulse and fall of blood pressure, which are a critical syndrome of prostration of *Yang* deficiency, a doctor should be told immediately to give emergency treatment. The prescription based on *Sini Tang* (Decoction for Resuscitation) and *Shengmai San*(Pulse— Activating Powder) with modification should be immediately taken to recuperate depleted *Yang* and rescue the patient from collapse.

(2) Herbs for regulating and reinforcing *Yin* and *Yang*, benefiting *Qi* and nourishing blood should be taken. The selected prescription is *Zhigancao Tang* with modification (Modified Decoction of Prepared Licorice) or 1 pill of *Baizi Yangxin Wan* (Semen Biotae Pill for Nourishing Heart) is taken twice daily, 1 pill of *Jinkui Shenqi Wan* (Pill of the Golden Chamber for Invigorating Kidney Energy) is taken twice daily.

3.9 Chronic Pulmonary Heart Disease

Chronic pulmonary heart disease is in brief form known as

"cor pulmonale", a kind of heart disease following bronchitis, pulmonary or a pulmo—vascular chronic trouble. It is characterized by cough, dyspnea, palpitation, oppressed feelings in the chest and full sensation in the abdomen, inability to lie flat, edema of extremeties, cyanotic complexion and lips, which belong to TCM range of cough, phlegm retention, palpitation, etc. .

General Nursing

1. The ward should be well ventilated and the air regularly sterilized. On entering the ward, the work staff and visiters must wear gauze mask to prevent cross infection. The patients should attend to keeping warm especially in autumn and winter, and during changing weather to avoid catching cold.

2. The patients with good function of heart and lung should do proper exercises to build up their health but not be too tired. Those with functional exhaustion of heart and lung should take absolute bed rest. Those with palpitation, shortness of breath and inability to lie flat should take a semireclining position and reduce movement as much as possible.

3. Diet should be light, easily digested, peppery, raw, cold, salty and sweet foods being contraindicated. Smoking must be abstained from.

4. The patient's mouth cavity should be cleaned to prevent mycotic infection. The mouth may be rinsed with *Kushen Jian Ji* (Decoction of Flavescent Sophora Root) . or *Yinqin Tang* (Decoction of Honeysuckle Flower and Scutellaria Root) . Oral ulcer may be applied with ointment such as *Xilei San, Bingpeng San,* etc. .

5. Phlegm should be removed to keep the respiratory tract unobstructed. The patient should be encouraged to cough out sputum. If the patient is too weak to do so, he may be given a change of body position or tapped lightly on the back so as to facilitate expectoration. Those with difficulty in coughing out sputum should be given spray inhalation to make the sputum thinner and easily expectorated.

6. Patients with cough may take liquid made of bamboo juice, Laiyang pear pectoral syrup or needling such acupoints as Dingchuan(EXB1) , Fengmen(BL12) , Feishu(UB13) , Hegu(LI4) , to which Chize(LU5) , Lieque(LU7) are added for severe cough; Fenglong (ST40) is added for excessive sputum.

7. Observe such conditions as respiratory rate, rhythm, depth, etc. . Patients with dyspnea may be given constant oxygen supply of low flow and density. During oxygen therapy, note changes in the patient's conditions such as emotion, breathing and facial colour.

8. Observe feverish condition. Fever with chills, cough with yellowish, little but ropy sputum, red tongue with yellow and greasy coating, slippery and rapid pulse are mostly due to accumulation of pathogenic heat in the lung. Struggle between vital and pathogenic factors may not be obvious in the elderly and week patients due to exhaustion of vital energy and lack of power to fight against pathogens. Therefore, the cough gets severe, and there is yellow sputum and red tongue. In this condition, existence of external pathogen should be considered. Falling of the body temperation, cyanotic complexion, cold limbs, excessive perspiration, faint pulse tending to disappear shows the kidney—
Yang to be exhausted which should be reported to a doctor to

carry out emergency treatment.

9. Watch for changes of blood pressure. Fall of blood pressure can be caused by severe infection, exhaustion of heart—energy and breathing, hemorrhage of digestive tract, etc. . If abnormal phenomena are found, a doctor should be told immediately in order to take measures of treatment.

10. Observe such conditions as quantity, colour and smell of expectoration, difficuty or easiness in promoting sputum dischrge. Generally, little quantity of sputum with white colour shows that pathogen is milder; increasing amounts of sputum with yellowness and thickness shows that pathogenic heat is more severe.

11. Observe the changes of coating on the tongue, pulse condition and emotion. If the patient shows indifferent facial expression, somnolence, irritability and unclear speaking or unwillingness to speak, all of which are signs of pulmonary encephalopathy, a doctor should be informed and nursing given according to coma (refer to 2. 2 coma nursing) .

12. Usually, some foods and medicines for strengthening the body resistance or restoring normal functioning of the body to consolidate the constitution should be taken.

Nursing According to Syndrome Differentiation

1. Lung and Heart Attacked by Exogenous Wind—cold Evils and Water

Clinical Manifestations

Cough, thin white sputum, dyspnea, palpitation, heavy feelings and pain of the body, edema of limbs, more severe edema of the face, fever, chills, clear and profuse urination, thin and white tongue coating, superficial and light pulse.

Nursing

(1) Because of lung—deficiency and failure of the defensive *Qi* to protect the body against disease, aversion to wind and easy perspiration, patients should attend to keeping themselves warm, especially after sweating, to prevent the attack of pathogenic wind and exacerbation of the disease.

(2) Cough and dyspnea are made more severe by even slight work because of deficiency and weakness of lung—*Qi* and the accumulation of phlegm, so the patients should take bed rest.

(3) Herbs should be taken to relieve pathogenic factors from the exterior and to disperse cold, warm the interior to reduce watery phlegm. The selected prescription *Huayin Jiebiao Tang* with modification (Modified Decoction for Removing Fluid Retention and From the Exterior and Dispelling Wind and Cold From the Exterior) or *Zhikedingchuan Wan* 9 g (Pills for Treatment of Cough and Asthma 9 g) is taken twice daily.

2. Fluid Retention in the Heart and Lung due to Deficiency of the Spleen

Clinical Manifestations

Dyspnea, shortness of breath. palpitation, loss of appetite, loose stool, edema of limbs, pale complexion, cyanotic lips, pale and moist tongue with white and sticky coating, sinking wiry and rolling pulse.

Nursing

(1) Small intake of food and loose stool is due to hypofunction of the spleen—*Yang*, so food for warming the kidney, strengthening the spleen and inducing astringency to stop

diarrhea should be taken, such as mutton, sword bean, walnut, lotus seed, Chinese yam.

(2) Attention should be paid to the skin nursing for severe edema, and quantity of urination should be noted.

(3) Herbs should be taken for warming and strengthening the spleen *Yang*, removing obstruction and resolving phlegm, the selected prescription being *Ling Gui Zhu Gan Tang* with modification (Modified Decoction of Poria, Bighead Atractylodes, Cinnamom and Licorice) .

(4) *Erchen Wan* 9 g is taken each time, twice daily.

3. Adverse Rising of the *Qi* due to Failure of the Kidney in Receciving Air.

Clinical Manifestations

Cough, asthmatic breathing, more exhalation than inhalation, occasional paroxysm of asthmatic breathing, choking cough, palpitation, oppressed feelings in the chest with much phlegm, poor spirit, indifferent expression, somnolence, coma, dark red, or light purple tongue with sticky white or light yellow coating, thin, slippery and rapid pulse.

Nursing

(1) Attend to mental changes, when the patients show indifferent mind, hazy consciousness or somnolence, their function of respiration should be improved actively, secretion of respiratory, tract must be cleared away and oxygen inhalation must be given, Needling can be applied to shuigou(DU26) , Shixuan (EX–UE11) , Yongquan(K11) , etc. *Angong Niuhuang Wan* (Bezoar Bolus for Resurrection) or *Zhibao Dan* (Treasured Bolus) can be taken to remove heat from the heart to resuscitate. If restlessness and clonic convulsion appear, Xingjian(LR2) ,

Zhongwan(RN12) . Ganshu(BL18) , Xinshu(BL15) may be needled. *Chuanxie Fen* 3 g (Powder of Scorpio) and *Wugong Fen* 3 g (Powder of Scolopendra) are taken after being infused in boiling water.

(2) Herbs for clearing heat, cooling blood to stop bleeding should be taken for mucocutaneous hemorrhage, hemoptysis and hematochezia. Bleeding must be attended to.

(3) The case with failure of the kedney in receiving air may take *Jinkui Shenqi Wan* (Pill for Invigorating Kidney Energy of the Golden Chamber) 1—2 pills twice daily.

3.10   Acute Gastroenteritis

The disease is within the TCM range of " vomiting" "diarrhea" and "cholera morbus", characterized by nausea, vomiting, abdominal pain, diarrhea and fever. It occurs mostly in summer and autumn.

General Nursing

1. Keep a ward clean, air fresh and well ventilated to prevent patients from vomiting caused by reaction to dirty air.

2. The patients with severe fever, vomiting and diarrhea should take bed rest avoiding turning too frequently. They should rinse their mouths with warm water after vomiting, their excreta must be cleared, and contaminated clothing, bedclothes, etc. must be changed promptly.

3. Since irregular diet, excessive intake of food or over eating raw, cold, oil, greasy and dirty food can result in relapse due to impairment of the stomach and stagnation of the spleen— *Qi*,

dietetic nursing is very important.

A mild case may be given a fluid diet and a severe case with violent vomiting must completely refrain from intake of food. The severe case may gradually restore his diet as his condition improves. At the early stage, fluid, semi—fluid and soft diet may be taken after returning to normal, a more normal diet can be taken but it should be light, soft, easily digested with fat, oil, sweet, greasy and irritative food being contraindicated. Plenty of water should be taken at patient's discretion.

4. Note the time of vomiting, contents, quantity, colour and smell of vomitus, character, times, colour of feces. If necessary, the sample may be retained for testing.

5. Note the changes of patient's condition. If vomiting is sharp with spurting and accompanied by severe headache and unconsciousness, this is a severe syndrome of invasion of pathogenic factors in the heart and liver. Vomitus with fresh blood or a coffee colour is due to impairment of stomach—collaterals. Dizziness, restlessness, somnolence and hyperpnea are due to Yin—fluid depletion, frequently vomiting, pale complexion, cold perspiration, cool limbs, thin and frail pulse are the evidence of prostration syndrome. If the above condition are found, a doctor should be informed in order to take measures of treatment.

6. Herbal decoction should be taken little and frequently. If necessary, it may be concentrated, 3—5 drops of fresh ginger juice should be added to it or Neiguan (PC6) point can be punctured and auricular— plaster therapy can be given to the points of stomach and Shenmen(HT7) .

7. The patients with severe diarrhea should clean their anus

with warm water after defecation and apply talcum powder externally.

8. Both acupuncture and moxibustion are given to Tianshu (ST25), Neiguan(PC6), Zusanli(ST36). Guanyuan (RN4) is added for severe diarrhea, Jinjing (EX—HN12) for severe vomiting, Quchi(LI11) for fever, moxibustion should be put on for fever and Shenque (RN8) is added for a tendency of Yang—Qi to be exhausted.

9. Ear needling is given to the points small intestine, sympathetic, Shenmen (HT7), Stomach and Spleen.

10. The therapy of *Guasha* or salt compress on umbilical region may be taken.

Nursing According to Syndrome Differentiation

1. Summer—damp Type

Clinical Manifestations

Frequent vomiting and diarrhea, oppressed feelings in the epigastrium, nausea, abdominal pain accompanied by bad—odour vomits and discharge, vexation and thirst or accompanied by fever, yellow and sticky—coating, soggy and rapid pulse.

Nursing

(1) Watch for fever the patient's condition. When high fever appears, measures for lowering temperature should be taken (refer to 2. 2 nursing of high fever).

(2) Herbs should be taken to clear summer—heat, remove dampness, filthiness and regulate the stomach. The prescription is based on *Ranzhao Tang* and *Lianpu Yin* with modification.

(3) Needling is given to Zusanli(ST36), Neiting(ST44),

Tianshu(ST25) , Quchi(LI. 11) and Shixuan(EX-UE11) .

(4) *Liuyi San* (Six to One Powder) 30 g and Semen Dolichoris 9 g are given in decoction for oral use.

2. Cold—dampness Type

Clinical Manifestations

Nausea, vomiting, clear and thin vomitus and discharge, abdominal and epigastric distension and borborygmi, heavy feelings of the body, fatigue, headache, cold limbs or with chills, low fever, white and sticky tongue coating, soggy and moderate pulse.

Nursing

(1) Diet should be hot, light and easily digested, with replenishment of salt, raw and cold food being contraindicated.

(2) Herbs should be taken to dry dampness and disperse cold, resolve turbidity with aromatics, the selected prescription is *Huoxiang Zhengqi San* with modification (Modified Powder of Agastachis for Restoring Health) . The decoction should be taken warm.

(3) Needling is given to Zusanli(ST36) , Tianshu (ST25) and Dachangshu(UB25) .

3. Cold—insufficiency Type

Clinical Manifestations

Frequent vomiting and diarrhea, clear feces and vomitus, abdominal pain which may be relieved by pressure and warmth, pale complexion, cold limbs, pale tongue coating, sinking, slow or thin and minute pulse.

Nursing

(1) The patient's body should be kept warm from cold evils to avoid exacerbation of the disease.

(2) Diet should be hot, raw and cold food is contraindicat-

ed.

(3) Needling is given to the acupoints, Zusanli(ST36) , Dachang (Large Intestine) , Baihui(DU20) , Yongquan (KI1) . Moxibustion is given to Shenque (RN8) .

(4) When there is an abdominal pain, moxibustion is given to Zhongwan(RN12) or hot compress is used on abdomen.

4. Retention of Food Type

Clinical Manifestations

Acid fermented vomitus, belching, sensation of fullness, abdominal pain relieved after defecation, anorexia, acid fetid discharge, thick and sticky tongue coating, wiry and slippery pulse.

Nursing

(1) Food retained in the stomach should be regurgitated completely, if necessary inducing vomiting therapy can be used.

(2) Herbs should be taken, for promoting digestion, resolving food accumulation and regulating the stomach. *Bohe Wan* with modification (Modified Lenitive Pill) can be selected.

(3) Diet should be controlled depending on how serious the accumulation of food is. If necessary, eating is contraindicated for 24 hours.

(4) The case with abdominal distension may take *Muxiang Shunqi Wan* 9 g (The Saussurea Pills for Regulating *Qi*) twice daily.

(5) Acupuncture treatment is given to the points, Sifeng (EX-UE10) , Sanjiaoshu(BL22) , Zhongwan(RN12) , Zusanli (ST36) , etc. .

3.11 Peptic Ulcerative Disease

Ulcerative disease is also known as peptic ulcer, character-ized clinically by chronic, rhythmical, periodic pain in the epigastrium and specific complication. It is within the TCM range of "epigastralgia".

General Nursing

1. The patient's daily life should be arranged rationaly and over tiredness avoided. Those with more severe pain or with bleeding should take complete bed rest.

2. Emotional care is necessary. Since mental stress, stimuli and anxiety are all predisposing factors, the patient should be in-structed to avoid emotional stimuli, keep stable emotions and es-tablish confidence in treatment.

3. Suitable diet is very significant in treatment and preven-tion of a seizure of the disease and occurrence of complication. Diet should be nourishing and easily digested. Fluid, semi—fluid or soft food should be had depending on how serious a patient's condition is, the diet should be regular and suitable in the cold-ness and hotness, and small frequent meals should be had. Vora-cious eating should be prohibited; raw, cold, fatty, peppery and irritating food avoided; smoking and drinking forbidden.

4. Watch the region, character, time, regularity and concomitant symptoms of stomach—ache such as an acute severe pain in the epigastrium followed by pain in the whole abdomen, pale complexion, thin and rapid pulse, fall of blood pressure. If there appears the above symptoms, a doctor should be informed

and assisted in further examination so as to ascertain correct diagnosis. If perforation or bleeding appears, preoperative preparation should be made well.

5. Watch the character of vomitus and feces and concomitant symptoms such as coffee colour or dark red of vomitus, black feces or the colour like tar, accompanied by dizziness, palpitation, pale complexion, perspiration, etc. . It is necessary to watch for bleeding, careful notes being taken. Blood pressure should be taken and pulse felt regularly, etc. , the doctor should be reported and emergency work should be prepared well.

6. The case with milder and stable condition should do suitable exercises such as *Taijiquan, Qigong,* to build up the health but it is not appropriate to do strenuous exercise.

Nursing According to Syndrome Differentiation

1. Incoordination Between the Liver and Stomach
Clinical Manifestations
Epigastragia, hypochondriac distension and oppressed feelings in both sides, belching, acid regurgitation, irritability and sighs, emotional instability, acid and bitter taste in the mouth, thin and white tongue coating and wiry pulse.

Nursing
(1) Herbs should be taken to soothe the liver and regulate the circulation of *Qi* and the function of the stomach to alleviate pains. *Chaihu Shugan San* with modification (Modified Bupleurum Powder for Relieving Liver—*Qi*) should be used.

(2) Acupuncture and moxibustion treatment is given to the points, Zhongwan(RN12) , Ganshu(BL18) , Neiguan (PC6) ,

Yanglingquan(GB34) .

2. Stagnation of Fire in the Liver and Stomach

Clinical Manifestations

Epigastric pain without regular time, burning sensation in the stomach, acid regurgitation, vexation, irritability, bitter taste in the mouth and dry throat, thirst, preference for cool drinking, or vomiting of blood, black feces, redish tongue with yellow coating, wiry and rapid pulse.

Nursing

(1) Herbs should be taken for nourishing *Yin* and soothing the liver, regulating the stomach and purging heat. *Yiguan Jian* with modification (Modified Ever Effective Decoction for Nourishing the Liver and Kidney) should be used.

(2) Needling is given to the points, Zhongwan(RN12) , Liangqiu(ST34) , Neiting(ST44) , Qiuxu(GB40) .

3. Deficiency and Cold of the Spleen and Stomach

Clinical Manifestations

Long–recurrent stomachache with intermittent dull pain which occurs mostly before meals or at nights and responds to warmth and pressure, may be relieved by small meals and aggravated by cold, abdominal distension due to overeating, sallow complexion, lassitude, cold limbs, pale tongue with thin and white coating, soggy and thin pulse.

Nursing

(1) The patient should be kept warm, avoiding cold and cool. Diet should be hot; raw and cold food is contraindicated.

(2) The patient with stomachache may be given a hot medicated compress on the abdomen.

(3) Herbs should be taken for strengthening the spleen and

regulating the stomach, warming the middle—*Jiao* and dispelling cold. The selected prescription is based on *Fuzi Lizhong Wan* (Modified Bolus for Middle— *Jiao* Regulating with Aconite) and *Huangqi Jiaozhong Tang* (Decoction of Astragalus for Tonifying Middle—*Jiao*) with modification.

4. Impairment of Vessels due to Blood Stasis

Clinical Manifestations

Severe and constant pain in a fixed area which may be aggravated by intake of food and pressure, repeated black feces or hemoptysis, purple dark tongue with ecchymosis.

Nursing

(1) The patient should have complete bed rest.

(2) Herbs should be taken for hemostasis by removing the blood stasis, regulating *Qi* and the stomach. *Gexia Zhuyu Tang* with modification (Modified Decoction for Dissipating Blood stasis Under Diaphram) should be used.

(3) Watch for any vomiting of blood and hemafecia. Once it is found, a doctor should be told in order to take treatment measures.

3.12 Urinary Infection

The disease is mainly manifested as frequent, urgent and painful urination. Pyelitis is mostly accompanied by symptoms of lumbago. The disease includes " stranguria" and " lumbago" in TCM.

General Nursing

1. During the acute period, the patient should take complete

bed rest and during the chronic period, they may do suitable exercise but must not overtire themselves.

2. Note carefully the time, quantity and colour of urination. If necessary, a sample should be taken for testing. The case with lumbago can be given a hot compress on the renal region.

3. Diet should be light, nourishing, fruits mostly eaten, water or soup of red bean mostly taken to clear away heat and cause diuresis. Peppery and irritative food are contraindicated.

4. Give health advice and education, and instruct the patient to attend to progenital cleanliness and menstrual hygiene.

Nursing According to Syndrome Differentiation

1. Accumulation of Damp—heat Type

Clinical Manifestations

Frequent, urgent and painful urination, turbid or yellow urine, burning sensation in urethra, fall and distension in the lower abdomen, lumbago, chills and fever, yellow and sticky tongue coating, slippery and rapid pulse.

Nursing

(1) Observe and take note of feverish condition (refer to 2. 1 nursing fevers).

(2) The case with urgent, frequent and painful urination can be treated with sitz bath of decoction to clean their pudenda, Flos Lonicerae 30 g, Herba Taraxaci 30 g, Folium Artemisiae Argyi 30 g being decocted and used as a fumigant and lotion.

(3) Herbs should be taken for clearing away heat and promoting diuresis. *Bazheng San* with modification (Modified Eight Health Restoring Powder) may be used, the decoction being

taken warm.

(4) Needling is given to the acupoints, Dazhui(DU14) , Quchi (LI11) , Guanyuan(RN4) , Sanyinjiao(SP6) .

2. Insufficiency of Both the Spleen and the Kidney *Yang*

Clinical Manifestations

Pale complexion, soreness of lumbar region and cold limbs, fatigue, thirst with desire for hot drink, loss of appetite, loose stool, white tongue coating, deep and thin pulse.

Nursing

(1) Good emotional care should be given to prevent impairment of the spleen and kidney due to fright or anxiety, and the exacerbation of the disease.

(2) Herbs should be taken for strengthening the spleen, benefiting the kidney, and clearing away damp—heat. *Sijunzi Tang* with modification (Modified Decoction of Four Noble Drugs) can be used, the decoction being taken warm.

(3) Acupuncture and moxibustion treatment should be applied in combination to Shenshu(BL23) , Zusanli(ST36) , Zhongwan(RN12) , Yangguan(GB33) .

(4) The patients should be careful to keep warm and avoid cold and have plenty of hot drink.

3.13 Nephritis

Nephritis is an allergic disease with renal lesions as the domininant factor, being mainly bilateral, with diffuse glomerulonephritis. Its major clinical manifestations are edema, elevation of blood pressure, urinary changes such as oliguria, hematuria, proteinuria. The disease falls into acute and chronic

nephritis based on clinical manifestations and different pathological changes. It is within the range of "edema" in TCM.

General Nursing

1. During the stage of acute onset, the patients should take
bed rest until the symptoms and signs all disappear and the
urinary test shows normal results. The case with obvious changes
of urine, severe swelling or high blood pressure needs bed rest,
and that with choking sensation in the chest due to severe swelling should take semireclining position. The mild case or convales-
cent may do suitable exercises but should not be overtired.

2. The room temperature should be suitable, the patients
must not be affected by cool to prevent catching cold.

3. Intake of water and salt should be limited Sodium salt intake must be strictly limited to the patient during the acute stage
and with edema, low salt intake being permissable after swelling
disappears. The quantity of water to be drunk or fluid infusion
everyday is decided according to the amount of urine passed.
Generally, it is suitable that the total amount for drinking is
500cc more than that passed in urine the previous day.

4. Take good care of the mouth. *Yinqin Tang* may be given
for rinsing. Attend to nursing the patient staying in bed of his or
her skin to prevent occurrence of bed sores and infection.

5. Intake and output volume of liquid should be recorded every day. The abdominal perimeter of the case with ascites should
be measured according to demand. The body weight is measured
once a week. Those with high blood pressure should have their
blood pressure taken 1—2 times daily, the results being recorded.

6. Take care to watch the position, degree and pattern of growth and decline of edema, times, quantity and colour of urination, body temperature, blood pressure, tongue picture and pulse condition.

7. Be careful to watch for complications such as sudden appearance of headache, nausea, vomiting, somnolence, even unconsciousness, convulsion, etc. which are indicative of hypertensive cerebral syndrome. Palpitation, shortness of breath, spitting frothy sputum with pink colour are symptomatic of left ventricular failure. The symptoms mentioned above all belong to critical conditions and a doctor should be informed immediately in order to take emergency meassure.

8. The effect and reaction of administrating medicine should be watched for when herbs for eliminating retained fluid or purgation are used. Intake and output volume of liquid should be noted.

Nursing According to Syndrome Differentiation

1. Confrontation Between Wind and Water

Clinical Manifestations

Abrupt onset of edema with puffy face and eyelids, then limbs and even anasarca, scanty urination, intolerance of wind, fever with general pain, thin and white tongue coating, superficial and tight pulse.

Nursing

(1) The patient should be kept warm and not be affected by cool to prevent upper respiratory tract infection.

(2) The case with obvious symptoms caused by exopathogen

can have semi—fluid diet and is generally given easily digested and light food, Such food for inducing diuresis and alleviating edema as red bean, waxgourd, watermelon should mostly be eaten. The intake of high protein food should be suitably limited. Normal diet may be taken during recovery stage.

(3) Herbs for dispelling wind and promoting diuresis should be taken. *Yuebi Jia Zhu Tang* with modification (Modified Decoction with White Atractylodes Rhizome for Relieving Edema) is used, the patient should lie in bed well covered and the sweating should be watched. After sweating, the patient must avoid cooling to prevent the exacerbation of the illness.

(4) The changes of body temperature must be watched and feverish cases may be nursed according to 2. 1 Fever Nursing.

(5) Needling is given to the points, Dazhu(BL11) , Hegu(LI4) , Qihai(RN6) , Sanyinjiao(SP6) and moxibustion to Shuifen(RN9) .

2. Accumulation of Heat and Dampness

Clinical Manifestations

Edema over the whole body, enlarged abdomen with fullness, oppressed feelings in the chest, coarse voice, fever, dry mouth, scanty and dark urine, constipation, yellow and sticky tongue coating, deep and thin pulse.

Nursing

(1) The patient should have bed rest. The case with oppressed feelings in the chest and coarse voice should take a semireclining position.

(2) Special care should be taken of the skin to prevent occurrence of bed sores.

(3) The diet is the same as that used for symptoms of con-

frontation between wind and water.

(4) Needling is given to Dazhui(DU14) , Sanjiaoshu (BL22) , Qihai(RN6) , Zusanli (ST36) .

3. Water—dampness in the Spleen

Clinical Manifestations

Repeated onset of edema over the whole body, especially on the lower limbs aggravated after meals, severe edema upon rising in the morning, heavy feelings of extremities, loss of appetite, distension of abdomen, white and sticky tongue coating, deep and moderate pulse.

Nursing

(1) The case with severe edema should take semireclining position; the lower limbs being elevated above trunk to alleviate edema.

(2) The diet requires food for eliminating and promoting urination, such as coix seed, red bean, mung bean, carp, crucian carp.

(3) Herbs should be taken to activate *Yang,* dispel turbidity and promote diuresis. The prescription is based on *Wuling San* (Powder of Five Drugs) and *Wupi Yin* (Decoction of Peel of Five drugs) with modification.

(4) Needling is given to Qihai(RN6) , Guanyuan (RN4) , Yinlingquan(SP9) , Pishu(UB20) , Zusanli(ST36) .

4. *Yang* Insufficiency of Both the Spleen and Kidney

Clinical Manifestations

Prolonged edema over the whole body, especially remarkable below the lumber regions, accompanied by pitting edema, reduced clear urine output, small intake of food, loose stools, chills, cold limbs, white and moist tongue coating, deep and thin pulse.

Nursing

(1) The patient should have bed rest, those with severe edema should take a semireclining position. The skin should be taken care of to prevent bed sores.

(2) The patient's body should be kept warm with plenty of clothes to prevent catching cold.

(3) Food for eliminating dampness and promoting diuresis should be mostly eaten so as to increase nutrition, such as Chinese date, longan, eggs, beans, aquatic products.

(4) Watch carefully for any changes in the patient's condition. If there are symptoms such as anuresis, nausea, vomiting, which indicate urinaemia, a doctor should be informed to take measures.

(5) Needling is given to Pishu(UB20) , Shenshu (UB23) , Sanyinjiao(SP6) .

(6) Stigma Maydis 30 g and Herba Verbenaebog 60 g are decocted in water as a kind of tea to help swelling subside.

3.14 Urinary Calculus

The illness is mainly manifested as dull pain in the lower back and abdomen, hematuria, and dysuria. It is within the TCM range of "painful urination with blood" and "dysuria caused by calculi and sand".

General Nursing

1. Except for feverish cases which must have bed rest, others should do some exercises to promote stone discharge.

2. Encourage the case to drink plenty of water and to im-

prove his dietary habits according to the stone type. The case with urate calculus should have a purine diet. Those with phosphate calculus should have a high protein and fatty diet and eat mostly acidic food. Those wiht oxalate calculus should have small amounts of vegetables such as tomato, potato, spinach. Those with calcareous calculus should avoid eating beef.

3. Be sure to observe the urinary colour and quantity and whether there is a discharged stone.

4. The case with more severe pain and concurrently having hematuria should take Pulvis Medicinalis Albus produced in Yunnan or Qilisan (Anti—bruise Powder) .

5. Needling is given to Shenshu(BL23) , Baliao, Guanyuan (RN4), Zhongji(RN3) , Zusanli(ST36) . Electroacupuncture can be used.

6. "General attack therapy" (GAT) is suitable for the case with urinary calculus whose stones are within 1 cm diameter, without severe urinary infection and obvious accumulation of water in renal pelvis. At six o'clock in the morning, a form of *Pai shi Tang* (Decoction for Removal of Urinary Calculus) is taken and meanwhile 200 ml of water is also taken. At 6: 30, 50 mg of Dihydrochlorothiazide (DCT) is taken. At 7: 00, 0. 5 mg of Atropine is injected and meanwhile electroacupuncture is given to the points, Shenshu(BL23) , Pangguangshu(BL28) or the points selected in the calculus area of abdominal side, for 15—20 minutes and then the patients are instructed in doing jumping exercises.

Nursing According to Syndrome Differentiation

1. Calculi due to Accumulation of Dampness and Heat in the

Lower Warmer

Clinical Manifestations

Colicky pain in the lumbar region and abdomen, rediating to the lower abdomen or pudendum, frequent and urgent urination, dysuria, sudden interruption of urination, urine with blood or presence of calculi in the urine, yellow and sticky tongue coating, wiry and rapid pulse.

Nursing

(1) Observe carefully the condition of colicky pain in the kidney and explain to the patients that the onset of such pain in the abdomen usually indicates the possibility of lithecbole, reassure patients so as to keep them calm and carefully watch the condition of stone discharge.

(2) When the onset of colicky pain in the kidney is severe, electroacupuncture may be given to arrest pain to the acupoints, Shenshu (BL23) , Pangguangshu(BL28) Sanyinjiao(SP6) , Yanglingquan(GB34) . Ear needling can also be applied to kidney and urinary bladder areas.

(3) Herbs for clearing away heat and expelling dampness, treating stranguria and removing stones should be administrated. *Paishi Tang* with modification (Modified Decoction for Discharge of Stone) can be selected, the decoction being taken warm. Plenty of water should be taken. The removal of urinary calculus should be attended to.

2. Stagnation of *Qi* and Blood due to Long Retentio of Calculi

Clinical Manifestations

Soreness, pain and distension of the lumbar region, distension, fullness and dull pain of lower abdomen, hesitant urination with pain, dripping, hematuria or with blood clot, red tongue with thin coating, wiry slippery pulse.

Nursing

(1) Watch carefully any changes of body temperature and prevent multiple urinary infection.

(2) Observe carefully the condition of urine and hematuria and take a good note.

(3) Herbs should be taken to regulate *Qi* and remove the stagnancy and blood stasis in the channels. *Xiaoji Yinzi* with modification (Modified Decoction of Small Thistle) can be used.

(4) Supervise patients in doing jumping exercises.

3.15 Diabetes

Diabetes is a common disease, a kind of metabolic endocrinopathy with genetic predisposition. It is characterized by hyperglycemia or glyoresis, and manifested as polyuria, polydipsia, polyphagia, fatigue, emaciation, etc. . Complication of pyogenic infection, pulmonary tuberculosis, arteriosclerosis and pathologic changes of nerve, kidney, eye and others are mostly found. The illness is within the TCM ragne of " *Xiaoke*" or "*Xiaobi*".

General Nursing

1. The case with obvious complications should have bed rest, without such complications may do proper work but avoid over fatigue.

2. Diet should be regular, over hunger and overeating

avoided and dietetic amount of physiological requirement should be given according to the doctor's advice. Those with obvious hunger can eat such food boiled many times as thin meat, prepared beans, but should refrain from peppery, fatty and sweet food, smoking and alcohol.

3. The patient's skin should be kept clean to prevent occurrence of pyogenic infection. Once it happens, active treatment should be given.

4. Take good care of the mouth cavity in the severe case so as to prevent ulceration of oralmucosa and gum, *Yingqin Tang* being given for rinsing the mouth.

5. The body weight is taken twice a week, the weight is not decreased but gradually increased under the condition of controlled diet or medicinal treatment, which shows the patient is on the mend.

6. Take notes of the quantity of intake of water and urine discharge in twenty—four hours . A sample of urine should be set aside promptly and tested regularly.

7. Be sure to watch the patient's condition. If there is occurrence of such symptoms as dizziness, palpitation, perspiration, weakness, etc. , whether they are caused by hypoglycemia should be considered, and if so sugar—liquid should be taken immediately. If the symptoms persist, a doctor should be informed to give the patients an injection of 50%glucose solution. If the patients are found to have the symptoms of anorexia, vomiting, abdominal pain, apple smell in the mouth, which may be caused by acidosis, a doctor should be informed to take measures.

8. Medicine for lowering glucose should be used but the time of administration and the diet should be controlled seriously.

9. Give health advice and education to the patients, familiarise them with their condition and help them master the method of testing glucose in urine, administering medicine accordingly, prevention of complication, and common treatment.

Nursing According to Syndrome Differentiation

1. Impairment of Body Fluids due to Lung—heat

Clinical Manifestations

Thirst, polydipsia, dry throat and tongue, frequent urination, thin and yellow tongue coating and rapid pulse.

Nursing

(1) The patients should avoid mental stimuli and stress, eliminate anxiety and should actively cooperate in treatment.

(2) Herbs can be used for clearing away the lung—heat and moisturizing, and promoting the production of body fluid, *Xiaoke Tang* (Decoction for Relieving Diabetes) with modification is selected, being cooperated with taking porridge of spinach root.

(3) Needling is given to Feishu(BL13) , Taiyuan(LU9) , Shenmen(HT7) , Neiting(ST44) .

2. *Yin*—impairment due to Stomach—dryness

Clinical Manifestations

Thirst, polydipsia, polyphagia but easy hunger, emaciation, frequent urination, constipation, dry tongue coating, slippery and rapid pulse.

Nursing

(1) The case with constipation should eat plenty of vegetables and be given laxative such as *Daihuang Pian* (Rhubarb Tab-

let) and Folium Cassiae, etc. if necessary.

(2) Herbs for clearing away the stomach—heat, purging fire and nourishing *Yin* should be used, the selected prescription being *Yunu Jian* with modification (Modified Gypsum Decoction) , being cooperated with taking porridge of pork tripe.

(3) Needling is given to Weishu (BL21) , Zhongwan (RN12) , Zusanli (ST36) and Sanyinjiao(SP6) .

3. Dificiency of the Kidney Essence

Clinical Manifestations

Frequent urination with copious amounts like grease, dizziness, hazy eye, soreness of the lumbar region and weakness of legs, chills, cold, limbs, dry mouth, reddish tongue and rapid pulse.

Nursing

(1) The severe case should have bed rest and be advised agaist controlling sexual life.

(2) Herbs should be taken for nourishing the kidney and controlling nocturnal emission, the selected prescription is *Liuwei Dihuang Wan* with modification (Bolus of Six Drugs Including Rehmannia); the decoction being taken warm.

(3) Closely watch for the changes of patients, condition and give timely treatment to the case with complications.

(4) Needling is given to Shenshu(BL23) , Sanjiaoshu (BL22) , Guanyuan(RN4) and Taixi (KI3) . etc. .

3.16 Rheumatoid Arthritis

The illness is mainly characterized by arthralgia involving

one or several joints, local swelling, distension or deformation. It is within the TCM range of *"Bi—syndrome"*.

General Nursing

1. Keep the ward dry, the temperature suitable and the air fresh, and well ventilated keeping draughts off the patients to avoid the effect of cold and dampness causing recurrence or prolongation of the disease.

2. The case with fever, more severe arthralgia of limbs, obvious swelling and distension should have bed rest. During recovery, he can do proper exercises but must prevent over fatigue.

3. Usually, the patients may be given nourishing diet and those with excessive dampness and cold should refrain from eating raw and cold food. Those with fever may eat semi—fluid or soft food and with exhaustion of body fluid due to fever should have much water, but avoid eating peppery and irritative food.

4. The patients with excessive perspiration, general asthenia, weak immune system are easily affected by exopathogen, so they should be wiped with a dry towel after sweating and their clothes and bedclothes should be changed any time. Those with sweating at night should be given a compress of a suitable amount of *Wubeizi Fen* (Chinese Gall Powder) mixed with water, placed on the navel area before sleeping every night.

5. Take the body temperature regularly observing and noting any changes. Fever usually takes place in the afternoon and lower fever is generally not treated. Hot drinks are taken to promote sweating, causing the body temperature to lower. When the body

temperature is 38. 5℃, medicine for reducing fever and relieving pain may be taken and physically lowering temperature is not used.

6. Observe the relationship between the patient's onset factors, painful location, nature of symptoms, time and climate.

7. The onset of the illness is closely related to vital organic energy, climate conditions and living environment. Therefore, the upper respiratory tract infection must be given prompt effective treatment. The patients should take care to avoid cold and dampness, especially during seasonal changes and be ready to add extra clothing and bedclothing at any time, and should do exercises to build up their health. If there is an infectious nidus, early treatment should be given to prevent the onset of valvular heart disease.

Nursing According to Syndrome Differentiation

1. With Wind and Heat

Clinical Manifestations

Fever with excessive perspiration, reddish swelling and painful joints, feverish sensation when touching, desire for cold, aversion to heat, mostly occurring in the joints of hands and feet, limitation of movement, yellow and greasy tongue coating, thin and rapid pulse.

Nursing

(1) Watch carefully for changes of fever, joint swelling and pain, palpitation and others.

(2) Watch for the swelling condition, the case with excessive perspiration should have his wet clothes and bedclothes changed

promptly to prevent the effect of wind.

(3) Herbs should be taken for clearing away heat and dispelling wind and concurrently expelling toxin and removing wetness. The selected prescription is *Baihu Jia Guizhi Tang* with modification(Modified White Tiger Decoction with Cinnamon) .

(4) Needling is given to Quchi(LI11) , Waiguan(SJ5) and the surrounding points of the painful area.

(5) When the joints are red, swollen and feverishing painful, Chinese herbal paste can be applied externally.

a. *Fengxian Gao*: A suitable amount of fresh Canlis Impatientis is broken into pieces to be applied externally to the local area or *Fengxiancao Gao* is applied externally.

b. *Furong Gao*: A suitable amount of Folium Hibisci is ground into powder mixed well with castor oil for external application.

(3) *Chuanjinpi Gao*: Equal amounts of Cortex Hibisci, Semen Persicae, Rhizoma Seu and Radix Notopterygii, are ground together into powder mixed with castor oil for external application.

2. With Cold and Dampness

Clinical Manifestations

Affected distension in the back and loin, deformity of big joints, severe pain, limitation of movement and dyskinesia in a severe case, contracture of limbs, poor appetite, white and sticky tongue coating, deep and slow or deep and rolling pulse.

Nursing

(1) For the case of arthralgia relieved by warmth and aggravated by cold, the local area should be carefully kept warm. The treatments may be given as a hot compress with a bag of hot

water or with *Kanlisha,* or field effect healing if necessary. The joints must not be exposed to cold or rain.

(2) Encourage and assist the patient to carry on the limb dirigibility.

(3) Herbs should be taken for dispersing cold and removing wetness and concurrently dispelling wind and removing obstruction in the channels. The selected prescription is *Yiyiren Tang* with modification (Modified Decoction of Coix seed) , being taken warm with small amount of millet wine.

(4) Needling is given to Fengfu (DU16), Waiguan (SJ5) , Fuliu(KI7) and Ah shih points.

3. Obstruction of Vessels due to Accumulation of Phlegm

Clinical Manifestations

Prolonged obstruction of vessels, local joint swelling and pain aggravated by pressure or cyanosis, limitation of movement, joint deformity, subcutaneous nodules or ecchymosis, thick and sticky tongue coating, thin and choppy pulse.

Nursing

(1) Instruct and assist the patient in doing limb exercises to build up the movement of joints.

(2) Massage, acupuncture, physical or external therapy should be coordinated.

(3) The case with deformation of the spinal column should lie on the board bed, with arthralgia or deformed joint may be given a special cage so as to avoid pressing the wounded limbs and adding to suffering. Those with stiff joints or stiffness can be treated coordinating with therapies—massage, acupuncture and others to dredge the channels and regulate *Qi* and blood.

(4) The patient with arthralgia, swelling and distension of

limbs can be treated by combining steaning with washing. *Huoxue Zhitong San* (Powder for Promoting Circulation of Blood and Alleviating Pain) is often used or Chinese herbs used orally by the patient are decocted again to steam and wash the affected areas. Steaming and washing is given 1—2 times daily, 30 minutes each time. Care should be taken of the temperature which must be suitable so as to avoid scalding. After washed, the joints are wrapped well with dry towels to avoid catching wind.

(5) The case with grotesquely shaped joints may be given orthopedic traction but the strength must not be too great nor sudden so as to avoid causing fracture. Make sure the weight and angle of traction are suitable and observe condition of blood circulation in the limbs, correcting immediately any abnormal condition. Take care of the skin.

4 Nursing For Commonly Encountered Surgical Diseases

4.1 Furuncle

Furuncle is an acute suppurative infectious disease produced in a single hair follicle and its sebaceous glands, often occurring on the face, neck and back. It is common in the summer and autumn months. The early symptom of the disease is a red, small and hard lump with whitish yellow pus point. In a few days the pus will erupt and the lump disappear. The systemic features, such as fever and a version to cold, are the frequent complications in severe cases. In Traditional Chinese medicine furuncles can be classified as summer boil, boil of face and " mole cricket" furuncles according to the seasons and causes of their attacks or their forms.

General Nursing

1. The patient should keep the skin clean and dry, have frequent baths and hair cut, and change clothes regularly to prevent and reduce the incidence of furuncle.

2. The hair around the boil should be shaved to facilitate not only changing the dressing and external application, but also keeping the local area clean and avoiding repeated attacks.

3. Carefully observe the patients, temperature and the other conditions in the affected area.

Nursing According to Syndrome Differentiation

1. The Stage of Painful Swelling of Skin

Clinical Manifestations

In the early stage local rising becomes red small lump with whitish yellow pus point, which is swelling hot and painful. Severe cases often have systemic features such as fever and aversion to cold.

Nursing

(1) A case acompanied with fever should have bed rest, raising the affected part, which should be kept clean and given *Badu Gao* (adhesive plaster for drawing out of the pus) or *Daqing Gao* (Isatis Indigotica Fort) for external application. In addition, same amount of Herba Taraxact, Herba Portulacae and Flos Chrysanthemi Indici can be cleaned and pulverized for external application or boiled in water for drinking in order to promote its own detumescence.

(2) It is important to avoid pressing and compressing the boil, especially that close to the nose or lip so as not to cause intracranical infection or pyemia which results from pathogenic toxin attacking *Zong—Fu* organs.

(3) Give acupuncture and bloodletting to dredge the *Du* chennel and to clear away the blood heat. The acupuncture points are Lingtai (DU10), Hegu (LI4), Weizhong (BL40) etc. Lingtai (DU10) and Hegu (LI 4) needled with reducing method and bloodletting is often done by pricking Weizhong (UB40). In a case with fever, needling Dazhui (DU14) and Quchi (LI11) is added.

(4) A milder case can take *Jiedu Xiaoyan Wan* (Pills for

Clearing Away Toxin and Inflammation), *Liushen Wan* (Pills of six Ingredients with Magical Effects) or *Wanshi Niuhuang Qingxin Wan* (Wan's Bezoar Sedative Bolus). In addition, *Liushen Wan* (Pills of six Ingredients with Magical Eaffects) may be ground with a little water for external application. The case with boil on face acompanied by fever and aversion to cold may be given herbs for clearing away heat and toxin and subsiding swelling. *Wuwei Xiaodu Yin* (Antiphlogistic Decoction of Five Herbs) is a suitable prescription. The decoction should be taken cool. Plenty of water should be drunk. the case with summer boil should also take heat—clearing and detoxifying herbs or wetness—clearing herbs. *Qingshu Tang* (Decoction for Clearing Away Summer—heat) is a suitable prescription.

(5) The patients should have a vegetarian and common diet. A case with boil on the face or close to the nose or lip may be provided with a vegetarian diet or liquid diet. For a case with summer boil, heat—clearing diet is indicated, including watermelon, muskmelon, mung bean juice and tea, or *Liu Yi San* (six to one powder) infused in water. Pungent or bitter and irritative diet should be avoided.

2. The Stage of Ulceration

Clinical Manifestations

Abscess has developed, the centre of which has become soft with fluctuation. When the sore runs itself or be cut open, yellow and thick pus will be discharged and then the pain and swelling will subside.

Nursing

(1) The abscess is festered by itself or cut open. Drainage must be adequate. Opening the boil on the face in the early stage

is usually contraindicated.

(2) Oleo-gauze with rheum is applied to the festered sore. The top of the sore and necrotic tissue are not easily removed. *Jiuyi Dan* (Nine to one pill) and *Jiuhuang Dan* are given to the patient without adequate drainage to discharge the pus. The festered abscess with much pus and serious inflammation should be washed with detoxicating herbs before a dressing change. In milder cases, the sore with granulation should be covered with *Shengji San* (Power for Promoting Tissue Regeneration) and then coated with *Shengji Yuhong Gao* oleo-gauge.

(3) During a dressing change, the skin around the sore must be thoroughly cleaned and the dressing carefully fixed. In addition, it is necessary to note whether any other boil has appeared.

4.2 Carbuncle

Carbuncle can be defined as an acute pyogenic infection caused by pyogenic bacteria invading more hair follicles in neighbourhood and sebaceous glands. At the begining the local part is red, swelling, hot and painful with a honeycomb-like pus point. As the necrosis of the skin around the pus piont develops, the ulcer comes into being. The carbuncle can heal from gradually granulating, systemic symptoms such as fever, anorexia, etc. are often accompanied. It is classified into "*Youtou Ju* "(carbuncle) in Traditional Chinese Medicine.

General Nursing

1. The patients with light or severe systematic symptoms should be kept in bed in a comfortable posture according to the locality of the furuncle. A patient with carbuncle on face should

speak little and should be kept from chewing in order to relieve pain.

2. It is necessary to note the patients' conditions, and the changes of temperature, blood pressure, coating of the tongue and type of pulse. those with fever should be nursed according to the high fever nursing (2.1).

3. The incidence of the disease is higher in old people. Considering their characteristics, it is necessary to nurse their, life well and help the weaker turn over in bed and move their limbs. It can promote vital energy (*Qi*) in motion rendering and blood circulation normally, and be away from complications. The patient with diabetes should be treated at the same time.

4. Hairs round the carbuncles of a neck must be shaved. The sore area must be kept clean and dry for a change of dressing.

5. *Mahuang Ding* (Semen Strychni 30 g Rbizoma Coptides 30 g are pulverized then immersed in 75% alcohol 300 mg. for 3−5 days, and hermetically sealed for use) is applied to the skin round the festered part so that the pathologic change can be prevented from extending unaffected areas.

Nursing According to Syndrome Differenfiation

1. The Stage of Painful Swelling on the Body Surface
Clinical Manifestations

In the local diseased part, there appears lump which is red, swollen, hot and painful with several puspoints, in the shape of a honey−comb. In excess syndrome, the red lump projects extremely and the fasciculation of the patient sfoot appears. In the deficiency−syndrome, the sore is not protuberant and festers slowly. Accompanied complications are fever, aversion to cold, excessive thirst, constipation, yellow urine, pale or red tongue with yellow and dry coating and rapid pulse.

Nursing

(1) The affected area must be cleaned. Patients with red swelling, hot and pain can be given heat—clearing and toxin—removing soft plaster for external application, for example, *Daqing Gao* (Isatis Indegotica, Fort) and *Jinhuang Gao* are used to promote internal absorption.

(2) Medicine for oral administration: Herbs for heat—clearing and toxin—removing, promoting blood circulation and removing blood stasis are provided for a patient with excess syndrome. The prescribed medicine is *Qingre Jiedu Yin* (Decoction for Heat—clearing and Detoxifying) of *Xigxiao Wan* can be applied for a accompaning drug. The decoction should be taken warm. A patient with deficiency—syndrome is given herbs for nourishing *Yin* and promoting the production of body fluids, and clearing heat and removing toxin. The prescribed medicine is *Zhuye Huangqi Tang* (Lophatherum and Astragalus root Decoction). Patients having difficulty in taking medicine by themselves should be helped. But medicine for clearing heat, removing toxin, and loosening bowel should be prescribed to those who have interior heat syndrome of excess type accompanied by fever, excessive thirst, constipation, yellow—dry tongue coating, strong and rapid pulse. *Neishu Huanglian Tang* (Coptis Decoction for Removing Internal Heat) should be prescribed. A cold compress is applied to those with high temperature. If the temperature remains high, *Angong Niuhuang Wan* 1 pill (Bezoar Bolus for Resurrection) or *Zixue Dan* 0.9 g (*Zixue* Powder, Purple Snowy Powder) is effective for oral use. Listlessness or fidgeting, rapid

pulse and execusion of local red swelling are the signs of fire—toxin invaginations. Doctors should be informed in order that they may take effective measures and prepare for emergency.

(3) A light, digestable vegetarian diet should be given to the patients. A vegetarian and liquid or semi—liquid diet is good for a case with high temperature. The patient should have melons, beans, spinach, pineaple, banana and water, plenty of which are helpful to clearing away heat and toxic matterals. Those with slow suppuration of deficiency type may be recommended fresh fish, shrimp or cock's head soup, etc. Which are helpful to promoting the drainage of pus and removing toxin. The diet for a patient suffering from diabetes must be carefully supervised. They are given proper amount of milk, tremella, towel gourd (vegetable sponge), etc. to nourish *Yin* and clear away heat. Rich fatty diet, pungent food, and alcohol should be avoided to prevent phlegm—wetness and fire—toxin from being formed inside the body, which leads to a severe condition.

2. Stage of Ulceration

Clinical Manifestations

Abscess has developd. The pus pionts break and look like a honeycomb, from which yellow and thick or thin pus is discharged. As the pus is discharged, the toxin is removed and the systemic symptoms are alleviated.

Nursing

(1) When the abscess is featered by itself or cut open, Drainage must be adequate. Washing medicinal herbs for clearing toxin are applied to the opening of the sore. Then *Jiuhuang Dan* and *Zhuidu Dan* (Pellets of Toxin—removing Medicine) are used for external application to let out the pus, or medicated thread placed

into the opening of the sore is effective for drainage and to clear away necrotic tissue promptly. Oleo–gauze with rheum is used for a change of dressing. *Zhenzhu Shengji San* is applied for granulation tissue, covered with *Shengji Yuhong Gao* (Powder for Regeneration of Tissue) oleo–gauze to assist the healing of the sore.

(2) The skin round the sore must be clean and dry. The bed must be covered with oil cloth for a running sore. It is essential that the topical application of drug should be changed promptly in case the bedding is stained with pus.

(3) If the sore is extensive and slow to heal, Vitamin B_1 100 mg, should be injected into Zusanli (ST36) on both sides alternately to promote healing.

(4) Patients with excessive syndrome are often given clearing–heat–toxin and discharging–pus medicine. *Oingre Jiedu Tang* (Decoction for clearing heat, and Detoxifying) is prescribed to be taken cool. *Tuoli Xiaodu San* (powder for Tonify *Qi* and Blood and Detoxifying) is effective for a patient with fever and deficiency. A patient suffering from deficiency of both *Qi* and blood may be given medicine to supplement the vital energy and nourish blood, such as *Bazhen Tang* or *Shiquan Dabu Tang* (Eight Becious Ingredients Decoction or Decoction of powerful Tonics). Careful observation sbould be made of the syndrom's change during applying the medicine and a doctor should be informed promptly to change the prescription.

(5) The proper diet must be nourishing. Patients with deficiency of both *Qi* and blood are usually the aged. The digestive system of old patients is badly functioning so it is good for them to take warm cooked, soft, nourishing and digestible dilicious

food with the function of supplenmenting *Qi* and nourishing blood, for instance, meat, eggs, milk, bean curd, gruel made of milkvetch root, etc.. But nourising food is harmful to patients with pathogenic heat. Fried and roasted food should be avoided.

4.3 Infection of Hand

Pyogenic infection of hand known as nail–like boil in TCM is mostly associated with a mild injury, which brings in pyogenic bacteria. In TCM according to different parts of the body, there are different names, for example, paronychia is called nail–like boil around fingers; the pustule of the finger tip is called snake–head–like boil; the suppurative tenosynovitis is called thecal whitlow; an infection of inner part of the hand is palmar pustule, of which the nail–like boil around fingers and the snake–head–like infection are more common.

General Nursing

1. The treatment of infection of hand includes elevation of the affected part, restriction of activities, and triangular bandage for suspending the forearm to relieve pain. Those who have constitutional symptoms must be kept in bed.

2. The injury or foreign body in the hand require early treatment.

3. Observe the patient's condition carefully. The local affected part requires proper and prompt treatment.

Nursing According to Syndrome Differentiation

1. The Painful Swelling Stage

Clinical Manifestations

The local part is red, swollen, hot and painful or complicated by fever, headache, drymouth anorexia reddened tongue or whitish–yellow tongue coating, wiry and rapid pulse.

Nursing

1) In the early stage, dissipating the swelling is most important and heat–clearing and detoxifying herbs are suitable. Medicine for subduing swelling and alleviating pain is used for external application. Usage:

(1) Realgar 10 g, alumen 10 g, Venenum Bufonis 1 g, one Scolopendra are ground into fine powder. Put 3 g of the powder into a gall bladder of the pig or an uncooked egg with the drugsin if through one brokenend and stir it well and immerse the infected finger in it and it should be changed until it becomes dry.

(2) *Daqing Gao* or *Jinhuang Gao* can be applied to the local part. Herba Taraxact 60 g and Herba Porulacae 60 g. are cleaned, pulverised and mixed with a suitable amount of egg white for external application.

(3) Wash herbs (Flos lonicerae, Radix Sophorae Elavecentis, Cortex Phellodendri, Herba Violae, Herba Taraxact, Fructus Forsythiae, Herba lycopi, Herba Schizonepetae, Radix Ledebouriellae, Radix Glycyrrhizae, 10 g. each) are decocted and used as a lotion for the affected part.

(4) 50% Natrii Sulfus liquid is used for immersion.

2) Medicines should be administered to clear away heat and toxin, to activate blood flow and to reduce swelling. *Wuwei Xiaodu Yin* (Antiphlogistic Decoction of Five Drugs) is the drug of choice. A patient with fever or chill can be prescribed 3 pills of *Chansu Wan* (Pill of Toad Venom) for oral administration.

3) A patient with severe pain in the infected part is usually recommended to have acupuncture analgesia (corresponding

channel point selection) or auricular–plaster therapy (points of selection: hand, wrist, Shenmen (HT7), Sympathetic, etc.

4) The patients should have a vegetarian diet and light drink, and avoid pungent and dryness–heat–causing food.

2. The Stage of Ulceration

Clinical Manifestations

The local infected part is red, swollen with severe shooting pain and tenderness. General symptoms are aversion to cold, fever and poor appetite.

Nursing

(1) Carefully observe the infected part. Promptly open the abscess to drain the pus for prevention of swelling and medullitis due to the circulatory disturbance of *Qi* and blood. (Follow the method for a dressing change shown in the chapter of Furuncles)

(2) *Wuwei Xiaodu Yin* (Antiphlogistic Decoction of Five Drugs) may be administered to those who have systemic features such as fever and chill. It is necessary to observe the patients 'conditions. The infection accompanied by lymphagitis lymphadenitis or osteomyelitis should be delt with promptly. Once lymphagitis is established with sequester in it, the sequester should be removed after it becomes less crowded to facilitate healing of the injury.

(3) Exercise must be done to prevent from dysfunction of hands.

(4) In restoration stage, nourishing diet is necessary.

4.4　Acute Cellulitis

Acute cellulitis is an acute suppurative infection caused by suppurative bacteria invading the subcutaneous area, the lower part of the pleura intramuscular spatia or the deeper cellular tissue. It is usually accompanied by systemic features such as fever, chill and headache, it is classified as carbuncle and inominate inflammatory swelling in TCM.

General Nursing

1. A patient with severe pain and other systemic features must have complete bed rest. The preferable posture in bed depends upon the various sites of infection.

2. Observe carefully the patients'conditions. Acupuncture treatment is suitable for a patient with headache. The points selected are Baihui (DU20), Yintang (EX−HN3), Touwei (ST8), Taiyang (EX−HN5) and so on. The nursing method for the cases with high temperature shown in Chapter 2.1 is available.

3. Keep the patients under observation and check for any complications. Lymph nodex of axillary fascia, groin or cervical part may become swollen and painful of the extremities or the neck involved. Nursing shown in Chapter Furuncle at the Stage of Painful Swelling of Skin is available. Edema of the larynx is as sociated with submaxillary phlegmon. Severe cases having dyspnea must abstain from food, be kept quiet and may be prepared for a tracheotomy if necessary.

Nursing According to Syndrome Differentiation

1. The Painful−swollen Stage
Clinical Manifestations
The local affected part is red swollen, hot and painful. There is a fever, chill, yellow tongue coating and wiry and rapid pulse.
    Nursing

(1) In the early stage, detoxifying medicine can be used to fumigate and wash the local infection. Fresh Radix Et Rhizoma Rhei 9 g. Folium Isatidis 9 g Rhizoma Pleionis 6 g. are pulverised and mixed with honey for external application.

(2) Acupuncture: Acupuncture points are established according to the affected areas by corresponding channel point selection in order to dredge channels, to reduce swelling and alleviate pain. Dazhui (DU14), Quchi (LI11), and Hegu (LI4) may be used for the patients with fever.

(3) Medicine for clearing heat, removing toxin, activating blood and eliminating stasis should be given. *Wuwei Xiaodu Yin* (Antiphlogistic decoction of Five Herbs) is the best prescription.

(4) Light food, heat–clearing and detoxifying vegetables, fruits, melons, beans, banana, pineapples and so on are suitable. Peppery food must be avoided.

2. The Stage of Ulceration

Clinical Manifestations

Swelling pain becomes severe with marked tenderness. The abscess has progressed to softening and wary in central part of the affected area. The sore will be healed gradually as it is ulcerated and opened. If the pathogenic factors can not be removed, the pus will not be expelled freely and the swelling does not subside.

Nursing

(1) Observe carefully the affected part which is still swollen with pus after ulceration. Medicine for eliminating the pathogenic factors and strengthening the body resistance is given. *Tuoli Xiaodu San* (Powder for Eliminating the Pathogenic Factors and Detoxifying) is prescribed. Give special attention to the patients who have taken the medicine. When the symptoms are not re-

lieved and the patient's temperature is running high with septicemia, let the doctors know immediately so as to give an emergency treatment.

(2) The local affected part must be kept clean. Adequate drainage should be used in those whose abscesses has been ulcerated or opened. The cases with excessive pus and more necrotic tissue can be provided with washing drug for removing toxic substances and oleo–gauze with rheum is applied to the affected part. The opening of the sore with necrotic tissue is smeared with *Wuwu Dan* (Five to Five Pills) to eliminate putrefaction. When the granulation tissues have developed, *Shengji Yuhong Gao* (Plaster for Remoting Tissue Regeneration) should be applied until the infection is healed.

(3) Nursing the patients of their diet: Provide nutritive food for the patients. The patients with decreasing fever and deficiency of both vital energy and blood, whose wound fails in promoting tissue regeneration may take high–protein and vitamin–rich food, such as meat, eggs, fresh vegetables and fruits. Pungent food, smoking, drinking and seafoods are abstained from.

4.5 Erysipelas

Erysipelas is an acute infectious inflammation caused by homolytic streptococus. In the early stage a patch of red appears on the local skin which fades when pressed and is restored when loosened. The edge of the affected area with blisters is distinct and irregular, and a little higher than the skin surface. It can spread rapidly. Blisters appear after the sense of severe hot. Chill, fever, headache and thirst are the common complications. Severe cases are usually accompanied by invagination with pathogenic toxin. Different terms are given according to different affected parts. The infection of craniofacial part is called "erysipelas of the head", erysipelas in the lower part of the trunk refers to the infection of the truneal part, and erysipelas of the lower limb is called erysipelas of the shank.

General Nursing

1. The patients should be kept in bed. Take good care of those who have a fever (Consult the nursing method shown in 2.1).

2. Pay close attention to the patient's condition and the change of temperature. When invagination occurs, nursing care must be coordinated with prompt treatment. (Consult the nursing outlined in the chapter of general pyogenic infection).

3. Give light and semi—liquid diet. A patient with high temperature should drink plenty of water, rice juice, water—melon juice, mungbean juice, etc.. Pungent—hot diet cohich can cause dryness—heat must be avoided.

4. Give prompt treatment to those who have mucosa damaged with tinea pedis in order to prevent further in fection.

5. The instrument used to treat the sore and the used drug for topical application should be disinfected strictly or incinerated to prevent the cross infection.

Nursing According to Syndrome Differentiation

1. Erysipelas of the Head
Clinical Manifestations
The local part of the skin is red with a feeling of burning and edema followed by blepharal swelling. Eyes become red and extremely sensitive to light, the ala nasi swells, destending pain in

the head develops. It is difficult for the head to move.

Nursing

(1) The patient must be kept in bed with the head of the bed elevated. The room temperature must not be high. Humid air and dark light in the room is necessary.

(2) The face is kept clean. *Huanglian* is boiled in water for external application to the eyelid palpebra and the ala nasi in order to clear away heat and relieve swelling.

(3) A case with headache can be given acupuncture at the points Lieque(LU 7), Waiguan(SJ 5), Hegu(LI 4), or auricular–plaster therapy (using mung bean or vaccaria seeds) and the ear points of face, nose, eyes are selected.

(4) Heat–clearing, detoxifying and reducing swelling drugs should be taken. *Puji Xiaodu Yin* (Universal Relief Decoction for Disinfection) is suitable. The patient should drink plenty of water.

(5) The affected area must be cleaned. *Daqing Gao* (isatis, Jinhuang Gao Indigotica Fore plaster) or *Jinhuang Gao*, or *Shuangbai San* is mixed with some honey for external application to clear away heat and toxin, reduce swelling and relieve the pain.

2. Erysipelas of Lower Limbs

Clinical Manifestations

It occurs on feet or shank, sometimes involving the femur. Most cases of erysipelas on lower limbs are considered as downward flow of damp–heat and have repeated attacks.

Nursing

(1) Keep the patients in bed with the affected part raised to reduce swelling and relieve pain.

(2) Washing drug: Natrii Sulfas 10 g.Alumen 10 g, *Yueshi* 10

g are infused with boiled water and then used to fumigate and wash the local part. Fresh Herba Taraxaci 90 g, Alumen 10 g, Indigo Naturalis 10 g are pulverized for external application to the affected part.

(3) Medicines for clearing away heat, promoting diuresis and blood circulation by removing blood stasis should be taken. *Simiao Yongan Tang* (Decoction of Four Wonderful Drugs for Quick Restoration of Health) is suitable. *Longdan Xiegan Wan* (Pills of Gentiana for Purging the Liverfire) and *Huoxue Tongmai Pian* (Tablet for Promting Blood Circulation) are also beneficial. Watch carefully for any adverse reaction after administration of these medicines.

(4) When the symptoms vanish after the treatment, the medicines must be applied for 5—7 days to prevent recurrence.

(5) Erysipelas on lower limbs is susceptible to repeated attacks. Symptoms become severe time by time. *Baihua Danshen* (White—flower Radix Salviae Miltiorrhizae) injection 10 mg with 5% glucose injection 500 ml can be given for intravenous drip. The course of treatment is 15 days. A case with elepantiasis crus caused by repeated attacks must be applied with washing herbs to promote the circulation of blood and relieve pain, one or two times a day. It is also necessary to use compression bandage for diseased limbs. The course of the disease is much longer. Such patients require reassurance to maintain their confidence. Successful therapy is ensured if the treatment continues over a long period of time.

4.6 Acute Mastitis

Acute mastitis is the suppurative inflammation of the

mammary gland, most commonly occurring within the first few weeks of lactation (Ist—4th weeks) of primipara. In the early stage the local affected part is red, swollen, hot and painful, or there is a mass with jumping pain. Abscess develops, acampanied by such general symptoms as fever, chill and dry mouth, which is known as acute mastitis in TCM.

General Nursing

1. A patient with general systems must be kept in bed and the surrounding should be quiet and comfortable avoiding ill stimulation.

2. Acute mastitis occurs due to stagnation of the liver—*Qi*. So patients must be nursed carefully and kept in good spirits. Show great concern to them, have an intimate understanding of what they think and remove all harmful factors to make them happy and gay. Any melancholy and rage can lead to a severe condition.

3. The nipple should be often cleaned with warm water and soapduring breast feeding. If the nipple is pressed in, draw it out. Sesame yolk or oil can be applied externally to the rupturedarea.

4. Disseminate knowledge of hygiene concerning feeding. Feeding child must also be regular. All the milk must be drunk when feeding. The remained milk should be pumped or pressed out with hand in order not to be stagnated. An infant should not be left asleep with the nipple in his mouth. The mother should have ease mind, be careful to prevent violent rage or sadness, and have a regular diet to protect her from dyspepsia dysfunction of the spleen and stomachin transport and digesting and stagnation of stomach—heat to result in occurrence of a disease.

Nursing According to Syndrome Differentiation

1. The Early Stage

Clinical Manifestations

The affected breast is swollen and tender with abscess accompanied by aversion to cold fever, thirst, restlessness, anorexia, constipation, yellow coating on the tongue and wiry—rapid pulse.

Nursing

(1) Refer to the nursing method shown in Chapter 2.1 for a case with fever.

(2) Apply massage to a breast with stasis by pressing and rubbing gently with fingers from all sides towards the nipple. While rubbing, draw the nipple softly several times, or use a wooden comb by moving it from the upper pant of the breast to the nipple and rub the mass of the breast tissue to press the stagnated milk. Stop breast feeding when there is severe inflammation. Herba Menthae 30 g. Pericarpium Citri Reticulatae 30 g are boiled in water for warm compress. The milk should be pumped out after the warm compress *Daqing Gao* (Isatis Indigotica Fort) or *Jinhuang Gao* are used for external application. Opuntia Dillenii How 90 g. Alumen 15 g are pounded into pieces for external application. Natrii Sulfas can be given to those who have excessive milk.

(3) In the early stage of acute mastitis insert *Dingxian* powder (powder of Flos Caryophylli) packed in cotton balls into nostrils, 1—2 hours each time, 3—4 times a day.

(4) Apply herbs for soothing the liver and clearing away the stomach heat and promoting lactation by regulating the nutrient system. *Gualou Niubang Tang* with modification (Modified

Decoction of Trlchosanthes Fruit and Arctium Fruit) is suitable. The warm decoction should be taken.

(5) Acupuncture is recommended for promoting the secretion of mammary gland and clearing away heat and toxin. The selected points are Danzhong (RN17), Rugen (ST 18), Shaoze (SI 1), Neiguan (PC 6)etc.. The points for auricular—plaster therapy are mammary gland, Shenmen (HT 7) and adrenal gland Subcortex.

(6) A bland diet is necessary. Pungent greasy food, meat and fish are prohibited in order to prevent promotion of fire and impairment of *Yin*, or injury to the spleen and stomach. Those who have excessive and thick milk must avoid drinking too much soup. Those who have stomach—heat nausea, poor appetite and thirst should take plenty of water. Radix Trichosanthis 9 g, Radix Ophiopogonis 9 g and Herba Lophatheri 9 g may also be taken after being infused in hot water to clear away heat and promote appetite.

2. The Stage of Inflammation

Clinical Manifestations

Abscess may be festering or cut open with fever coming down and pain being relieved. Because of the different winner in the struggle between the vital energy and the pathogenic factor, there appear different sumptoms, such as yellow thick pus, persistant swelling and pain, or unsmoothly discharging or light pus, pale and slowly—growing granulation.

Nursing

(1) The patient must have plenty of rest. Use brassiere or triangular bandage as a support to relieve pain and to make drainage effective.

(2) When the abscess becomes diabrotic with profuse pus and necrotic tissues, squeeze oleo—gauze with rheum with a little *Jiuyi Dan* (Nine to One Powder), *Baer Dan* (Eight to Two Powder) or *Huafu San* (Powder for Removing Putrefaction) is inserted in the opening of the sore to expel the pus. *Shengji Yuhang Gao* (Plaster for Promoting Tissue Regeneration) oleo—gauze is applied to the sore with less pus and new granulation tissue. *Lurong Shengji San* (Cornu Cervi Pantorichum Powder) for promoting tissue regeneration or *Zhenzhu Shengji San* is given for external application to the sore with slow tissue regeneration. If breast sinus has developed, put a *Hongsheng Fiao* into the sinus to promote tissue regeneration.

(3) Pay careful attention to changes of the patients' condition and the different symptoms in the transformation of disease, and give medicines according to the differentiatiation of syndrome and medical orders. The toxin has not been removed completely if the inflammation becomes diabrotic, the fever comes down and the pain subsides but the pus is whitish yellow and thick, and the body is weak. The medicines for supplementing and restoring vital energy and blood and removing toxin are prescribed. *Simiao Tang* (Decoction of Four Wonderful Herbs) should be selected. If the pus is not expelled effectively and the pain is not relieved, the body resistance weakened while pathogenic factors prevail, medecines for supplementing and restoring vital energy and blood, and for clearing toxin, subsiding swelling should be prescribed. *Tuolixiaodu San* (Powder of Promoting Vital Energy and Clearing Toxin) is suitable. When the granulation is whitish with slow regeneration, the pus becomes thin and the sore is slow to heal, there is deficiency of both vital

energy and blood, medicine for supplementing and restoring vital energy and blood must be given. The best prescription is *Shiquan Dabu Tang* (Decoction of Ten Powerful Tonics) or *Bazhen Tang* (Eight Ingredients Decoction) which is boiled in water and taken as a warm drink.

(4) Diet for nursing health and recuperation: The appropriate diet depends on the symptoms of different stages of the disease. For example, in order to supplement and restore vital energy and blood, fish, meat, poultry, eggs etc, should be given to those who are deficient in both vital energy and blood, and in *Yang* of the spleen with difficulty in the sore healing. But not all nourishing food is beneficial for those with pathogenic heat.

4.7 Acute Suppurative Infection

Acute suppurative infection is caused by suppurative bacteria with their toxin invading blood circulation. It is classified into 3 types: toxaemia, septicemia and pyemia., which is known as *Zouhuang Neixian* in TCM.

General Nursing

1. Give moral support and encouragement and ease the patient's mind. An active cooperation with the doctor during the treatment is necessary.

2. Pay attention to the patients' condition, and the changes of his temperature, tongue coating, type of pulse and manner. The patients with high fever should be nursed referring to 2.1 High Fever Nursing.

3. Observe the conditions of all parts of the body. If local infection exists, it should be treated as early as possible. In the early

stage *Jinhuang Gao* and *Furong Gao* (Plaster of Cottonrose Hibiscus) may be given for external application to promote internal absorption. When the infection becomes diabrolic, dressing changes should be made carefully. Assist the doctor to clear the primary focus away in the operation on the patient whose infection is caused by acute abdomen.

4. As the patient's resistance is weak, and there is susceptibility to infection, acupuncture or injection is recommended with skin disinfection and strict aseptic manipulation. Help and encourage those with weakness to turn over in order to promote the free flow of *Qi* and blood and prevent bed sores.

5. Keep the oral cavity clean, rinse out before and after meals. A patient with aphthae may be given *Bingpeng San*, *XiLei San* (tin—group powder) or *Shishuang* (Persimmon frost) for external application. Sesame oil is applied to dry and cracked lips.

Nursing According to Syndrome Differentiation

1. Heat in *Qi* and *Ying* Systems
Clinical Manifestations
The onset is abrupt with chills, high fever excessive thirst, sweating, anuria, constipation, red tongue with yellow dry or thin yellowish coating, and taut and rapid or full and rapid pulse.
Nursing
(1) The patient should stay in bed. Those with profuse sweating must have the clothes and quilt changed frequently and keep the skin dry and clean to clear away cold.

(2) Patients with high fever and convulsions may be given acupuncture. The points needled are Dazhui (DU14), Quchi (LI11), Hegu (LI 4), Taichong (LR3), Sanyinjiao (SP6). Cold

compress may be applied to reduce the temperature, or *Lingyang Fen* 0.5−1.5g (Powder of Antelope's Horn) is taken orally.

(3) Medicines for clearing *Qi* and purging heat, and clearing toxins should be administered. *Baihu Tang* and *Huanglian Jiedu Tang* (Antidotal Decoction of Coptis) with modification should be selected and the decoction taken cold. Take note of the tongue coating and defecation after the patients take medicines. When the tongue coating becomes thin and there is free movement of the bowels, the patient is in the recovery stage.

(4) Those with constipation should take honey−water, or Folium Cassiae 6−9 g after being infused in hot water and served as tea. Acupuncture treatment is recommanded. The points for needling are Dachangshu (BL 25), Sanjiaoshu (BL 22), Yinlingquan (SP 9) and so on.

(5) Light vegetarian and liquid or semi−liquid diet should be available. Since the body fluid is consumed due to high fever, the patient should have plenty of water or light drinks. Flos Lonicerae 9 g, Radix Trichosanthis 9 g and Radix Ophiopgonis 9 g, are taken as tea after being infused in hot water in order to remove heat and toxin, nourish *Yin* and promote the production of the body fluid. Radix Astragali seu Hedysari, Radix Adenophorae or Radix Panacis Quinguefolii decocted in water are given to patients with deficiency of *Qi* and profuse sweating in order to invigorate *Qi* and reduce sweating. Hot, pungent and fried food and alcohol must be prohibited.

2. Invasion of Blood Systems By Heat

Clinical Manifestations

High fever, unconsciousness, mania, spots, apostaxis (epistaxis), bright red tongue, dry and thin coating on the tongue, thready and rapid pulse.

Nursing

(1) Pay careful attention to the patient's condition and changes of expression, breath, blood pressure and pulse. Use bed balustrade for those with anxiety to keep them from falling to the ground. Cooperate with the doctor in management of the patients who are invaded by toxin and pathogenic factors, and have shock and decreasing blood pressure. (Refer to the nursing method of syncope shown in Chapter 2.3).

(2) Drugs to remove heat and toxin and cool blood and to clear up the *Ying* system are available. *Xijiao Dihuang Tang* (Decoction of Rhinoceros Horn and Rehmannia) and *Huanglian Jiedu Tang* (Antidotal Decoction of Coptis with modification) are suitable. It should be taken warm, frequently but in small amounts. If necessary, they can be administered nasally.

(3) Acupuncture treatment is used for the patients of coma and delirium. The points to be needled are Shuigon (DU 26), Shixuan (EX—UE11) or Yongquan (KI1). Sometimes, *Angong Niuhuang Wan* (Bezoar Bolus for Resurrection) or *Zixue Dan* (Zixue Powder, Purple Snowy Powder) may be given by feeding.

(4) The patients with epistaxis should be managed promptly according to the condition of epistaxis, and those with nose bleeding should stay in bed with cold compress on the forehead. Fresh Radix Rubi Parvifolii is decocted for oral administration as tea. Carefully observe the blood color and amount of bleeding.

(5) Supporting treatment is given to the severe cases, for example, fluid infusion, blood transfusion, oxygen inhalation or antibiotics injection.

(6) The disease is often produced by carbuncle complication

by septicemia or by invagination of heat and toxin. So patients' conditions must be carefully attended to. There will be signs of *Yin* and *Yang* exhaustion if the patient's pulse becomes thready, rapid and weak. Cooperate with doctors in first—aid treatment of the patient (Consult the nursing method shown in the section of Syncopy).

4.8   Gastro—duodenal Ulcer Perforation

The disease is one of the severe complications associated with gastric and duodenal ulcers. It is characterized by tearing sudden pain in the mid—upper abdomen, subsequently spreading over the entire abdomen. It is called epigastralgia or precordial pain with cold limbs in TCM.

General Nursing

1. Give patients moral support and encouragement, dispel. their fear so that they can cooperate with doctors during the treatment.

2. The patient must be kept in bed in semireclining position. The horizontal position is suitable for a patient with unstable blood pressure. The posture with crooking arms and bending knees must be avoided in order to prevent subphrenic abscess or interintestinal abscess.

3. Pay attention to the changes of the patient's spirit, blood pressure, temperature, coating on the tongue, pulse and reaction after treatment.

4. Take good care of the oral cavity. After applying nasalgastric tube, give patients *Yinqin Tang*, normal salt water for gargling their mouths, or lubricant for lips.

Nursing According to Syndrome Differentiation

1. The First Stage (The stage of stagnation of vital energy and blood in the middle—*Jiao*)

Clinical Manifestations

There are continual severe rebounding pains, tenderness and tension in the abdomen. Gurgling sound becomes weak or subsides, accompanied by nausea, vomiting, vexation, cyanosis, sweating, cold limbs, rapid respiration, weak pulse, whitish–thin coating on the tongue.

Nursing

(1) Give acupuncture treatment to relieve spasm and pain in the light of the rule of relieving the secondary symptom in an acute case. Explain the operating method and the curative effect to patients so that they may cooperate better with doctors. Keep patients warm and in comfortable posture. Having observed condition of the abdomen and auscultated the gurgling sound, give acupuncture treatment. Acupuncture points consist of Zhongwan (RN12), Liangmen (ST21) (double); Zusanli (ST26) (double); Neiguan (PC6) (double) is added for those with vomiting, and Tianshu (ST25) (double) for those with abdominal distention. The needles are retained for 30–60 minutes and manipulated every 10–15 minutes. The needles are twirled with the fingers, or acupuncture with electric stimulation may be given and manipulated every 4–6 hours. Note carefully any changes of pain, fullness, and gurgling sound in the abdomen. Drug injection therapy: Vitamin B 100 mg should be administered at one Zusanli (ST26) point after another. Selection of the point must be precise, so that an obvious needling sensation may be felt and the pain re-

lieved, and the ulcer healed.

(2) Fasting: Decompress the gastric intestine, aspirate the gastric contents, relieve obstruction in the middle Jiao, assure the effective decompression. Observe the discharge and its color and quantity.

(3) Clyster with Chinese Medicine: In order to disperse the stagnation and nelieve pain, the Medicine for purgation and promoting the intestinal channel can be used to promote the function of the spleen and stomach and the activities of *Qi*. *Dachengqi Tang* with modification should be selected and is decocted into 500 ml. After being filtered, the decoction is poured into an infusion bottle and suitable temperature is 39−40c. The patient is kept in the left lateral position or horizontal position with one end of thick urinary catheter inserted into the anus at 25−27 cm. The other end of the catheter is connected with the glass tube of the infusion bottle. Drops of the decoction are put in the colon slowly at 80−100 drops per minute. Observe the patient's reaction. If the peristaltic movement of the intestines is quickened, the patient desires to defecate, and has a pain in the abdomen before defecation, which is normal phenomenon. The patient should be advised to keep calm.

(4) As the patient has incoordination between the spleen and the stomach, absorption of foodstuff and refined nutritious substances is weakened and the vital energy is injured with general debility. So during a fast, supporting treatment must be given, for example, fluid infusion, blood transfusion, etc..

2. The Second Stage (The heat−transmission due to prolonged stagnacy in middle−*Jiao*).

Clinical Manifestations

Abdominal distention and pain are weaked, muscular tension has disappeared or localized in the right upper abdomen, epigastrium tenderness is alleviated and gurgling sound restores, and passing gas and stool occur. Remaining symptoms, such as fever, rapid pulse, redden tongue with yellowish coating and dark yellow urine are found.

Nursing

(1) The relaxation of acute symptoms is indicative of closed perforation. In this stage herbal medicine is essential. Heat—clearing and toxin—removing medicine and this for dredging the intestines should be given. A suitable prescription is *Fufang Da Chaihu Tang* (Composite Major Bupleurum Decoction). The usage: at the early stage, the dose of decoction should be injected from the stomach tube after filtered and concentrated to 150 ml with 39—40℃. 50 ml is injected gradually for the first time. (The powder can be used together with the decoction). The contents of the stomach should be evacuated before injection Douche the stomach tube with some warm water in order to prevent the tube from blocking. After injecting, the tube is clipped for 1—2 hours, then symptoms and signs in the abdominal region should be observed closely. When abdominal pain is not intensified and the gurgling sound occurs, take the tube out and stop gastrointestinal decompression. Give herbal medicine for oral administration, 100 ml for the morning and another 100 ml for the evening. Those with bad general symptoms should be given two doses 4 times a day.

(2) Cases with heat symptoms caused by exopathogen can be given external treatment. A suitable prescription is antiinflamatory powder (Folium Hibiscl 300 g, Radix Scutellariae

250 g, Radix Et Rhizoma Rhei 300 g, Cortex Phellodendri 250 g, Rhizoma Coptidis 250 g, Herba Lycopi 250 g, Borneolum 10 g ground into powder for external application). A suitable amount of the powder and the millet wine (or decoction of the Chinese onion and wine) are pounded into paste for external application to the right upper abdomen so as to accelerate the limitation or disappearance of inflammation in the abdominal cavity.

(3) After stopping reducing gastrointestinal pressure, supply patients with liquid diet. At first, they should take frequent but small amount of meals. Overeating is harmful. Semi—liquid diet and full diet may be given gradually. Observe reactions after meals and investigate the condition of passing flatus,and defecation.

(4) Pay attention to the systemic features and complications such as subphrenic infection and abscess, or interintestinal abscess and pelvic abscess. After abscess has developed, there may be continuous fever and abdominal distention with tenderness and a mass touched in the local part. When the subphrenic abscess develops, reactive symptoms of the thoracic cavity such as cough and expectoration may occur. The pelvic abscess may be associated with such rectal symptoms as rectal tenesmus and mucus in stool. Doctors should be assisted in taking proper measures. Those without complications, should be encouraged to do appropriate exercises.

Most patients will recover from the illness after treatment in the first or second stage. But there are occasional cases who require operation. Special care is needed for such patients before and after the operation.

3. The Third Stage (The stage of Recovery)

Clinical Manifestations

Subjective symptoms vanish; diet, temperature and bowel movements normalize; muscular tension in the abdomen or rebound tenderness is relieved, or remains as slight tenderness in the lower part of xiphoid process and right upper abdomen. Nursing is carried out according to the different symptoms. The disease can be clinically divided into three types.

(1) Cold of Insufficiency Type

Clinical Manifestations

Epigastric vague pain relieved by pressing, emaciation with sallow complexion, loss of appetite, dyspepsia, light thin coating on the tongue.

Nursing

1) Regulation of diet: It is necessary to warm the middle—*Jiao* (stomach) and invigorate the spleen. Warm, cooked, soft and nourishing food and food with warm in nature and cold—dispelling function should be taken, eg. stewed mutton, porkliver soup, soft—shelled turtle, milk, sheep milk, Chinese—date, lotus seed gruel, Chinese yam gruel, fennel, gruel, carrot gruel, hawthorn, sugared ginger and so on. Raw and cold food should be avoided.

2) Keep the patient warm: The room must be kept warm. Hot medicated compress is used for the affected area, e. g. bran, salt or heated brick compress Ericarpium Citri Reticulatae 6g, Ginger 6g are heated in water for drinking.

3) Analgesia: Acupuncture treatment: Zhongwan (RN12), Zusanli (ST36), Neiguan (PC6), moxibustion snould be given to Zhongwan (RN12).

(2) Stagnation of the Liver—*Qi* Type

Clinical Manifestations

Cardiac distending pain involving hypochondria, eructation, acid regurgitation, anorexia, bitter taste, susceptibility to anger, stringy pulse.

Nursing

1) Give morale boosting care so that the patients can be in good spirits and in a calm, unruffled mood. Prevent anger which may result in impairment of the liver, and protect the stomach from the liver—Qi.

2) Taking nourishing food: Supply food for soothing the liver and regulating the flow of Qi to promot digestion. For example, radish, spinach, haw orange, or carrot gruel, chicken's gizzard—skin gruel, candied radish, and *Fo shou* 3 g (fingered citron) steeped in hot water for drinking.

3) Analgesia: Needle the points of Zhongwan (RN12), Qimen (LR14) (double), Taichong (LR3) (double) etc. or use auricular—plaster therapy to the points of Liver, Gallbladder, Spleen, Stomach, Sympthetic, etc..

(3) Blood Stasis Type

Clinical Manifestations

Localized painful area, stabbing pains, dark and gloomy appearance around the eyes, black and sticky stool, uneven pulse.

Nürsing

1) Keep patients from over exertion. Carefully observe patient's condition.

2) Give moral care and set the patient's mind at rest. Those with vomiting and hematochezia must lie quietly avoiding exercise, tension and fear.

3) Analgesia: Needle the points Zusanli(ST36) and

Zhongwan (RN12) or apply Radix Notoginseng 1.5 g, Rhizoma Corydalis 1.5 g for oral administration with warm boiled water.

4) Observation of stools: When there is melena, apply specimen for examination in order to find out the bleeding level and assist doctors in administing medicine according to the patient's condition.

5) Give nourishing food: It is beneficial for the patient to have nourishing, well cooked, light food, and diet for promoting the flow of *Qi* (vital energy) and blood circulation, such as black edible fungus, sea cucumber, jellyfish, *Xiangu* mushroom, Chinese—datas, carot, taro, etc. Avoid fried, roast and cruder cooked food.

4.9 Acute Appendicitis

Acute appendicitis is a commonly encountered abdominal disease. It may occur in adolescence and early adult life. The first symptom of the disease is pain in the upper abdomen, or about the navel. After a few hours or a day pain shifts to the right lower quadrant and becomes localized there. Pain becomes severe in paroxysmal way and is usually followed by such systemic features as nausea, vomiting, heat and constipation. It is called intestinal abscess in TCM.

General Nursing

1. Pay close attention to the patient's condition and the character of the pain. Check for signs of peritoneal irritation and note changes of the temperature, tongue coating and pulse, which is favourable to nursing according to syndrome differentiation.

2. Patients should usually take bed rest. Those who develop

peritonitis or appendiceal abscess should take semireclining position so as to avoid subphrehic abscess or interrintestinal abscess.

3. In TCM the cause of the disease is considered to be associated with emotional stimulation. Moral support must be given to free patient's mind of apprehensions so that patients can cooperate well with the doctors during treatment.

Nursing According to Syndrome Differentiation

1. Stagnating Type

Clinical Manifestations

Normal or low fever, fullness in the stomach; nausea; anorexia; migrating pain round the navel in the cases with severe stagnation of *Qi*; localized pain in those with blood stasis regular bowel movement or constipation; yellow or clear urine, local tenderness, mild musular tension, local mass by pressing, thin light tongue coating, wiry and rapid pulse, which belongs to simple appendicitis.

Nursing

(1) A moderate amount of physical exercise is beneficial for patients but overfatigue must be avoided.

(2) Acupuncture treatment: Selection of points: Appendix, Zusanli (ST36) can be chosed. Meburney's point can be added to those patients with severe blood stasis, Tianshu (ST25), and Daheng (SP15) are used for those with stagnation of *Qi*, Neiguan (PC6), Shangwan (RN13) for patients with nausea and vomiting and Quchi (LI11), Hegu (LI4) for patients with fever.

(3) External treatment: Use hot medicated compress. Grenular salt 1 kg is parched in a pot to cracking. After adding vinegar, stir it well. Put the mixture in a cloth bag and apply it to

the part of tenderness in the right lower abdomen and change the bag after it becomes colder, once or twice a day.

(4) Medicine for relieving constipation, clearing stagnation of food and exelling heat and excessive fluid through purgation, for promoting blood circulation by removing blood stasis and for clearing away heat and toxin should be taken. A suitable prescription is *Lanwei Huayu Tang* (Removing—blood—stasis Decoction). The patient with stagnation of *Qi* should be given *Yuanhu—Fen* (Corydalis Tuber Powder). Defecation should be observed after the patient takes the medicine. It is normal for the patient to defecate 2—3 times a day. If the defecation becomes too frequent, the dosage must be decreased. The same dosage must be given if the drug is vomited so as to guarantee the drug effection.

(5) Pay careful attention to the patient's condition, check for any changes of abdominal pain, temperature, the tongue coating and pulse. The patient is on the way to recovery when the pain is relieved and the temperature comes down. If there remains constipation and symptoms, let the doctors know promptly so that they can give appropriate treatment as soon as possible.

(6) The diet must be light, bland, soft and semiliquid, moderate amounts of food may be taken avoiding pungent and fried food.

2. Damp—heat Type

Clinical Manifestations

Pain in the right lower abdomen, rebound tenderness, tension of abdominal muscles, or local mass, fever, anorexia, constipation or loose stool, scanty dark urine, red tongue with yellow—greasy coating, slippery or wiry and rapid pulse, localized peritonitis associated with suppurative appendicitis, periapendix abscess.

Nursing

(1) Medicines for relieving constipation, expelling heat and excessive fluid through purgation and medicines for clearing away heat and toxin should be taken. A suitable prescription is *Lanwei Qinghua Tang* (Decoction for Clearing Away Heat from Appendix). Those with anorexia and vomiting can be given more frequent dosages.

(2) The points for acupuncture treatment are the same as those mentioned in Stagnating Type. If there is a local mass in the right lower abdomen, 3—4 points around the mass may be punctured.

(3) External treatment: Natrii Sulphas is usually used for external application, that is, Natrii Sulphas 150—200 g ground into fine powder is put in a gauze pocket and applied to the painful part of the right lower abdomen. Several hours later the medicine hardens by absorbing water and must be changed, 2 times a day.

(4) Pay attention to the patient's condition and investigate any changes of the illness. The patient is on the mend if the abdominal pain is relieved, the tenderness is localized, the temperature becomes normal, the movement of the bowels is free, the urine is clear and free, the coating on the tongue is thin and the pulse becomes slow after treatment. If the patient's condition has worsened, doctors should be told in order to prepare for operation.

(5) Light and liquid or semi—liquid vegetarian diet should be taken. The patient with high temperature and thirst must have more light drink. The patient with dampness must be given Flos Lonicerae 12 g, Herba Lophatheri 9 g, Fructus Herba

Germinatuss 9 g, soaked in water for gargling, in order to stimulate the appetite. Fruits should be available. Those who must be operated on should abstain from eating.

3. Toxic—heat Type

Clinical Manifestations

Severe pain in the abdomen; rebound tenderness; abdominal muscular tension; high temperature; chill; flushed face and red eyes; dry mouth and coating tongue; nausea; constipation; dysuria with dark urine; crimson tongue with yellow or dry coating; full and slippery, or wiry and rapid or strong pulse. Impairment of the *Yin* fluid by intense heat, deficiency of *Yin* affecting *Yang*; listlessness and cold limbs; spontaneous perspiration; shortness of breath; fall of blood pressure, etc..

Nursing

(1) This is the highest heat stage at which deteriorated case can appear easily, so the patients must be kept in bed and the patients without shock are kept in semireclining position. Observe changes in the spirits, temperature, blood pressure and abdominal sign. Nurse the patients with high temperature and shock according to High Fever Nursing in Chapter 2.1 and Syncope Nursing in Chapter 2.3.

(2) Medicines for clearing away heat and toxin, relieving constipation, promoting flow of *Qi* and removing heat from blood should be taken. When the patients have the symptoms of abdominal distension, vomiting, persistant high temperature and dry tongue without coating because of deficiency of body fluid they should be given fluid infusing so that the water and electrolyte balance can be maintained boosting the efficacy of the medicine.

(3) Acupuncture treatment is recommended in stagnating Type. In addition, otopoint: appendix, Large intestine Shenmen (H7) point and Sympthetic, etc, can be used.

(4) External treatment: 6—8 cloves of garlic (peeled) and Natrii Sulphas 15—30 g are pounded to paste which is mixed with powder of Rhubarb (Radixet Rhizoma Rhei 60 g and some vinegar. Spread the mixture on vaseline gauze (12 × 10 cm) which is applied to the painful part of the right lower abdomen. To prevent the paste from draining away and stimulating the skin, fold the edges of two pieces of gauze. The surface is covered with plastic film and bound up with an abdominal belt for two hours. The powder of Radix et Rhizoma Rhei and vinegar are mixed into paste and used for enternal application to the same part after the gauze is removed. To keep the paste damp, the surface is covered with plastic film. The paste can be used for external application for 8—10 hours. If the paste of Bulbus Alii and Natrii Sulphas is applied to the skin (usually for about 15 minutes).

(5) After treatment the abdominal pain is relieved, the temperature comes down and the movement of bowels becomes free. But the patients must be kept in bed and continue taking medicine for 5—7 days. If the symptoms can not be relieved, and the patient has cold limbs and deep pathogenic heat, the operation should be performed. Good preoperative care of the patients is necessary. They are encouraged to get up and take exercise as soon as possible, so as to promote vital energy and blood flowing and to cause the function of the intestine to return to normal.

4.10　Intestinal Obstruction

Intestinal Obstruction is considered as the symptoms and

pathologic change produced by the impairment of the movement of the intestinal tract due to various of causes. Vomiting, abdominal distension and constipation are the main clinical features followed by high temperature. Loss of body fluid can bring about extreme thirst, parched lips, skin without elasticity, apathy and *Yin* and *Yang* depletion. It is called "obstuction and rejection" and "knot of intestines" in Chinese Medicine.

General Nursing

1. Ease the patient's mind and make him activily, cooperate with the doctor during the treatment.

2. Pay attention to the changes of spirits, temperature, tongue coating, pulse condition, blood pressure and abdominal symptoms such as the nature and location of abdominal pain, times, feature and quantity of vomiting; the severity of abdominal distention and the conditions of defecation and flatulence in order to nurse according to syndrome differenciation.

3. Abstain from eating. Gastrointestinal decompression can relieve flatulence, promote *Qi* and blood flowing of intestinal wall recover peristalsis and function of intestinal absorption. Gastric evacuation is beneficial to the absorption of medicine and can prevent vomiting. Keep the stomach tube unobstructed during gastrointestinal decompression. It is beneficial to observe the color and quantity of the aspirate in ascertaining the progress of the patient. When the aspirate turns to pale yellow from grass green, the patient is on the way to recovery.

4. The patient should be given fluid infusion in order to be prevented from extreme thirst, dysphoria, dry mouth with cracked lips, skin without resitience, weak pulse, headache, dizzi-

ness and dehydration caused by loss of body fluid due to vomiting and difficulty in taking food.

5. Oral hygiene is necessary. While using the stomach tube, clean the mouth with physiological saline. The patient should rinse out the mouth with *Yinqin Tang* Lubricating oil is applied to the dry lips. The patints with ulcerative stomatitis may be given *Bingpeng San* or *Xilei San* for oral application.

Nursing According to Syndrome Differentiation

1. Cold of Insufficiency type

Clinical Manifestations

Mild pain in the abdomen but severe abdominal distension, intermittent pain without a fixed place. abdominal tenderness but no abdominal muscular tension, no fever or low fever, pale or swollen tongue with tooth prints, thin—pale or greasy coating, deep and thready pulse.

Nursing

Keep the patient warm

(1) Patients need peace and quiet and the room must be warm. Take good care of the patient's daily life. Close attention and adequate rest is essential for the patients.

(2) Medicines for warming *Yang*, strengthening the spleen, promoting the circulation of *Qi* and removing stagnancy and obstruction should be taken. A suitable prescription is *Wenpi Tang* (Decoction for Warming Spleen), or *Liqikuanchong Tang* (Decoction for Regulating the Flow of *Qi* and Relieving Depression). The decoction must be injected through the stomach tube (consult the details on usage shown in the chapter Gasro—duodenal Ulcer Perforation). The dosage is 100—200 ml

each time, attention must be given to the reaction of the patient after injecting the medicine.

(3) Acupuncture and moxibustion the acupuncture points: Shangwan (RN13), Guanyuan (RN4), Tienshu(ST25), double Zusanli (ST36) double are used to relieve flatulence and pain. Moxibustion is applied to Shenque(RN8) to expel pathogenic cold from the channel, Point—injection therapy: Zusanli (ST36) (double) is injected with neostigmine 0.25 mg for promoting peristalsis.

(4) External treatment: Wheat—baran hot medicated compress is available. Wheat baran 500 g and two Bulbu Allii Fistulose (diced) are fried in an iron pan and a suitable amount of vinegar is added and mixed up. The mixture is then wrapped in a piece of cloth or put into a bag for external application on the abdomen.

(5) Enema: *Dacheng Qi Tang* or Fructus Gleditsiac Sinensis 30 g, Herba Asari 10 g are decocted and used as enema. (consult the instructions shown in Chapter 4.8).

(6) Pay attention to the patient's condition. When the abdominal pain and abdominal distension are gradually relieved, the anus breaks wind and has a bowel movement, the stomach tube can be removed and orally administered medicine taken Other treatment may be given until the patient feels well.

(7) Regulating the patient's diet: After the stomach tube has been removed the patient should take liquid, or semiliquid, or soft diet. The food should be warm, nourishing and easily digested. Avoid greasy and irritating food.

2. Heat of Excess Type

Clinical Manifestations

Severe pain in the abdomen, jactitation, pain of fixed location, visible intestinal peristalsis and peristaltic wave, excessive bowel sound, abdominal tenderness, rebound tenderness, muscular tension and other signs of peritoneal irritation, accompanied by fever, dry mouth, constipation, oliguria, dark red tongue, with dry—yellow and greasy—yellow coating, wiry rapid and strong pulse.

Nursing

(1) Medicine for clearing stagnation of food and expelling internal heat, promoting flow of Qi and blood circulation and eliminating extravasated blood by catharsis should be taken. A suitable prescription is Fufang Dachengqi Tang or Gansui Tongjie Tang (Decoction of Gansui for Removing Intestinal Obstruction). The decoction is injected through the stomach tube. In the course of taking medicine if the patients have the symptoms of aversion to cold, tastelessness, hiccup, pale tongue, white—sleppery coating, weak—deep thready pulse, abdominal pain relieved by pressing and by warming up and desire for warm drink, the syndrome has transformed into an interior cold one, thus the puring heat drugs should be stopped using.

(2) Acupuncture treatment: The points of selection are: Zhongwan(RN12), Tianshu(ST25) (double), Zusanli(ST36) (double) and Dachangshu (BL25) (double).Quchi (LI11) (double) and Hegu (LI4) (double) are the additional points to those with fever Point—infection therapy: Zusanli (ST36) is injected with atropine 0.25 mg for relieving the severe pain and preventing vomiting after taking the medicine.

(3) Enema: Use Dachengqi, Tang. In addition, physiological saline 500 mg and atropine 1—2 ml can be used for retention

enema to relax enterospasm and to ease the patient's suffering.

(4) Intestinal obstruction caused by twisting of bowel may be treated with massage therapy or toss therapy, and that caused by intussusception is treated with finger—press—reposition method or air—enema—reposition method. Cooking—oil method is available to the obstruction caused by ascarides. Soya—bean oil or sesame oil (200—250 ml for adults, 80—150 ml for children) is heated for oral administration or injection through a tube. Before using the method, reassure the patients that there will be no suffering caused by it. Care must be taken to observe the effect of the treatment and the patients must be kept in bed after taking the oil.

(5) After treatment the patients begin to recover and are able to sleep restfully. The symptoms of abdominal pain, vomiting and abdominal distension are obviously relieved. The anus breaks wind and there is bowel movement. The obstruction is relaxed. The patients may take liquid or semi—liquid diet: Otherwise, the patient's condition will worsen. There appear a fall of blood pressure, severe abdominal pain and distension with signs of peritoneal irritation. Care is needed for the patient who must be operated on.

4.11 Infection of the Biliary Tract and Cholelithiasis

Infections of the biliary tract and cholelithiasis are common acute abdominal syndromes. The main clinical feature is dull or paroxysmal pain in the right upper abdomen or the lower part of the xiphoid process, accompanied by fever, rigor, nausea, vomiting, anorexia, abdominal distension and dry throat with bitter taste, etc.. The disease is classified as hypochondraic pain and jaundice in Traditional Chinese Medicine.

General Nursing

Psychological Nuring

1. Emptional Care: Chronic infection of the biliary tract may result in concretion which is further complicated by the infection of the biliary tract. The two conditions aggravate and complicate each other, and exist simultaneously. The gallbladder and the liver are externally and internally related and have the same function of promoting the free flow of *Qi*. The liver—energy inclines to grow freely and not to be depressed and stagnated. The induced or worsened symptoms result from emotional upsets, leading to stagnation of liver—energy and sluggishness of the vital energy and blood. So it is necessary to give emotional care and ease the patient's mind to remove the stagnation and alleviating pain.

2. Pay close attention to the condition of the illness, the characteristics of the pain, temperature, the existence of jaundice, the changes of coating on the tongue and pulse condition so as to ascertain the degree of seriousness of the illness and its clinical development. If there is a pink to bright red tongue with thin white to dry yellow coating accompanied by fever, rigor, full rapid pulse and a descent of blood pressure, it indicates excessive damp heat, failure of *Qi* inresisting pathogens and toxins of suppurative infections entering the body. The doctors must be summoned to give immediate treatment.

3. The patient with dry throat and bitter taste which affect his appetite should rinse out the mouth repeatedly or be pre-

scribed Flos Lonicerae 9 g, Radix Ophiopogonis 9g and Radix Trichosanthis 9 g which should be taken as a drink after being infused in hot water in order to clear away heat, purge fire, benefit the stomach and promote the production of body fluid. Gargling with *Yinqin Tang* (Decoction of Lonicera and Forsythia) and more light drink are also acceptable. The oral cavity must be given good care, particularly in serious cases.

4. Observe seriously the clinical development of the patient after taking *Pai Shi Tang* (Decoction for Expelling Stones) or combined therapy. If exacerbation of abdominal pain, fever, rapid pulse and even jaundice appear, it suggests the stones are being discharged. The abdominal pain disappears as soon as the stones are discharged, the temperature descends and jaundice subsides. At this time, feces should be collected so as to monitor the passing of stone. If there is an abdominal pain without any signs of relief, abatement of high fever, the attacks alternating between chill and fever and exacerbated jaundice, the surgeons must be summoned and an operation should be prepared.

Nursing According to Sydrome Differenciations

1. Stagnation of *Qi* Type

Clinical Manifestations

Colicky or jumping pain in the right hypochondrium, or dull pain and distension in the hypochondrium and the epigastric region which affect the shoulder and the back, often accompanied by bitter taste, dry throat, dizziness and anorexia, pink tongue—peak with thin—white or light—yellowish coating, wiry and tight or wiry and thin pulse.

Nursing

(1) The patients should be kept in a calm, unruffled mood and as cheerful as possible to avoid depression. Plenty of rest and avoidance of strenuous exercises are needed.

(2) They should have a regular diet including melon, spinach, aubergine and radish gruel. 3–6 g of Fructus Citri Sarcodactylic should be taken as tea after being infused in hot water, to relax the liver and dispel depression, promote the circulation of Qi and release the pain. The patients with choleolithiasis may frequently have Herba Lysimachiae gruel which is helpful to expelling the gall stone.

(3) Zhong wan (RN12), Qimen (LR14) and Dannang (EX–LE6) points are needled. If there is a colicky pain, Hegu (LI 4) point should be needled besides the acupoints above. In the case of dizziness, Yintang (EX–HN3) and Fengchi (GB20) points are needled, and for anorexia, Zusanli (ST36) point is needled.

(4) External therapy: A piece of Zhenjiang plaster which is covered with 0.25 g of borneol after having been made pliable by heat, is applied on the area of gall bladder or the place of the shoulder and back pain. It must be warmed every day after the plaster is taken away and covered again with the same amount of borneol for the next use. Zhenjiang plaster has the functions of removing stagnant Qi and moving Qi by means of aromatics, dredging the channel and alleviating pain.

(5) Herbs should be taken to relax the liver and regulate the circulation of Qi and relieve pain. The prescription Qingdan Xingqi Tang (Decoction to Clear the Gall Bladder and Promote the Circulation of Qi) should be selected. It is appropriate to take hot.

(6) It is essential for the patient to live a regular life and

dress appropriately according to weather conditions to prevent the disease from recurring or becoming more severe because of a sudden change of weather.

2. Damp—heat Type

Clinical Manifestations

Continued distending pain in the right—upper abdomen, which often radiates to the right shoulder, muscular tension in the right—upper abdomen, pressing pain, swelling gallbladder which can be palpated sometimes, accompanied by alternative attacks of chills and fever, dry throat with bitter taste, nausea and vomiting, loss of appetite, yellow brown pigmentation of skin and eyes, constipation, yellowish—turbid urine in small amount, red tongue with yellowish greasy coating, wiry and slippery or wiry and thin pulse.

Nursing

(1) The patient must stay in bed and can gradually develop the capacity for exercise after the symptoms disappear.

(2) Herbs for relaxing the liver and normalizing the function of the gallbladder, clearing away heat and promoting diuresis should be taken, *Qingdan Lishi Tang* (Decoction for Clearing Away Gallbladder—heat and Promoting Diuresis) should be selected. The warm decoction is indicated. 60—100 g of Herba Hysimachiae should be decocted and taken in several small doses or 60 g of Stigma Maydis should be taken as a drink after being infused in hot water, which can clear away heat, promote diuresis and remove gall stones.

(3) Acupuncture:Dannang (LE6), Yanglingquan (SP9), Zhongwan (RN12), Taichong (LR3) and Danshu (BL19) points are needled. In addition, if jaundice appears, Zhiyin (BL67) and

Riyue (BB24) points are added; for vomiting Neiguan (PC6) point should be added.

Auricula–plaster therapy is given to the points: Liver, Gallbladder, Duodenum, Shenmen, Sympathetic and stomach. A piece of *Zhenjiang* plaster with borneol can also be applied to the part to relieve pain.

(4) The patients should have a nutritious and digestible vegetarian diet. They should eat plenty of fruit and little glutinous food and avoid eating pungent and greasy food. The patient with cholithiasis can frequently take shelled walnuts which have the function of inducing decomposition of calculi.

Eating method: 5–6 shelled walnuts, crystal sugar and some sesame oil are steamed together in the pot. It is taken once a day.

(5) For those whose skin itches so severely that they can not sleep because of jaundice, antipreritic, soda solution or boric acid lotion should be used to clean the skin. Frequent baths should be taken to keep skin clean.

3. Fire of Excess Type

Clinical Manifestations

Severe persistent abdominal pain which can not be relieved and can involve other parts, regidity of abdominal muscle, tenderness with throbbing pain or with a mass, unreduced high fever, flushed face and blood–shot eyes, dry mouth and tongue, yellow–brown pigmentation of skin, constipation, dark yellowish coloured urine; The severe cases may have coma and delirium, cold clammy limbs, ecchymosis of skin, epistaxis, gingival hemorrhage, dark red tongue with dry and yellowish coating which is rough and prickly, and wiry, slippery and rapid pulse or sinking, thin and weak pulse.

Nursing

(1) The developments of consciousness, blood pressure and temperature should be observed seriously because of the severe condition caused by fire transmission due to damp—heat pathogen, and internal damage caused by toxic heat. The cases with fever must be given essential supporting treatment such as fluid infusion and blood transfusion or antibiotics. (Referring to high—fever nursing 2.1)

(2)In preparation for operation, the patients should take medicine for clearing heat and purging fire, soothing the liver and normalizing the gallbladder. A suitable prescription is *Qingdan Xiehuo Tang* (Decoction for Clearing Away Gallbladder—heat and Purging Fire), which should be decocted and taken cool. Those who vomit severely and have difficulty in taking the medicine may be given it in injected form by means of inserting an esophageal. Acupuncture and external therapy may also be chosen as supplementary measures.

(3)If the symptoms are relieved after the treatment above, the same nursing may be continued. If the result is contrary, an emergency operation is necessary and intensive nursing before or after the operation should be given.

4.12　Ascariasis of the Biliary Tract

Biliary ascariasis is the obstruction and infection of the biliary tract, caused by ascaris'getting into the biliary tract, and is a common complicating disease of intestinal ascariasis. It is characterized by the sudden severe colicky pain which feels like drilling under the xiphoid process in the upper abdomen. The patients are restless or accompanied by nausea vomiting, chill, fever and cold limbs. The jaundice may appear in severe cases. It is called colic by ascaris in traditional Chinese medicine.

General Nursing

1. Observe the condition carefully, understand the characteristics of abdominal pains and help the doctors to relieve the patient's pain. The first choices of relieving spasm and pain are as the following:

(1) Acupuncture Therapy

a) Body acupuncture: The following group points can be chosen: Zhongwan(RN12) through–Liangmen(ST21), Yingxiang (LI20)–through–Sibai(ST2); Yight Danshu (BL19) of both sides, Dannang (EX–LE6), Taichong (LR3) and Neiguan (PC6). The needle method is used for a strong stimulation. The needles are retained for 30 minutes.

b) Ear acupuncture; sympthetic, Shenmen(HT7), Liver, gallblodder, pancreas, duodenucm points, etc. , are needled, or auricular–plaster therapy can be used.

c) Electric needling (Electro–acupuncture): Two needles are connected to each of the electrodes after they are inserted into right Danshu (BL19) (–)and Zhongwan (RN12) (+) and needling sensation has been stimulated. By means of continuous wave the electric current is gradually increased to a level just unover the patient's threshold of tolerance.

d) Point–injection Therapy: 1 ml of Atropine or Vitamin K3 is injected into one or two points of Dannang (EX–LE6), Danshu (BL19), Zhongwan (RN12), Jiuwei (RN15), etc. . per injection.

(2) Vinegar therapy: 100 ml of edible vinegar with a small amount of Chinese prickly ash is boiled and the liquid is taken as

draught.

(3) Back tapping therapy: The operator taps the right spinal costal angle of the patient with the right root of the palm while the patient is in a sitting position or left lateral position. The purpose of relieving pain can be reached when the strength of the tapping is consistent.

(4) Cupping therapy: A cup is applied on the pressure pain area under the xiphoid process. The treatment may last 30 minutes.

2. Preventive treatment of disease: The patients must be advised to have a regular diet and living habit, keep themselves in a comfortable temperature, pay attention to the hygiene of food and beverage, avoid crapulence, have good personal health habits and wash hands before meals and after passing stools. Ascariasis of the biliary tract must be treated as soon as it appears. Ascaris can be expelled according to the doctor's advice. The methods are as the following:

(1) 5—10 g of peeled roasted Fructus Quisqualis should be chewed and taken on an empty stomach for an adult, half the dose for a child.

(2) Acupunctare: The fallowing pionts can be chosen: both sides of Guanyan (RN4), Taichong (LR3), Xuehai (SP10) and Fenglong (ST40).

(3) 30 g of Chinaberry root bark without the outer cover should be decocted and taken after adding some brown sugar as correctives. In order to ascertain the effectiveness of driving out the ascarides, the condition of parasite elimination should come under the patient's observation.

Nursing According to Sydrome Differentiation

1. Cold of Insufficiency Type

Clinical Manifestations

The patient feels abdominal colicky pain which occurs spasmodically and is relieved by pressure and warmth. In the intervals between pains the patient feels as well as a normal person. The other symptoms: Vomiting clear water or ascarides, cold clammy limbs, pale complexion, cold sweat accompanied by anorexia, normal or loose stool, polyuria with clear urine, thick and tender tongue with white and greasy coating and wiry—tight or deep—sited pulse.

Nursing

(1) The patient should be advised to get plenty of rest, keep his living quarters at suitable temperature and dress appropriately for the weather conditions in order to prevent the disease from worsening due to exopathogens'invading to impaire *Yang—Qi*. A hot medicated compress (i,e. bran or salty compress) should be used to keep the abdomen warm or moxibustion can be used over Shangwan (RN13) to expel pathogenic cold from the channel.

(2) Diet regulation: The principle of recuperation is to build up the patient's health, protect acquired constitution and strengthen the body. Warm—hot and rich nutritive food with the function of warming middle—*Jiao* to dispel cold should be given to promote the recovery of the transporting and transforming function of the spleen and the stomach. In addition, according to the ascarid's characteristics, i. e. being immovable when smelling sour or having pungent flavour, some edible vinegar, Chinese prickly ash and other condiments of acrid and tart flavour should

be added to cooking. The patient should often take Chinese hawthorn and haw slice (jelly), drink sweet—sour plum juice or smoked plum gruel and avoid eating raw or cold and greasy food.

(3) The most efficacious medicine to relieve colic by ascarids and warm the middle—*Jiao* to expel ascarids is hot *Wumei Tang* (Black Plum Decoction) which should be taken when the abdominal pain stops temperarily. After it's application, the patient's abdominal pain can usually be relieved and he sleeps quietly. If the colic can not be relieved and shows continuous megalgia accompanied by alternating bouts of chills and fever, the doctor should be summoned to treat it.

2. Damp—heat Type

Clinical Manifestations:

Continuous distending pain in the abdomen, which becomes severe paroxysmally, tenderness accompanied by alternating bouts of chills and fever, dry throat with bitter taste, anorexia, red tongue with yellowish and greasy coating, wiry pulse.

Nursing

(1) The patient should be kept in bed and have quiet and comfortable surroundings. The fever cases should be nursed according to high—fever nursing (2.1).

(2) The most efficacious medicine for clearing away heat and promoting diuresis and regulating the flow of *Qi* is *Qingdan Lishi Tang* (Decoction for Clearing Away Heat from the Gallbladder and promoting diuresis). It is beneficial to take it warm. After taking it the patient's conditions of parasite elimination and stool passing should be recorded. In addition, it is important to observe the development of the case. It suggests that the patient is well again if the fever is reduced and the pain is relieved. If high fever

appears accompanied by chill, yellowish eyes and body, dark red tongue with dry and yellowish coating, sepsis should be taken into consideration. Pay close attention to the patient's spirit and variance of blood pressure, inform the doctor and prepare for operation.

(3) Nursing the patient's diet: The patient should have a vegetarian and liquid or semi–liquid diet and food mainly for clearing away heat and promoting diuresis, such as adsuki bean, broad bean, celery, and drink plenty of tea to boost the efficacy of the medicine. Those who have a dry throat with bitter taste and anorexia should rinse out the mouth or be accordingly prescribed Honeysuckle Flower 9 g, Tuber of Dwarf Liluturf 9 g and Radix Trichosanthis 9 g which are infused in hot water and taken as a drink to clear away heat, purge fire, reinforce the stomach, and promote the production of body fluids.

4.13   Thrombophlebitis (Thrombotic Phlebitis)

Thrombophlebitis often occurs in superficial veins of the limbs. It is characterized by pain, swelling and high fever with a feeling of burning in local venae superficiales and a felt hard node or band–like object. Periphlebitis may even appear. It is accompanied by general constitutional symptoms like fever. It is classified as rheumatism with the blood vessels involved in traditional Chinese medicine.

Genneral Nursing

1. Do a good prevention job: Most cases are caused by toxic pathogenic factors' invasion due to trauma infection and intravenous infusion. So a proper and prompt treatment must be

given for local trauma and infection. It is very important to use only sterilized needles, not reusing them until they have been sterilized and to avoid the use of irritative medicine when possible.

2. Pay close attention to the development of the case. If intermittent migratory thrombophlebitis occurs in the limbs repeatedly, nurses should assist doctors to determine whether the patient suffers from other diseases such as thromboangiitis obliterans, (Buerger's disease) or potential visceral cancer.

Nursing According to Sydrome Differentiation

1. Damp—heat Type

Clinical Manifestations

Local inflammatory with a feeling of burning, swelling, edema of limbs caused by severe dampness, sense of heaviness, a touched hard rode or band—like object and distinct tenderness.

Nursing

(1) The patient with a high fever should stay in bed with the affected limb raised, and the limb should be moved as seldom as possible during the course of treatment.

(2) Dyer's Woad Leaf Plaster, *Maogu* Plaster or Fresh Portulaca is pounded into paste and applied topically on the affected part. *Mahuang Ding* (Tincture of Seed of Strychnos and Ephedra Used to Reduce Swelling and Resolve Masses) can also be smeared on the affected part.

(3) The hot decoction of antiseptic wash drug or the wash drug of nitro—vitrial which has been infused in boiling water can be applied to the affected area as hot compress.

(4) Jiaguan (on each side of the infected vein with an interval of 1 cm, Geshu (BL17) Taiyuan(LU9) points may be needled. Ex-

tra points which may be treated are Neiguan(PC6) and Yanglingquan(GB34) for the inflammation of venae thoracoepigastrica superficiales, Hegu(LI4) for the inflammation of the superficial vein of the upper limbs, Yinlingquan(SP9) and Sanyinjiao(SP6) points for the inflammation of venae superficiales of the lower limbs.

2. Stagnation of blood Type

Clinical Manifestations

Local damp and heat retreating gradually, blood stasis stagnated channels and collaterals forming hard nodes or band—like objects left, pigmentation left in the local skin.

Nursing

(1) The steam of hot decoction of *Zhitong San* (Blood—activating and Pain—stopping Powder) is used to heat the affected part.

(2) *Sanjie Pian* (Mass—resolving tablet) or *Huoxue Quyu Pian* (Blood—Activating and Stasiseliminating Tablet) can be taken for a long period of time.

(3) Eating plenty of kelp, clam and laver, etc. is beneficial for activating blood and eliminating stasis.

4.14 Thrombosis of Deep Vein of lower Limbs

The thrombosis of deep vein of lower limbs often occurs in iliofemoral vein. The most common case is the thrombosis of the left iliofemoral vein, which is characterized by intensive swelling and pain of the lower limbs. It is classified as rheumatism with the blood vessels involved, swelling and blood stasis in traditional Chinese medicine.

General Nursing

1. The onset is acute with sudden swelling and pain of the immovable limbs. Most patients are in a state of dread and anxiety. So nurses should do their best to free the patient's mind of the tense feeling, keep him in good spirits and assist the doctor with the treatment.

2. The patient should stay in bed with the affected limb raised, which is helpful to the venous return and relieving the swelling and pain of the affected limb.

3. Pay close attention to the development of the case. The thrombosis of iliofemoral vein scales easily within 4 weeks after its appearance. It is possible that pulmonary infarction may appear with pectoralgia, hemoplysis, and fever, etc.. In the other hand, the thrombosis may spread upwards and into the inferior vena cava. The renal veins may be even involved in complicating posthepatic high portal venous pressure. Jaundice and ascites follow. So the nurse should take special care of the patient, observe the development of the condition at all times and assist the doctor to treat the case as soon as the abnormal condition appears.

4. The cause of the disease is associated with a long stay in bed after an operation or giving birth. So doctors and nurses should encourage awareness among people, and advise the patients and parturients to be up and about as soon as possible in order to reduce the incidence of the disease.

Nursing According to Sydrome Differenciation

1. Downward Flow of Damp—heat Type
Clinical Manifestations

In the early stage of the disease: inflammation, fever of the whole body, swelling and distending pain of the affected limb, white or yellowish greasy coating on the tongue.

Nursing

(1) The patient must be kept in bed for 3—4 weeks with the affected limb raised. Those with fever should be nursed according to the high fever nursing (2.1).

(2) Each dose of *Simiaoyongan Tang* with modification (Modified Decoction of Four Wanderful Drugs for Quick Restoration of Health) and *Huoxuetongmai Yin* (Drink of Promoting blood Circulation to Remove Obstruction in the Channels and Vessels) may be taken to clear away heat and promote diuresis, and promote blood circulation to remove blood stasis. They can be used interchangeably to concentrate the potency of the drugs in relieving swelling and removing obstruction in the channels. The decoction should be taken warm and the patients reaction must be observed after taking it. *Huoxie Tongmai Pian* and *Sichuong Pian* can be taken in addition to it.

(3) Nursing the Patients of Their Diet

Food with the function of clearing away heat and promoting diuresis and promoting blood circulation and removing obstruction in the channels should be taken, such as kelp, laver, the soup of red bean and Chinese waxgourd, etc.. Rich nourishing food is contraindicated.

2. Blood Stasis and Excessive Dampness

Clinical Manifestations

The appearance of thrombosis following the retreat of the inflammation of deep vein, accompanied by the distinct swelling of the leg, the varicosity of the superficial vein and the telangiectasis of the skin and the dark red tongue or the petechia of the tongue.

Nursing

(1) The proper exercise may be done with the affected limb. *Huoxue Zhitong San* (Powder of Promoting Blood Circulation to Stop Pain) can be applied to the affected limb as a hot compress in order to relieve swelling and pain, promote the forming of the collateral circulation and improve the blood circulation of the limbs.

(2) *Danshen Huoxue Tang* (Decoction of Red Sage for Promoting the Blood Circulation) or *Huoxue Tongmai Yin* (Decoction of Promoting the blood Circulation and Removing Obstruction in the Channels) should be taken to promote the blood circulation to remove blood stasis, promote diuresis and remove obstruction in the channels. *Sichong Wan* (The Pill of Four Worms) and *Dahuangzhechong Wan* (Pills of Rhubarb and Ground Beetle) can be taken as accompanying drugs.

(3) Because of the swelling, varicosity of the superficial vein and the telangiectasis of the skin, the affected limb must be protected from the injury and infection of the local skin. Elastic bandage can be used to wrap up the affected limb in order to alleviate blood stasis and telangiectasis.

(4) Nursing the patients of their diet: The patient has white greasy coating on the tongue due to the retention of damp—evil after the extinction of heat—evil. so in summer the patient should take such food as water melon, Chinese waxgourd and soup of gram of fresh mushroom, edible fungus and sea cucumber. He should often drink tea or corn stigma infused in boiling water which is beneficial for promoting blood circulation to remove blood stasis and damp.

3. Insuffi ciency Type of Both the Spleen and the Kidney

Clinical Manifestations

Swelling and distending pain of the affected limb, soreness and aversion to cold of the lumbar area which tends to be more severe in the evening; lassitude and weak state, eating little and no feeling of thirst; thin and white coating on the red tongue.

Nursing

(1) The patient must be given plenty of rest and kept warm and adjust his clothing and covering in order not to catch cold, etc. according to weather conditions.

(2) Protect the affected limb and raise it up when sleeping at night. Nitro—vitriol can also be used to wash the affected limb again.

(3) A hot decoction of *Wenshen Jianpi Tang* (Decoction for Warming the Kidney and Strengthening the Spleen) can be taken to tonify the kidney, invigorate the spleen, promote diuresis and remove obstruction in the channels.

(4) Nursing the patients of their diet: The food for warming and recuperating the spleen to promote diuresis should be taken, such as mutton, sea cucumber, soft shelled turtle, edible fungus, lotus seed, jujube or gruel made from chestnut, walunt kernel. Chinese yam and prepared rhizome of rehmannia and rice. Some condiment should be put in the food of the patient with anorexia during cooking, such as ginger, onion, garlic, Chinese prickly ash, fennel and vinegar, etc.. Zhongwan (RN 12) and Zusanli (ST 36) points may be needled to stimulate the appetite.

4.15 Varicosis Vein of Lower Limbs

Varicosis Vein of lower limbs occurs in great and small

saphenous veins. Varicosis of the great saphenous vein is commonly found in middle—age persons. It is characterized by a sense of heaviness of the shank, distending pain, fatigability, edema of leg and ankle caused by standing for prolonged periods, varicosis, projection and arcuation. In severe cases the vein may be curved into a ball. The disease may be accompanied by superficial thrombosed phlebitis and ulcer of the lower limbs. It is classified as ecthma in TCM.

General Nursing

1. The patient should take plenty of rest and raise the affected limb when sleeping, to assist the return of the venous blood.

2. Standing long and carrying heavy things should be avoided. Elastic polyamide fibre stockings or elastic bandage can be worn for a long time. The skin of the affected limb must be protected from injury and infection.

3. Careful pre—operative and post—operative nursing care is necessary for those needing operation. The methods of nursing the complications caused by varicosis Vein of lower limbs are as the following:

Nursing According to Sydrome Differenciation

1. Downward Flow of Damp—heat Type
Clinical Manifestations
Thrombotic superficial phlebitis in the lower limbs or infective ulcer swelling, heat and pain, a local itch in those with eczematoid dermatitis, a yellowish greasy coating on the tongue.
Nursing
(1) The patient should stay in bed with the affected limb

raised. The ulcer with much pus should be immersed and cleaned with the decocted lotion for detoxifying and washing and then the dressing should be changed with a piece of oleo–gauze with rheum. If the pus has been cleaned away and granulation has manifested itself, a small amount of *Shengji San* (Promoting Tissue Regeneration Powder) may be used to promote tissue regeneration.

(2) Decocted antipruritic or desiccant medicine can be used to fumigate and wash the eczematiod dermatitis. *Huangbai San* (Powder of Dried Bark of Phellodendron) and *Qing Ge San* (The Powder of Natural Indigo and Gecko) can be dusted on the wound area after mopping up the water from the skin. Scratching must be avoided to prevent infection.

(3) Those who have superficial thrombotic phlebitis must be nursed in reference to the nursing care of superficial thrombotic phlebitis.

2. Interior Heat Due to Yin Deficiency Type

Clinical Manifestations

Non–healing local, ulcer, light red or slight dark granulation, a little pus, swelling, and red tongue.

Nursing

(1) *Lurong ShengjiSan* or *Zhenzhu Shengji San* (Powder Made From Pilose Antler or Pearl to Promote Tissue Regenration) may be scattered on the local ulcer and then *Shengji Yuhong Gao* oleo–gauze should be used to cover it.

(2) 100 mg of VB_1 may be injected into Zusanli (ST36) and Yanglingquan (BL34) interchangeably to promote the healing of ulcers.

(3) While taking the medicine for replenishing *Yin* and re-

moving heat, the patient should eat more food with the same function, such as bean products, all kinds of melon, eggs, edible fungus and milk, etc, which are beneficial to the medicinal effect.

3. Deficicncy of Both *Qi* and Blood Type

Clinical Manifestations

Non—healing ulcer, light red or pale granulation, watery pus, general deficiency of *Qi*, pale tongue with thin white coating.

Nursing

(1) Local treatments is in reference to that of *Yin* deficiency and the interior heat—syndrome type. Moxibustion theropy can be used to the surface of the wound for the purpose of promoting healing.

(2) Because pathogen has been expelled and vital energy is asthemic, medicine for invigorating *Qi* and enriching the blood, and removing obstruction in the channels by regulating the nutrient should be taken, such as *Renshen Yangying Tang* (Ginseng Nutrition Decoction) and *Shiquan Dabu Tang* with modification (Modified Decoction of Ten Powerful Tonics)

(3) Dietetic Nursing: Food for invigorating *Qi* and enriching blood is suitable, such as pork, mutton, sheep and ox liver, soft—shelled trutle, sea cucumber and fresh vegetables and fruits.

4.16 Thromboangiitis Obliterans (Buerger's Disease)

Thromboangiitis obliterans is segmental inflammatory lesion of artery and vein. Because of hyperplasia of endagium caused by the inflammation of the full thickness vasculitis, thrombosis luminal obliteration appears, which leads to the ischemia of the extremities by the obstruction of the lumen. Gangrene of extremities develops at last. It is classified into "tuo ju" (gangrene of finger or toe) in TCM.

General Nursing

1. Emotional Care: The disease often occurs in young and middle—age adults. It is a longering disease causing aching all over and may lead to disability of affected limbs in varying degrees and bring about much mental suffering to the patient. A long term of melancholy may cause derangement of *Qi* and blood and lead to exacerbation of the disease or relapse. So sympathetic emotional care on the part of nurses is needed. The patient should be encouraged to build up faith in overcoming the disease and to cooperate with the doctor during the treatment. The patient should be urged to have plenty of rest and cultivate good living habits or guided to do exercises in *Qigong* which can build up resistance to disease by regulation of mental activities and respiration and adjustment of posture.

2. The observation on the usage of Chinese herbal medicine
One dose per day is required; two doses per day for serious cases. Because a long term of taking the drugs for promoting blood circulation to remove blood stasis and clearing away heat and toxic material may affect the digestive canal in varying degrees, the medicine at a moderate temperature should be taken but it is not so close to meal times in order not to induce nausea. The reaction after taking the medicine should also be observed. Those who suffer from anorexia may take the medicine for regulating the function of the spleen and stomach at the same time, or be given acupuncture to Zhongwan (RN 12), Zusanli (ST 36) to improve appetite.

3. Migrating superficial thrombotic phlebitis may easily appear in the early period of thromboangiitis obliterans or during the pathogenic process. Local changes of the affected limb must be observed. If any change appears, it must be treated so as to decrease the patient's suffering. The nursing should be in reference to that of superficial thrombotic phlebitis.

4. Forbidding Smoking: The patient should be made fully aware of the harmfulness of smoking which can not only cause malfunction of blood vessels but worsen the patient's condition or make relapse possible. Patients with this disease should permanently give up smoking.

Nursing According to Sydrome Differentiation

1. *Yin*—cold Type

Clinical Manifestations

Desire for warmth and fear of cold, cold limbs, local pale—white or flushed skin, light tongue with thin white coating, deep—faint or slow pulse.

Nursing

(1) Nursing the affected limb:

a) The patient should be sure to keep warm. The affected limb should be covered with soft, warm and comfortable cotton—padded shoes, socks or gloves. The patient should not be exposed to any coldness for prolonged periods. The bed—room should be kept warm.

b) The affected limb should be kept clean and often washed with warm water and soap. It should be dried with a soft towel to prevent possible injury to the skin. Nitro—vitriol solution may be used to wash feet infected with tinea. Breaking the skin of the foot when scratching an itch should be avoided.

c) Damage should be avoided while triming the patient's toe nails. They should be softened in hot-warm water before being trimmed. Corrosive ointment or medicinal power must not be used recklessly for ingrown nail and corn.

d) Prevent the affected limb from being touched and squeezed or further injury. Shoes and socks should be wide and soft so that the affected limb is free from pressure and the blood circulation is not disturbed.

(2) *Yanghe Tang* with modification (Modified *Yang*-activating Decoction) may be taken to expel pathogenic cold from channel and promote blood circulation to remove blood stasis or *Shengui Zaizao Wan* (Ginseng Antler Restorative Pills) and *Shenrong Dabu Wan* (Ginseng Antler Tonic Pills) may be chosen as the accompanying medicine. The patient's reaction after taking the medicine should be observed and the blood pressure taken regularly. Some cases will have symptoms of dry mouth or foreign-body sensation in the throat and dizziness, etc. after a long term of taking the medicine for warming and heating. The reason for such symptoms should be explained to the patients. Patients with normal blood pressure should persist in taking the medicine; the symptoms will eventually disappear. Those with severe dizziness will recover in 3-5 days after having stopped taking the medicine.

(3) The affected limb may be fumigated and washed with *HuiYang Zhitong Xiyao* (Washing Medicine for Recuperating Depleted Yang and Relieving Pain). The medicine temperature should be moderate and should not be over hot in case it cause extra pain.

(4) Acupuncture and moxibustion therapy: Acupuncture and moxibustion treatment has the functions of regulating *Qi* and blood, eliminating ateriospasm of limbs, promoting the forming of collateral circulation, etc.. The needles may be inserted into Quchi (LI 11), Hegu (LI 4), Neiguan (PC 6), Taiyuan (LU 9), etc. On the upper limbs, while Zusanli (ST36), Sanyinjiao (SP6), Chengshan (BL57), Kunlun (BL60), Yinlingquan (SP9) and Yanglingquan (GB34), On the lower limbs. Two or three points should be used each time. Ignited cones of moxa should be applied over Qihai (RN 6), Zusanli (ST36), Quchi (LI 11) etc..

(5) Pain in the affected limb: Taking *Tongmaian Pian* (Tablet for Promoting Circulation of *Qi*) and *Yuanhuzhitong Pian* (Tablet for Relieving Pain) or auricular−plaster therapy can relieve pain and alleviate the patient's suffering. As a prolonged term of dosage may lead to addiction, narcotics must be avoided.

(6) Direct the patient to train his affected limb.i. e keeping the patient lying on bed for 2−3 minutes with the affected limb raised to the height of 45 and then letting the limb fall down to the vertical of the edge of the bed for 3−5 minutes, putting it back on the bed for 2−3 minutes and doing this exercise repeatedly for 5−10 times. Such kind of exercise should be done three times a day in order to promote the circulation of *Qi* and blood.

(7) Dietetic nursing: Nutritious food with warm nature and promoting the flow of *Qi* and blood circulation should be taken such as mutton, chicken, carp crucian carp, grass carp, brown sugar, Chinese−date, hawthorn, orange, carrot and Chinese chives, etc.. The gruel made of Skullcap (foot) or the root of red−rooted salvia may be taken often. Fried food must not be eaten.

(8) Pay close attention to the varying of the circulation of the affected limb, e.g. the colour and temperature of the skin and the conditions of arteriopalmus of the femur, poplitea and the dorsum of foot. Understand the development of the disease to assist the doctor in prescribing according to the patient's syndrome.

2. Blood Stasis type

Clinical Manifestations

Continuous fixed pain in the affected limb, purplish red, dark red or black purple colour, petechiae and ecchymosis on the skin, bright red and purple tongue, petechia of the tongue with thin and white coating, deep, thin and uneven pulse.

Nursing

(1) The nursing of the affected limb is the same as that mentioned above. In addition, the affected limb should be stretched out and must not be in a suspended position. *Mahuang Ding* (Tincture of Seed of Strychnos and Ephedra Used to Reduce Swelling and Resolve Masses) can be used to smear the ecchymosis and petechiae on the local skin area.

(2) Severe continuous pain should be relieved to reduce the patient's suffering. The analgesic methods in clinic application are as following:

a) Acupuncture analgesia: The needles are usually inserted into the area of pain.

b) Injecting procaine: 3 ml of procaine (0.5%) should be injected into each point of Zusanli (ST36), Sanyinjiao (SP6), Juegu (LI 16), etc. for the upper limbs.

c) Blocking the peripheral of femoral artery: 20 ml of procaine (10%) and 100 mg of Vitamin B_1 can be used to block the peripheral femoral artery or the femoral nerve trunk.

d) It is effective to use Chinese medicinal narcotic to alleviate the suffering of serious pain, insomnia or letheomania. Method of application: 2—3 mg of *Zhongma* II or 2.5—5 mg of *Zhongma* I and 25 mg of chlorpromazine is diluted with 10 ml of normal saline and then is injected slowly into the vein. The patient will fall asleep after 3—5 minutes and generally remain asleep 6—8 hours. The injection is given once every two days. The pain will be relieved or disappear completely after 3—5 injections. Attentive nursing must be given and the changes of temperature, pulse, respiration and blood pressure must be observed carefully. If there is any abnormality, it can be dealt with according to the symptoms.

(3) The most suitable prescription is *Huoxue Tongmai Yin* (Drink for Promoting Blood Circulation and Invigorating Pulse—beat) to dredge the channel. The accompaning medicines are *Huoxue Huayu Pian* (Tablet for Promoting Blood Circulation to Remove Blood Stasis), *Sanqi Pian* (Tablet of Notoginseng) and *Fufang Danshen Pian* (Composite Red Sage Root Tablet).

(4) The patient should be encouraged to eat more and be given nourishing and easily digested food. Pungent and irrtative food must be avoided.

3. Downward Flow of Damp—heat Type

Clinical Manifestations

Flushed and purplish red swelling of the affected limb, acromelic light ulcer or gangrene, a red tongue with yellowish coating and wiry, thin and rapid pulse to the patient with inflammation.

Nursing

(1) The most suitable prescription is *Simiao Yongan Tang* with modification (Modified Decoction of Four Wanderful

Drugs for Quick Restoration of Health). The accompanying drugs are *Sichong Pian* (Tablet of Four Worms) and *Huoxue Quyu Pian* (Tablet for Promoting Blood Circulation to Remove Blood Stasis). After taking the medicine the patient's response should be observed. Diarrhea may appear in a few patients, but would soon disappear because of the diarrhea—relieving function of Radix Angelicae Sinensis and Scrophularia Root. Treatment is generally unnecessary. If the diarrhea is severe, the doctor should be informed. The patient will be well again as soon as stopping taking the medicine.

(2) Local treatment: The acromelic dry gangrene can be sterilized with alcochol—cotton wool and then dressed with sterilized dry gauze in order to keep it dry. Acromelic damp gangrene: If there is much pus or necrotic tissues in the wound, *Quanxie Gao* (Plaster of Scorpion) may be applied topically for removing slough to ease pain. The wound should be fumigated and washed with antiseptic and then dressed. The wound with little pus should be dressed with oleo gauze with rheum. The wound with little pus and fresh granulation can be dressed with *Shengji Yuhong Gao* oil—gauze (A Kind of Plaster for Promoting Tissue Regeneration) until its recovery. The whole operation must be done softly and gently in order not to increase the patient's pain.

(3) Dietetic Nursing: The patient should take nourishing and easily digested food and eat plenty of melons and beans which are helpful to clearing away heat and promoting diuresis.

4. Blazing Noxious Heat Type

Clinical Manifestations

Red swelling and hot pain in affected limb; much liquid of pus with fetid smell accompanied by high fever; chills; bright red tongue with yellowish greasy, yellowish dry, or even black coating; slippery rapid and full pulse.

Nursing

(1) Pay close attention to the patient's condition and the development of temperature, coating on the tongue, pulse condition and blood pressure. If there is any fever, it is due to blood stasis, which indicates the heat of excess type. Its symptoms are high fever, red complexion and conjunctival congestion, confusion and dysphoria. A cold compress may be used to reduce the temperature. Frequent inspections should be made of wards with such patients and bed fenders placed next to the bed in order to prevent the patient from falling out off the bed. The patients should be nursed according to the high fever nursing. (2.1).

(2) *Simiao Yongan Tang* with modification (Modified Decoction of Four Wonderful Drugs for Quick Restoration of Health) and *Hoxue Tongmai Yin* (Drink for Promoting Blood Circulation to Remove Obstruction in the Channels and Vessels) are suitable for clearing away heat and toxic material and promoting blood circulation to remove blood stasis. The two medicines can be taken interchangeably. Those who have difficulty in swallowing should be fed in small doses at frequent intervals and drink plenty of water after taking it. *Xihuang Wan* and *Niuhuang Qingxin Wan* (Bezoar Sedative Boluse) are accompanying drugs.

(3) Local Treatment: The dressing should be changed promptly for the patient with much pus and necrotic tissue in the affected area, or it should be changed after fumigating and washing the affected part with antisepticin order to reduce the fetid smell and prevent the bedding from being contaminated. If the secondary infection of gangrene spreads to the ankle joint or

above it and the patient has the symptoms of the continuous high fever and severe pain, amputation will have to be done. The nurse should assist the doctor in preparing for the operation. After operation, the stump should be laid flat. If the operation is done from the shank, the patient should avoid bending his knee joint in order that the amputated surface is not chafed on the bed. Meanwhile the condition of the patient's whole body should be observed. Hypokalemia can easily appear after the operation because of high fever and fasting before the operation. So the nurse should assist the doctor in the early treatment in case the hypokalemia happens. The time of removing stitches should be delayed because of the poor blood circulation of the affected limb and the slow healing of the amputed surface.

(4) Dietetic nursing: The patient should have a nourishing, easily digested and liquid or semi—liquid diet, eat plenty of fruits and fresh vegetables and drink plenty of water or light drinks. Flos Lonicerae 9g Radix Ophiopogonis 9 g and Radix Trichosanthis 9 g should be infused in hot water and be taken as a drink. The patient who can not take solid food should be given fluid replacement.

5. Deficiency of Both *Qi* and Blood Type

Clinical Manifestations

Emaciation and chloranemia, pathologic leanness and weakness, dryness and desquamation of the affected limb, drying and thickening of the unguis, growth retardation, muscular atrophy, long—term—disunion opening of wound, dark grey granulation, clear and dilute pus, light tongue with thin white coating, deep thin and weak pulse.

Nursing

(1) Exhaustion of *Qi* and blood and disharmony between *Ying* and *Wei* due to long–standing case lead to general asthenia. So a good dietetic nursing is necessary. According to the ability of transportation and digestion of the patient's spleen and stomach, food for nourishing blood and invigorating *Qi* should be given, such as meat, fish, eggs, sea cucumber, edible fungus, shrimp as well as apple, Chinese date, carrot, etc. . Or the patient should often have a mixed gruel made of rice and each of Chinese yam, Chinese angelica (root) and milkvetch (root). This is helpful to invigorate *Qi* and nourish blood, strengthen the spleen and reinforce the stomach.

(2) The nursing of the affected limb is the same as that for *Yin*–cold type. The patient with the opening of the wound should go on having the dressing changed. If the opening remains disunited for a prolonged period, 100 mg of Vitamin B1 should be injected into Zusanli (ST36) point (both sides). Moxibustion may be done at a suitable distance from the opening of the wound to promote healing.

(3) *Gubu Tang* with modification is a suitable prescription for invigorating *Qi*, nourishing blood and regulating *Ying* and *Wei*: *Shiquan Dabu Wan* (Bolus of Ten Powerful Tonics) and *Shenrong Dabu Wan* (Bolus of Ginseing and Pilose Antler) can be taken as the accompanying drugs. The change of the coating on the tongue should be observed during the taking of medicine. If the tongue coating changes from thin white to yellow, and anorexia develops, the patient should stop taking them.

(4) Because of the local pain and inaction for a prolonged period the patient will suffer from myophagism and have difficulty in moving the joint. So the patient should be directed to do

some dirigations at the restoration stage. It can promote the building—up of the vascular collateral circulation of the affected limb. The usual methods are as the following:

a) Massotherapy can be used on the local part.

b) *Huoxue Zhitong San* (Power of Promoting Blood Circulation to Stop Pain) should be used to fumigate and wash the local part and the joint should be exercised after being fumigated and washed.

4.17　Atherosclerosis Obliterans

Atherosclerosis obliterans is a local manifestation of the generalized atherosclerosis in the extremity. It often occurs in those over the age of 45. At the stage of onset, the extremity is cool, sensitive to cold, numb and swollen or has a burning sensation. As the exacerbation of the ischemic symptoms progresses dystrophy comes into being. An ulcer and gangrene can develop in severe cases. It is classified into gangrene of finger or toe in traditional Chinese medicine.

General Nursing

1. Emotional care: The disease happens mostly in the middle—aged and old people, accompanied by hypertension, coronary heart disease or cerebrouascular disease. The pain and gangrene of the affected limb can even cause disability and bring extreme suffering to the patients. So the nurse must give close attention to emotional care. According to the characteristics of the old people who fear loneliness and loss of respect, nurses should often provide companionship for them and encourage them to express themselves freely, in order to make them free from misgiv-

ings and cooperate actively with the doctor. In addition, the nurse should keep the patient's family or the relatives well informed and make them understand and cooperate with the doctors and nurses. It is especially important for the patient after amputation, that nurses should direct the relatives to help him in restoring the ability of providing for himself.

2. Dietetic nursing: The patient should eat warm, cooked, soft, nourishing and digestible food with the function of promoting flow of *Qi* and blood circulation to remove blood stasis in accordance with the character of hypofunction of the spleen and stomach of the old people. Besides the staple food: rice and cooked wheaten food, the patient should take plenty of spinach, carrot, black fungus, Chinese date, hawthorn and other vegetables and fruits. He should often have bean—curd, fresh mushroom, laver soup, kelp soup, lotus seed soup, Chinese angelica gruel and red rooted salvia gruel, etc.. The patient with coronary heart disease, hypertension and hyperlipemia, etc. should have a bland and low salt diet. Pungent and fried food must be avoided. In addition, the patient should cultivate good living habits and have meals at regular times. Over—satiation should be avoided. The patient should be encouraged to keep himself in a good mood, and avoid taking food after anger and being angry after meals. The patient should limit his intake of food and control his desire for more. He should avoid lying in bed after eating, and should have a walk for a proper time.

3. Avoiding smoking: Smoking can lead to the hypersecretion of adrenalin and novadrenalin, contraction of the blood vessels, injury of the arterial endothelia cell and hypercoagulability of the blood. This can worsen the condition of

the patient. So the patient with atherosclerosis obliterans should permanently give up smoking.

Nursing According to Sydrome Differentiation

1. Blood Stasis Type

Clinical Manifestations

Numb, cool and painful extremities; ecchymosis or purplish red colour of the extremity end; petechia of the dark red tongue; uneven wiry pulse.

Nursing

(1) Keep the affected limb from injury, and warm in winter. The local part can be fumigated and washed with *Huoxue Zhitong San* (Powder of Promoting blood Circulation to Stop Pain) which is decocted. During washing it the temperature of the decoction must not be too high. The ecchymosis of the extremity end can be smeared with *Mahuang Ding* (Tineture of Seed of Strychnos and Ephedra used to Remove Obstruction of the Channels and Relieve Pain).

(2) The medicine for promoting blood circulation to remove blood stasis should be taken. The best prescription is *Danshen Tongmai Yin* (Red SageDrink of Invigorating Pulse–beat) or *Huoxue Tongmai Yin* and *Huoxue Tongmai Pian* (Drink or Tablet for Promoting Blood Circulation and invigorating pulse). Additional medicine for regulating the function of the spleen and stomach can be used for the loss of appetite caused by taking the decoction for a prolonged period.

(3) Direct the patient to manipulate and massage himself. In the upper limbs, the methods are pressing and moving the cubital articular region, rubbing the elbow, holding and twisting the fin-

ger, kneading the palm and rubbing the back of the hand. In the lower limbs, pressing and moving Zusanli (ST36) point, grasping and kneading the leg, plucking Yanglingquan (GB34) point, rubbing Yongquan (KI 1) and rotating the ankle joint. The exercise for massage can relax muscles and tendons to promote blood circulation, remove blood stasis and obstruction in the channels, promote the building–up of the collateral circulation of the affected limb, improve the nutrition to the limb and release pain.

2. Downward Flow of Damp–heat Type

Clinical Manifestations

The infection of gangrene of the limb, red swelling pain, yellowish greasy coating on the tongue.

Nursing

(1) The patient should get plenty of rest and avoid over–fatigue.

(2) The affected limb should be given proper exercise in order that it be prevented from losing its function though lack of movement for a long period of time. The dressing of the opening should be changed according to its development. (Consult the Dressing Change of Downward Flow of Damp–heat Type of Thromboangiitis Obliterans)

(3) *Simiao Yongan Tang* with modification (Modified Decoction of four Wondenful Drugs for Quick Restoration of Health) are suitable for clearing away heat and promoting diuresis and blood circulation to remove blood stasis.

3. Blazing Noxious Heat Type

Clinical Manifestations

A severe gangrene infection of the extremity spreading up to the ankle and leg, etc. swelling. heat and pain ulcer with a lot of pus accompanied by fever, the severe ones with metal confusion and hypofunction of appetite.

Nursing

(1) The patient should be kept in bed for complete rest. Those with high fever should be nursed according to the nursing of high fever (2.1)

(2) Nurses should make frequent rounds of the wards, giving close attention to their patients and assisting them to turn over in bed, which can prevent the heat—transmission of the blood stasis due to a long period of local pressure from developing into the bed—sore. The pain of the affected limb can be dealt with according to the method of alleviating pain in Thromboangiitis Obliterans.

(3) The best medicine for clearing heat and toxic material and promoting blood circulation to remove blood stasis is *Simiao Huoxue Tang* (Decoction of Four Wanderful Drugs for Promoting Blood Circulation), *Sichong Pian* (Four Worms Tablet) can be used as accompanying medicine.

(4) Pay close attention to the patients condition and check the patient's consciousness, temperature and local change. If there is a severe gangrene infection in the local part, it should be treated according to the dressing change of blazing noxious heat type of Thromboangiitis Obliterans. If the gangrene speads soon, the patient's pyrexia can not abate and mental confusion may appear because of internal damage caused by pathogenic factors. Those who need amputation should be given careful nursing before and after the operation.

(5) The patient should have frequent drinks for clearing away heat and toxic material, such as *Yinhua Gancao Tang*

(Decoction of Honeysuckle Flower and Licorice Root) and *Xian Lugen Tang* (Decoction of Fresh Common Reed Rhizome). An injection, meanwhile, can be given as a supplemental treatment to maintain the equilibrium of water and electrolyte.

5   Nursing for Common Gynecologic Diseases

5.1   Irregular Menstruation

The abnormal changes in menstrual cycle, quantity, colour of flow and quality are known as irregular menstruation. Early and delayed menstruation, and irregular menstrual cycle are within the changes of menstrual cycle; the change of menstrual quantity includes the menorrhagia and scanty menstruation.

General Nursing

1. Emotional stimuli should be avoided and the patient should be kept at ease.

2. Observe the menstrual cycle, early and delayed menstruation, menstrual days of flow and the changes in menstrual quantity, colours, quality of flow, all of which should be made notes of and reported to the doctor for reference.

3. Be sure to observe the changes in abdominal pain, complexion, body temperature, pulse and blood pressure. If blood prostration occurs due to menorrhalgia, the doctor should be informed immediately to give emergency treatment.

4. The patient should be nursed carefully and kept warm. Cold baths, swimming, tub baths and sexual life are contraindicated during the menstruation.

5. The outer pudendum should be kept clean, and sanitary tissue should be soft and clean so as to avoid injuring the skin.

Sanitary belt sho 1 be frequently changed and washed, and then sun–dried so as to prevent the belt from being contaminated with pathogenic factors

6. Cold fruits, medicine and diet with cold and cool nature are contraindicated during the menstruation. Diet should be taken hot.

Nursing According to Syndrome Differentiation

1. Shortened Menstrual Cycle Due to Blood Heat
Clinical Manifestations
Shortened cycle, dark red and thick blood flow in large quantities or with blood stasis, lower abdominal distension and pain, restlessness, fullness in the chest, flushed face, feverish sensation in the palm, reddened tongue with slight yellow and dry tongue coating, thin and rapid pulse.

Nursing
1) Emotional care should be strengthened. Extreme anger, emotional excitement avoided and the patient's mind kept at ease. Emotional unease can cause disorder of the function of *Qi* resulting in derangement of *Qi* and blood.

2) Observe and note the time, quantity and colour of menstruation in shortened cycle and abdominal pain, etc. , and report the details to the doctor. Hot compress is contraindicated when the abdominal pain occurs so as to prevent profuse menses due to blood–heat.

3) Herbs for clearing heat and cooling blood should be taken; the selected prescription is *Qing Jing Tang* with modification (Modified Decoction of Clearing Heat and Arresting Uterine Bleeding), which should be taken warm.

4) The patient with dry mouth and constipation may take decoction of Radix Ophiopogonis, Radix Scrophulariae to nourish *Yin* and promote the production of the body fluids.

5) The patient should mostly eat black edible ear fungus, the juice of lotus root, etc. to clear away heat and cool the blood, refrain from eating raw onion and garlic, alcohol and peppery, warm and dry food.

2. Shortened Menstrual Cycle Due to Deficiency of *Qi*

Clinical Manifestations

Profuse, thin and light red menses in shortened cycle, lassitude, poor appetite, palpitation and shortness of breath, sinking sensation in the lower abdomen, pale tongue with coating, feeble and weak pulse.

Nursing

(1) The patient should rest and avoid tiredness during the menstruation. The patient with menorrhagia should have bed rest.

(2) Herbs should be taken for strengthening the spleen and nourshing the heart, benefiting *Qi* and replenishing blood. *Guipi Tang* with modification (Modified Decoction for Invigorating the Spleen and Nourishing the Heart) should be selected.

(3) The patient with deficiency of *Qi* caused by deficiency and weakness of the body due to prolonged illness should eat nourishing foods such as milk, eggs, soya—bean milk, pork liver, fresh vegetables.

3. Delayed Menstrual Cycle Due to Blood Cold

Clinical Manifestations

Scanty and dark coloured mensis in delayed cycle, colic pain in the lower abdomen, slightly alleviated by warmth, pale complexion, cold limbs and aversion to cold, white tongue with thin coating, thin and rapid pulse.

Nursing

(1) The patient must keep the body warm, rest and avoid tiredness during menstruation.

(2) Herbs should be taken for expelling pathogenic cold from the channels, *Wenjing Tang* with modification (Modifed Decoction for Warming Channels) should be selected and taken warm.

(3) The patient with lower abdominal pain during menstruation may be given a hot—water bag compress, or moxibustion over the points, Tianshu, (ST25) Qihai, (RN6), Guanyuan (RN1).

(4) The patient with insufficiency of *Yang—Qi* and deficiency of both *Qi* and blood due to the prolonged disease, and preference for warmth, which indicates the cold and deficiency type, should take 6 g of *Aifu Nuangong Wan* once with warm water on empty stomach, three times daily.

(5) The diet should be rich in nutrition. Raw and cold fruits are contraindicated.

4. Delayed Menstrual Cycle Due to Deficiency of Blood
Clinical Manifesstations

Scanty and light red menses in delayed cycle, painful feeling in the lower abdomen, pale complexion, dizziness, palpitation, light tongue with white coating, weak and thready pulse.

Nursing

(1) The patient should be sure to rest during the menstruation. The changes of quantity and colour of mensis should be observed and noted.

(2) Herbs for tonifying the blood and supplementing *Qi* should be taken, the selected prescription being *Renshen Yangrong Tang* with modification. (Modified Decoction for Ginseng Nutrition).

(3) Close attention should be given to the dietetic regulation and nutrition; tonic food can be mostly taken such as pork liver, Chinese date and longan and fresh ginger and Chinese date can be decocted to be taken in order to regulate the function of the stomach and promote digestion.

5. Delayed Menstrual Cycle Due to Stagnation of *Qi*

Clinical Manifestations

Scanty and dark red menses in delayed cycle, distending pain in the lower abdomen, mental depression, stuffy chest, distension in the breast and pain in the hypochondriac region, thin and yellow tongue coating, wiry and uneven pulse.

Nursing

(1) Emotional care should be strengthened. Explanation, encouragement, and comfort should be given to the patient so as to free her mind of misgivings and help her build up confidence to conquer the disease and cooperate positively with the doctor.

(2) Herbs for relieving mental depression and stagnation of *Qi* should be taken, the selected prescription being *Qizhi Xiangfu Wan* with modification. (Modified Pills of Seven Drugs Including Cyperus Tuber).

(3) Ordinarily the patient should drink liquid as tea made of Fructus Citri Sarcodactylis, Pericarpium Citri Reticulatae soaked in boiling water and keep a kumquat cake in her mouth, or take 3 g of *Xiaoyiao Wan* (Ease pill), three times daily, in order to relieve the depressed liver—*Qi*.

6. Irregular Menstrual Cycle Due to *Qi* Stagnation In the Liver

Clinical Manifestations

Alternation of menstrual cycle and quantity of blood flow, or scanty mensis, distending pain in the lower abdomen, oppressed feeling in the chest, distension and pain in the hypochondriac region and breast, frequent signing, thin and white tongue coating, wiry pulse.

Nursing

(1) Keep the ward quiet and clean to keep the patient calm, help her take good care of herself and have ease of mind to avoid emotional stimuli.

(2) Herbs should be taken for soothing the liver and regulating the circulation of *Qi* and blood, the selected prescription being *Xiaoyao San* with modification. (Modified Ease Powder).

(3) *Xiaoyao Wan* (Ease pill) should be taken, 6 g each time, twice daily and with warm boiled water so as to relieve the depressed liver—*Qi*.

7. Irregular Menstrual Cycle Due to Kidney—deficiency

Clinical Manifestations

Scanty, light red blood flow in varying cycle, subjective sinking sensation in the lower abdomen, soreness in the lumbar region, frequent night urination, pale tongue with thin and white coating, deep and thready pulse.

Nursing

(1) The patient should pay attention to rest, and not take part in any strenuous physical labour or activities during the menstruation, so as to prevent consumption of *Qi* and blood, resulting in irregular menstruation.

(2) The patient should be advised to have full sleep, so as to maintain vigour and feeling of stability and also control sexual life so as to avoid impairment of *Chong* and *Ren* channels.

(3) Herbs should be taken for tonifying the kieney—*Qi* and regulating the function of *Chong* and *Ren* Channels, the selected prescription being *Dingqi Yin* with modification.

(4) 20 cc of *Yimu Caogao* (Soft Extralt of Motherwort) with suitable amount of brown sugar should be taken in each morning and evening to promote blood circulation and remove blood stasis.

8. Menorrhagia Due to *Qi* Deficiency

Clinical Manifestations

Profuse, thin and light red menses without stopping after menstrual period, pale complexion, palpitation and shortness of breath, sinking sensation in the lower abdomen, weakness of limbs, pale tongue with thin and white coating, feeble and weak pulse.

Nursing

(1) The patient should have bed rest and avoid tiredness and sexual life.

(2) Herbs for supplementing *Qi* and blood, and restoring *Yang* should be taken, *Juyuanjian* with modification being selected.

(3) The patient with general debility and weakness of the limbs due to menorrhagia should be careful with diet regulation and intake, and should be nourished with food for warming and tonifying the spleen and stomach such as pork liver, soft—shelled turtle, Chinese date, longan, juice of lotus rhizome, black Jews—ear fungus, and fresh vegetables. Alcohol, peppery and

irritative food is contraindicated.

(4) The menstrual quantity, colourness, and amount of sanitary tissue used should be observed and noted. If blood prostration due to excessively profuse menses occurs, the doctor should be informed and the points, Shuigou (DU26), Shixuan (EX−UE11), Hegu (LI 4), Yongquan (KI 1) should be punctured or moxibustion is given to Baihui (DU20), or 3 g of Redix Ginseng Rubra powder may be taken orally in order to recuperate *Yang* and restore normal menstruation.

9. Menorrhagia Due to Blood Heat

Clinical Manifestations

Profuse, red and thick menses with purple clot without stopping after period of menses, distending pain in the lumber region and abdomen, restlessness, thirst, flushed face and dry lips, yellow urine and constipation, red tongue with yellow coating, slippery and rapid pulse.

Nursing

(1) The patient should have rest and prevent tiredness during the menstruation. The patient with menorrhagia should have bed rest.

(2) Herbs for clearing away heat and cooling the blood should be taken, the selected prescription being *Qingjing Siwu Tang* with modification (Modified Decoction for Clearing Channels with Four Drugs).

10. Hypomenorrhea Due to Deficiency of Blood

Clinical Manifestations

Scanty, light red and thin menses, dizziness and tinnitus, severe palpitation, soreness and lassitude in the lumbar region and knees, empty and painful feelings in the lower abdomen, sallow complexion, dryness of skin, pale tongue with thin coating, feeble and thready pulse.

Nursing

(1) The patient should boost nutrition. The patient with scanty menses due to irregular diet injurying the spleen and stomach resulting in their weakness and insufficiency of the source of blood and *Qi* and with deficiency—cold syndrome during the menstruation should refrain from raw, cool, bitter, cold and astringent food.

(2) The patient should take rest, avoid overtiredness, and control sexual life during the menstruation.

(3) Herbs for enriching the blood and invigorating *Qi*, and strengthening the spleen should be taken, the selected prescription being *Renshen Zixue Tang* with modification. (Modified Decoction of Ginseng for Nourishing Blood).

11. Scanty Menstruation Due to Blood Stasis

Clinical Manifestations

Scanty and dark menses with blood clots, lower abdominal distending pain aggravated on pressure and alleviated by discharge of blood clots, purple and dark margin of the tongue, deep and thin pulse.

Nursing

(1) The patient should have ease of mind and must prevent over anxiety so as to avoid effect of *Qi* activities causing decrease of the menses.

(2) Needling is given to the points Xuehai (SP10), Shaohai (HT 3), Guilai (ST29), Zusanli (ST36) for abdominal pain aggravated on pressure and auricular—plaster therapy given to the points,, uterus, sympathetic, edocrine, to promote blood stasis

discharged to relieve the pain.

(3) Herbs for promoting blood circulation to remove blood stasis should be taken, the selected prescription being *Guo Qi Yin* with modification.

(4) The patient with stagnation of *Qi* and blood stasis due to external invasion of cold—evils may take a decoction of a suitable amount of Fructus Foeniculi and Rhizoma Zingiberis or liquid of brown sugar and millet wine, to warm the channels and remove blood stasis.

5.2   Dysmenorrhea

Dysmenorrhea refers to the pain appearing in the lower abdomen and lower back before, after or during menstruation. The pain, sometimes intolerable, accompanied by nausea, vomiting, headache or coma and sustained attack during the cycle of menses is known as painful menstruation.

General Nursing

1. The patient should have rest. The severe case should have bed rest, the ward should be kept quiet and clean, well ventilated and the temperature should be suitable.

2. Take care of the patient's emotions encouraging the patient to have emotional stability, avoid emotional stimuli and keep the mind at ease. The patient's sexual passion should be controlled.

3. The patient should be sure to keep the lower abdomen warm, not even washing the lower limbs with cold—water and refraining from eating raw, cool and cold, sour and puckery food during the menstruation in order to prevent the invasion of

cold—evil.

4. Observe the time, region, characteristics, and degree of pains and the condition of the menses discharged. If necessary, a sample should be retained to be seen by a doctor or tested.

5. The patient with pale complexion, very cold hands and feet, cold—sweating, etc. due to sharp pain, should lie on her back immediately, be made warm and the doctor should be informed to give immediate emergency treatment.

6. Acupuncture is given to the acupoints Zhongji (RN3), Qihai (RN6), Sanyinjiao (SP6) or massage to the lower abdominal, lumbosacral portion and Qihai (RN6), Guanyuan (RN 4), Shenshu (BL23), Baliao, etc. , or pills of corydalis tuber, tablets for relieving pain, etc. are given. The patient with dysmenorrhea due to cold and dampness may be given a hot compress with a hot—water bag on the lower abdomen.

Nursing According to Syndrome Differentiation

1. The Stagnancy of *Qi* and Blood Stasis Type

Clinical Manifestations

Distending pain in the lower abdomen before and during menstruation, scanty and impeded and dark purple menses with clots, abdominal pain aggravated on pressure, alleviated by passing out the clots, distending pain in the hypochondriac region and breast, purple and dark tongue with purple spots on its edge, deep and wiry pulse.

Nursing:

(1) The patient must take bed rest during menstruation, avoid tiredness and control sexual life.

(2) The patient needs emotional care. Nurses should talk

with the patient to ease the patient's minds so as to encourage the patient to take good care of herself.

(3) Rich, light, easily digested food should be taken. Raw, cold and peppery food is contraindicated.

(4) Herbs should be taken for regulating *Qi* and promoting blood circulation to stop pain. *Xuefu Zhu Yu Tang* with modification (Modified Decoction for Removing Blood Stasis in the Chest) can be selected. The patient should have bed rest after taking it.

(5) The patient with abdominal pain aggravated on pressure should take the tablet of *Yuanhu Zhitong* pills (*Yuanhu* pills for Relieving pain), three times daily and two pills each time, or black soybean 15 g, brown sugar 30 g, safflower (Flos Carthami) 9 g are decocted, the decoction being taken warm.

(6) Acupuncture and moxibustion can be used. Two days before the menstruation, acupuncture and moxibustion are given to Zhongji (RN3), Sanyinjiao (SP6), Ciliao (BL32), Guanyuan (RN4), Mingmen (DU4), Zusanli (ST36) Qihai (RN6), ear needling is given to endocrine, uterus, subcortex, etc. In order to regulate menstruation and alleviate pain.

2. Stagnation of the Cold and Dampness Type

Clinical Manifestations

Cold pain in the lower abdomen before and during menstruation, aggravated on pressure, and alleviated by warmth, scanty and thin menses, darkness with clots, purplish tongue with white and greasy coating, deep and tense pulse.

Nursing

(1) The patient is advised to take hot diet or to have drinks of fresh ginger and brown sugar decocted in water (Decoction of

Several Pieces of Fresh Ginger with Brown Sugar) instead of tea, in order to disperse cold, promote blood circulation and relieve pain.

(2) The patient with abdominal cold pain should be given a warm compress, suitable amount of Folium Artemisiae Argyi and Rhizoma Zingiberis Recens are parched hot to be put on the navel area, moxibustion may be given. Be sure to keep the lower abdomen warm at any time.

(3) The Herbs for expelling pathogenic cold from channel, relieving pain and removing blood stasis should be taken, the selected prescription being *Wen Jing Tang* with modification (Modified Decoction for Warming Channels). The decoction is taken hot. After administration the patient should have bed rest.

(4) The patient with dysmenorrhea due to cold and wetness should be given acupuncture to Zhongji (RN3), Qihai (RN6), Sanyinjiao (SP6) or moxibustion is given to the points, Qihai (RN6), Sanyinjiao (SP6) in order to expel pathogenic cold from channel and relieve pain.

3. Deficiency and Weakness of *Qi* and Blood Type

Clinical Manifestations

Dull pains in the lower abdomen during or after menstruation alleviated by pressure, pink and thin menses, pale complexion, mental lassitude, small amount of menstruation, pale tongue with thin coating, thready and weak pulse.

Nursing

(1) The patient should have plenty of rest and keep warm, being sure not to catch cold, in order to prevent the evils from invading.

(2) Herbs for invigorating *Qi* and enriching the blood should

be taken. The selected prescription is *Huangqi Danggui Tongjing Tang* with modification (Modified Decoction for Restoring Menstrual Flow of Astragalus and Chinese Angelica). The decoction should be taken hot.

(3) The patient with deficiency of *Qi* and blood should be advised to take nutritious food. Powder of Chinese yam, pork liver, mutton, etc., should be often eaten, in order to invigorate *Qi* and enrich blood.

(4) The patient with abdominal pain due to cold and deficiency alleviated by warmth should be given a hot compress or tonifying acupuncture. Acupuncture and moxibustion are given to the acupoints, Mingmen (DU 4), Shenshu (UB 23), Guanyuan (RN 4), Zusan li (ST 36), Da He (KI 12), in order to regulate and tonify *Qi* and blood, and relieve pain with the warming and tonifying.

4. Impairment of liver and Kidney Type

Clinical Manifestations

Dull pain in the lower abdomen after menstruation, pink and scanty menses, soreness and distension in the lumber region, dizziness and tinnitus, light red tongue with thin coating, deep and thin pulse.

Nursing

(1) The patient should keep a good balance between work and rest, and moderate sexual life in order to reduce the wastage of *Qi* and blood to avoid injuring the liver and kidney.

(2) Herbs for regulating and tonifying liver and kidney should be taken, *Tiao Gan Tang* with modification (Modified Decoction of Regulating the Liver) can be selected.

(3) The patient with soreness in the lumber region and ab-

dominal pain may be given massage, particularly kneading, pushing, and digital acupoint pressure, to Sanyinjiao (SP6), Gui lai (ST29), Tai chong (LR3), adding Gan shu (BL18), Shen shu (BL23), Zusanli (ST36) so as to promote blood circulation and relieve pain.

5.3 Amenorrhea

Menstrual flow begins at about fourteen in healthy girls. Menstruation that does not come over 18 is called primary amenorrhea; suppression of menstruation for over three months, except during period of pregnancy and lactation and climacterium, is known as secondary amenorrhea.

General Nursing

1. Good emotional care should be given to avoid various bad irritations and encourage the patient to set up confidence of recovery and to actively cooprate with the doctor during treatment.

2. The patient with pubertal amenorrhea should properly increase the nutrition and take care to maintain a good combination of work and rest.

3. The patient with obesity should be encouraged to do physical activities in order to lose weight.

4. The woman with prolonged breast feeding period should be advised to wean the baby from the breast on time.

Nursing According to Syndrome Differentiation

1. The Insuffeciency of Liver and Kidney Type
Clinical Manifestations

Delayed menstrual period, amenorrhea after menstruation occurring, old complexion, dryness of skin, soreness and weakness in the lumber region and knees, dizziness and tinnitus, loss of weight, feverish sensation on the palm and sole, night sweat, pale tongue with thin yellowish coating, feeble, thin and rapid pulse.

Nursing

(1) Diet should be regular and food nourishing for liver and kidney should be eaten, such as tremella, soft—shelled turtle, donkey—hide gelatin, in order to nourish the liver and kidney.

(2) Life style should be regulated properly, and the patient should be sure not to be overtired and to control sexual life.

(3) Herbs for invigorating the liver, replenishing the kidney, nourishing the blood and regulating menstruation should be taken. *Guishen Wan* with modification (Modified pills for Invigorating the Kidney) may be selected.

(4) Auricular—plaster therapy may be given to the acupoints, endocrine, ovary, uterus in order to recuperate *Chong* and *Ren* channels.

2. The Deficiency and Weakness of *Qi* and Blood Type

Clinical Manifestations

Scanty and pink menses, gradual decrease of menses and amenorrhea, pale and sallow complexion, lassitude and weakness, dizziness, palpitation and short breath, pale tongue, thready and weak pulse.

Nursing

(1) The patient should be comforted to avoid emotional stimuli in order to strengthen the confidence of defeating the ailment.

(2) Cold food and drink should be avoided in order to pre-

vent injuring the spleen and stomach and Chinese date, longan, vegetables, pork liver, chichen broth, etc. can be often eaten to invigorate *Qi* and tonify the blood.

(3) Herbs for replenishing *Qi*, invigorating the spleen, nourishing the blood and regulating menstruation should be taken, *Liu Junzi Tang* with modification (Modified Decoction of Six Ingredients) may be selected.

3. The Stagnancy of *Qi* and Blood Stasis Type

Clinical Manifestations

Menoschesis, green and yellow complexion, depressed spirit, mental rashness, oppressed feeling in the chest and pain in the hypochondric region, lower abdominal pain aggravated on pressure, dark purple tongue coating with petechia on its borders, wiry and choppy pulse.

Nursing

(1) The patient should be given comfort and emotional care. The nurse should make her to get rid of her worries in order to assist in cooperating with the doctor during treament.

(2) Herbs for promoting blood circulation, removing blood stasis, regulating *Qi* and stimulating the menstrual flow during amenorrhea should be taken. The *Wuyao San* with modification (Modified Powder of Lindera) may be selected.

(3) The patient should drink Safflower—Millet Wine, the safflower 15 g infusing in the proper amount of millet wine for 5 days, taken 2—3 times each day, in order to promote blood circulation and remove blood stasis.

4. Accumulation of Phlegm and Dampness Type

Clinical Manifestations

Obesity after menolipsis, oppressed feelings in the chest with nausea, abundant sputum, abdominal distention, loss of appetite, leukorrhagia, whitish and greasy coating on the tongue, wiry and smooth pulse.

Nursing

(1) Give special attention to dietetic nursing, the food should be light, nutritious, and easily digested. Fat and sweet food should be eaten little to prevent putting on weight, restoring wetness and promoting sputum, and worsening the patient's condition.

(2) The patient should do suitable physical exercises to build up her resistance to disease and to get rid of excessive weight.

(3) Herbs for promoting the circulation of *Qi* and reducing phlegm, invigorating the spleen to eliminate dampness should be taken, *Cangfu Daotan Wan* with modification being selected.

5.4 Metrorrhagia and Metrostaxis

Vaginal hemorrhage beyond menstrual period, either copious or continuously dripping, is generally defined as metrorrhagia and metrostaxis. The copious bleeding with a sudden onset is referred to as profuse metrorrhagia, and the scanty bleeding with a gradual onset as continuous scanty uterine bleeding. Although they are different in manifestations, the two are intertransmutable during the process of the disease course and their etiology and pathogenesis are virtually the same, so they are known respectively as metrorrhagia and metrostaxis.

General Nursing

1. The patient's daily life should be taken care of. The ward should be kept quiet, clean and well ventilated. The temperature

and the humidity should be suitable.

2. Emotional care should be done well and the patient comforted to dispel emotional stimuli, and build up confidence of defeating the disease by cooperating with the doctor's treatment.

3. The diet should be nourishing and easily–digested. Pungent, peppery, fried and greasy foods are contraindicated.

4. Observe carefully any changes in the patient's condition, quantity, colour, quality, smell of vaginal bleeding, the tongue coating, pulse condition, blood pressure and manner, then make a note and report them to the doctor.

5. If the patient has continous scanty uterine bleeding or copious bleeding with a sudden onset and with stasis clots, the specimen is taken to a doctor or sent to the laboratory.

6. If the patient has pale complexion, cold sweat, fall of blood pressure, vaginal copious bleeding with a sudden onset and hollow pulse, the doctor must be informed to take emergency measures. Fluid infusion, blood transfusion and oxygen therapy should be prepared well.

Nursing According to Syndrome Differentiation

1. The Blood–heat Type

Clinical Manifestations

Sudden onset of profuse or prolonged continuous vaginal bleeding in deep red colour, or dark purple with blood clots in viscid and thick quality, flushed face, dry mouth, irritability, thirst with preference for cool drink; red tongue with yellow coating, slippery and rapid pulse.

Nursing

(1) The patient with copious bleeding should take plenty of

rest and little physical activity, avoid emotional stimuli, keep ease of mind in order to facilitate treatment.

(2) The patient should be provided nutritious and light food, such as duck, fish in order to enrich the *Qi* and blood, and eat plenty of fruits, vegetables and food for removing pathogenic heat from blood. Pungent, irritating, warm–dry and *Yang*–reinforcing food is contraindicated.

(3) Herbs for removing pathogenic heat from blood and arresting bleeding should be taken. The selected prescription is *Qingre Gujing Tang* with modification (Decoction for Clearing Heat and Arresting Uterine Bleeding). The decoction should be taken cool.

(4) Massage or finger pressure can be applied for abdominal pain, the points, Sanyinjiao (SP 6), Zusanli (ST36), Neixue, etc. to alleviate pain. Hot compress and moxibustion should not be used to avoid bleeding more seriously.

(5) The patient should pass stools smoothly. Those with dry stool may take an infusion of 5 g senna leaf in water as tea or eat banana, peach, honey, etc. in order to nourish the intestine and relax the bowels.

(6) Needling can be applied for copious bleeding to points, Guanyuan (RN4), Sanyinjiao (SP6), Yinbai (SP1), Xuehai (SP10), Shuiquan (KI5), etc. in order to purge heat from blood.

2. The Blood Stasis Type

Clinical Manifestations

Prolonged continuous vaginal bleeding or sudden onset of profuse bleeding with blood clots, lower abdominal pain aggravated on pressure and alleviated by discharge of blood clots, dark red or ecchymosis on the tip and border of the tongue as a sign of blood stasis, deep and choppy pulse.

Nursing

(1) The patient should be sure to rest and avoid overtiredness.

(2) The diet should be easily digested and nutritious. Raw, cold, sour and puckery, pungent and irritating food is contraindicated.

(3) Herbs for promoting blood circulation by removing blood stasis should be taken. The selected prescription is based on *Si Wu Tang* (Decoction of Four Ingredients) and d *Shi Xiao San* with modification (Wonderful Powder for Relieving Blood Stagnation).

(4) The patient with lower abdominal pain aggravated on pressure may be alleviated by hot compress on the lower abdomen with herbal medicine for promoting blood circulation, which is ground into powder, then mixed in boiling water, to promote the discharge of blood stasis.

(5) Needling is applied to Qihai (RN6), Sanyinjiao (SP6), Xuehai (SP 10), Zigong, etc. for copious bleeding.

3. Insufficiency of the Spleen Type

Clinical Manifestations

Sudden profuse bleeding or continuous scanty bleeding marked by light red and thin blood, pale complexion, lassitude, cold limbs, shortness of breath, apathy, oppressed feelings in the chest, poor appetite, loose stools, pale tongue with thin and white coating, feeble thin and weak pulse.

Nursing

(1) The patient should remain in bed, avoiding anxiety and overtiredness. Warm should be kept for general weakness and

chills.

(2) The patient should have a carefully regulated nutritious diet, particularly eating food for invigorating the spleen and benefiting *Qi*, such as the powder of Chiness yam, the Job's—tears seed gruel and the root of membranous milk vetch and *Dangshen* gruel, etc. . Raw, cold, hard and solid food is contraindicated.

(3) Herbs for invigorating the spleen to control the blood, nourishing the blood and arresting bleeding should be taken. The selected prescription is *Gui Pi Tang* with modification. (Decoction for Invigorating the Spleen and Nourishing the Heart). The decoction should be taken warm.

(4) When the patient is suddenly attacked with metrorrhagia, blood prostration must be prevented. If necessary, the decoction of *Du Shen Tang* (Decoction of Single Ginseng) is taken in order to supple *Qi*, to promote the restricting function of *Qi* and stop uterine bleeding.

(5) Needling is applied to Guanyuan (RN4), Sanyinjiao (SP 6), Yinbai (SP1), Zusanli (ST36), Pishu (BL20), etc, in order to promote the function of the restriction of qi on blood. Baihui (DU20), Qihai (RN6), should be given moxibustion for blood prostration in order to recuperate depleted *Yang* and stop uterine bleeding.

4. The Deficiency of the Kidney Type
Clinical Manifestations
Continuous and scanty uterine bleeding, dizziness and tinnitus, dysphoria with feverish sensation in chest, palms and soles, insomnia and night sweat, soreness and weakness in the lumber region and legs, red tongue with little coating, thready, rapid and weak pulse due to deficiency of kidney *Yin*; profuse

and continuous bleeding with pink colour, pale complexion, cold sensation and pain in the lower abdomen, lassitude, soreness and pain in the lumber region and back, frequent and excessive urine, loose stools, pale tongue with thin and white coating, deep and thin pulse due to the deficiency of kidney *Yang*.

Nursing

(1) The patient with deficiency of kidney *Yin* must keep comfortable clothing and bedding and stable feeling.

(2) A diet of nourishing *Yin* should be taken, such as duck, soft—shelled turtle, eggs, black Jews—ear fungus, fruits, and vegetables, etc. Fried and peppery food is contraindicated to prevent impairing *Yin* and supporting fire.

(3) Herbs for nourshing the kidney and reinforcing *Yin* should be taken. The selected prescription is *Zuo Gui Wan* with modification which should be taken warm.

(4) Acupuncture with the reinforcing method is applied to Shenshu (BL23), Guanyuan (RN4) San Yinjiao (SP6), Neiguan (PC6), Taixi (KI3) to regulate and nourish the heart and kidney and relieve the asthenic heat.

(5) Lumber and abdominal region should be kept warm for the patient with *Yang*—deficiency and the patient may go outdoors for activities after she is in a stable condition with less bleeding.

(6) Herbs for warming the kidney and arresting bleeding should be taken. The selected prescription is *Yougui Wan* with modification (Modified the Kidney—*Yang*—Reinforcing Bolus) and the decoction should be taken hot.

5.5 Menopausal Syndromes

Menstruation may stop at about 49, which is known as menopause or menoschesis. A short time before or after menopause, there appear irregular menstruation, dizziness and tinnitus, palpitation and insomnia, irritability, cold sweating, dysphoria with feverish sensation in the chest, palms and soles, or general edema and loose stools, soreness of lumber region, lassitude, abnormal emotions in some women. These symptoms mentioned above may be severe or light in different women and continue 2—3 years, and are known as menopausal syndrome, or menoschesis syndrome, known as climacteric syndrome in modern medicine.

General Nursing

1. The wards must be comfortable, safe, tidy, quiet and have enough sunlight, good circulation of air, suitable temperature and humidity.

2. It is necessary to have a good understanding of the patient's condition and thoughts. Nurses must be concerned about the sufferings of the patient and her daily life, feeling and diet.

3. Explain the condition to the patient patiently, make her understand the process of physiological changes during menopausal period and dispel her misgivings to let her cooperate with the doctors during treatment.

4. The patient should be careful to balance work with rest, avoid any strenuous activities, take part in meaningful social activities, live a regular life in order to heighten enjoyment of life.

5. The diet should be carefully regulated, light, digestible

and nutritious.

6. Advise the patient to take the medicine on time and then observe and nurse carefully and note the changes of nausea, vomiting and other conditions after administration especially decoction and report them promptly to the doctors.

Nursing According to Syndrome Differentiation

1. The Deficiency of the Kidney—*Yin* Type

Clinical Manifestations

Paroxysmal flushed cheeks, irritability or melancholy, feverish sensation over the palms and soles, dizziness and headache, tinnitus and hyperhidrosis, dry mouth and lips, poor appetite, soreness of lumber region and bone pain, constipation, scanty and red or purplish menses, red tongue with little coating, wiry, thready and little rapid pulse.

Nursing

(1) The patient should have plenty of rest. The patient with dizziness and headache should have bed rest in repose with her eyes closed, and may not walk about until the symptoms are relieved.

(2) Pay close attention to any changes of patient's feelings and attempt to give their confidence to boost their cooperation with the doctors.

(3) Changes of blood pressure should be carefully noted in those with dizziness. The hypertensive patient should limit the intake of table salt, eat plenty of kelp, celery, tremella, light food, etc. Pungent, fatty, sweet, greasy foods are contraindicated.

(4) Herbs for nourishing *Yin* and suppressing hyperactive *Yang*, tonifying the liver and kidney should be taken. The selected

prescription is *Liuwei Dihuang Tang* with modification. (Modified Decoction of Six Drugs Including Rehmannia).

(5) The patient with breakdown of the normal physiological coordination between the heart and the kidney should take *Buxin Dan* on an empty stomach, three times daily, 9 g each time with warm water or auricular—plaster therapy can be used to heart, kidney, Shenmen (HT 7), subcortex to relieve mental stress.

(6) The patient should do more physical exercises, such as *Taijiquan*, *Qi gong*, etc. in order to build up the health.

2. The Insufficiency of the Kidney—*Yang* Type

Clinical Manifestations

Profuse bleeding with light red blood, listlessness, intolerance of cold, soreness and weakness in the lumber region and knees, lassitude, poor appetite and general edema, loose stools, pale tongue with thin coating, deep, thready and feeble pulse.

Nursing

(1) Refer to the nursing of deficiency of kidney—*Yin*

(2) Diet regulation is important. Suitable foods are lotus seed, hyacinth bean, Job's tears, powder of Chinese yam and gorgon euryale, taken with bark of Chinese cassia tree and lesser galangal to reinforce the kidney and support yang. Raw and cold food is contraindicated.

(3) Herbs for warming the kidney and reinforcing *Yang* should be taken. The selected prescription is *Yougui Tang* (the Kidney—*Yang*—Reinforcing Decoction) with modification. The decoction should be taken warm before bed time.

(4) Massage is given to Guanyuan (RN4), Qihai (RN6), Pishu (BL20) Weishu (BL21), Shenshu (BL23), Changqiang (DU1), etc. or needling to Mingmen (DU4), and Guanyuan

(RN4) and Shenshu (BL23) reinforcing.

5.6 Morbid Leukorrhea

The vagina is often moistened by small amounts of uncoloured and transparent secretion, usually called leukorrhea. It is normal for the secretion to increase in the premenstrual and gestational period. Morbid leukorrhea called in TCM is a disease symptomized by excessive mucous vaginal discharge, and some changes of colour, quality and smell accompained by general symptoms.

Genernal Nursing

1. Pay attention to nursing the patient's daily life, keep ward clean and well ventilated.

2. The patient should be made aware of the importance of hygiene. The outer-pudendum should be kept clean. Fumigate and wash with the decoction of *Fufang Shechuangzi* (Composite Cnidium Decoction) every day.

3. The patient should be particularly attentive to menstrual hygiene. Use clear, soft sanitary tissue and change underwear regularly. Avoid tiredness, wind, cold and sexual life during menstruation because of weak resistance of the body.

4. The diet should be nutritious, light and mostly digestible, plenty of fresh vegetables and fruits should be taken such as Chinese yam, gordon fruit, hyacinth bean, tremella, etc. to invigorate the spleen and eliminate damp-evil. Raw, cold, pungent, greasy and fried food is contraindicated.

5. Observe the quantity, colour, quality, smell of morbid leukorrhea and general symptoms, take notes and report to the

doctor or sent samples to be tested.

6. Vulva-pruritus patients should be treated as early as possible, so as to prevent scratching resulting in infection.

Nursing According to Syndrome Differentiation

1. Insufficiency of the Spleen Type
Clinical Manifestations
Profuse thick, white or light yellow vaginal discharge without smell, pale or sallow complexion, cold limbs, lassitude, poor appetite, loose stools, edema in the lower limbs, pale tongue with white or greasy coating, slow pulse.

Nursing
(1) The patient should take plenty of rest and keep warm. Patients with cold limbs should stay in a warm and sunny ward with mantained temperature 20℃ or so. Over-tiredness should be avoided.

(2) Take good care of the patient's emotion, helping ease her fears.

(3) Herbs for strengthening the spleen, replenishing *Qi*, ascending *Yang* and removing dampness should be taken. The selected prescription is *Wan Dai Tang* with modification. (Modified Decoction for Morbid Leukorrhea). The decoction should be taken warm.

(4) The patient with loose stools should eat little of such food as raw, cold and fruits, and eat more hot millet gruel, the gruel of milk vetch and *Dangshen*, the Job's-tears seed gruel, the powder of Chinese yam, etc. to strengthen the spleen and remove dampness.

(5) 7 pieces of gingko nut peeled and broken are taken daily

after being infused in a bowl of boiling soyabean milk.

2. Deficiency of the Kidney Type

Clinical Manifestations

Profuse and continuous discharge of thin and transparent white liquid, soreness and weakness in the low back and knees, cold sensation in the lower abdomen, frequent and excessive urine, especially during night, loose stools, pale tongue with thin, white coating, deep and slow pulse.

Nursing

(1) Refer to the nursing of the insufficiency of spleen.

(2) Herbs for warming and reinforcing the kidney—*Yang*, removing dampness to stop leukorrhea should be taken. The selected prescription is *Neibu Wan*, which should be taken with warm boiled water, 2 pills (9 g of each pill) each time, twice daily.

(3) The patient should be sure to have good rest and control sexual life after taking this medicine.

3. Toxic Damp Type

Clinical Manifestations

A large amount of foul—smell yellow—green leukorrhagia like pus or with blood or as sticky as rice water, itching in the vulva, lower abdominal pain, scanty and yellow urine, dry throat with bitter taste, red tongue with yellow coating, smooth and rapid pulse.

Nursing

(1) The patient should have proper rest, avoiding overtiredness, and try to maintain ease of mind.

(2) The patient should eat nutritious food, especially that high protein. Pungent, irritative and greasy food is contraindicated.

(3) Herbs for clearing away heat and toxic materials, removing dampness to stop leukorrhea should be taken. The selected prescription is *Zhidai Fang* with modification. (Modified Decoction for Arresting Leukorrhagia).

(4) The patients with itching in the vulva should avoid tub—bathing and sexual life. The washing herbs, composite cnidium fruit can be selected as external use, which can be decocted and used for fumigating first and washing afterwards or needling may also be used to Baichongwo, Ligou (LR 5), Qugu (RN 2), Taichong (LR 3) Sanyinjiao (SP 6), etc.

5.7 Vaginitis

The vaginae of healthy women have the function of selfpurification, which can form naturally defensive power to inhibit the growth of bacterium. If the defensive function is destroyed, the invasion of bacterium may lead to inflammation of vagina, i. e. vaginitis. Senile vaginitis and trichomonal colpomycosis are common diseases.

General Nursing

1. Ensure that the patient has adequate rest, and that the ward is clean, quiet and well ventilated.

2. The patient should be kept calm, and her emotions should be nursed well. The nurse should familiarize herself with the patient's condition and daily routine, and regulate the patient's diet. Pungent and heavy food should not be eaten.

3. The patient should cultivate good hygienic habits, The vulva should be kept clean and underpants changed regularly. During menstrual period, sanitary tissue must be clean and soft

and the sanitary belt must be washed and changed frequently, and should be well sterilized before use. If secretion increases, the sample should be collected for doctor's observation or laboratory examination.

4. The decoction of washing herb can be used for fumigation and washing. Tub baths and sexual activity are contraindicated. The patient with trichomoniasis must not swim in swimming pool in order to prevent cross infection.

5. In order to prevent infection, those who have a severe itch and pain should attempt to refrain from scratching. Acupuncture and moxibustion therapy may be used as supplementary treatment.

Nursing According to Syndrome Differentiation

(1) Senile Vaginitis

Clinical Manifestations

A burning sensation in the vagina, a stabbing pain in the vulva and vagina after urination, sometimes watery or bloody mucous leukorrhea, red vaginal wall and cervical mucosa with light edema, tenderness and different sizes of patchy hemorrhagic spots, red tongue without coating, wiry and rapid pulse.

Nursing

(1) The patient should have a quiet rest during the acute stage. Since old patients can easily get into choleric mood, the pathogenic fire will cause impairment of *Yin*. Nutrition should be supplied to them for their general asthenia, anorexia and weak resistance. They should be given a bland and light diet and should not eat too much tonic food. Intake of pungent food and alcohol are prohibited.

(2) Herbs for removing heat and toxic material, invigorating the spleen and kidney should be taken. The prescription is *Zishen Liangxue Jiedu Tang* with modification (Modified Decoction for Nourishing the Kidney and Removing Pathogenic Heat from the Blood and Toxic Substances From the Body.)

(3) Hot decoction of Radix Sophorae Flavescentis 9 g and Cortex Phellodendri 9 g and Fructus Cnidii 15 g may be used to fumigate first and then wash the affected part once a day.

(4) Acupuncture and moxibustion therapy:

Baichongwo, Qugu (RN2), Henggu (KI11), Yinfu, Zusanli (ST36), Taixi (KI3) and Sanyinjiao (SP6) points, etc. are needled. Otopoints such as Shenmen (HT7), External genital organs, lung and Endocrine, etc. are needled. A point injection of 2 ml of *Didinghuangqin* Injection may be needed to alleviate pain and relieve itching.

2. Trichomonal Vaginitis and Colpomycosis

Clinical Manifestations

Itching in the vulva with leucorrhea manifested as, scanty yellow urine and irritation in vulva, yellow–green leucorrhea due to trichomonad, which is in great quantity, watery and foamy or rice–watery and of foul smell; creamy white mycotic leucorrhea due to mycete in the shape of lumps and beandregs; divergent hemorrhagic spots on the swelling vagina and cervical mucosa, with severe itching and a burning sensation.

Nursing

(1) Give wide publicity to prophylactic hygienic knowledge and advise the patient on building up physical strength and resistance. If the husband suffers from infection of truchomonad or mycete, the husband and wife may be treated together. Sexual ac-

tivity should be refrained from during the period of treatment to prevent infection from each other.

(2) The patient with trichomoniasis should take *Sanmiao San* with modification (Modified Powder of Three Wonderful Drugs) as the medicine for clearing away heat, removing diuresis, destroying parasites, removing toxic substances and relieving itching.

(3) 2% lactic acid solution can be used to wash vagina. After drying it, put *Xiongshe Wan* (Pill made of male snake) in it before sleeping and remove it after getting up. Five days is one course. Another five days should be prescribed for the patient who has not yet healed.

(4) The prescription of Chinese external wash prescription: Radix Sophorae Flavescentis 9 g and Cortex Phellodendri 9 g, Fructus Cnidii 30 g, Meliae Toosendan 6 g, Radix Lycii 15 g and dried alum 15 g are decocted and dripped into the vagina after the drugs are removed. The decoction may also be used to wash the vulva twice a day.

(5) Acupuncture and moxibustion therapy is the same as that for senile vaginitis.

(6) *Huashi Tang* with modification (Modified Decoction for Removing Diuresis) may be used as the medicine for clearing away heat and removing diuresis to the patient with mycosis.

(7) The prescription of Chinese external wash prescription: Fructus Cnidii 15 g, Cortex Lycii Radicis 6 g, Pericarpium Zanthoxyli 6 g and alum 6 g and Radix Sophorae Flavescentis 9 g are decocted, the decoction is used to fumigate and wash the affected part once or twice a day.

(8) A suitable amount of *Bingpeng San* and little glycerin are

well mixed, then ᴄoated the inside of vagina with it once every morning and night after washing vulva.

(9) The severely itching patient with colpomycosis should have a bloodletting at the blood vessel on the cross striation of the middle segment on the side of the fourth finger palm. This can stop itching for several hours and can be repeated several times.

5.8 Morning Sickness

Symptoms including nausea and vomiting, dizziness and anorexia, body indolence and preference for sour and salty food can appear in the early stage of pregnancy. It is called morning sickness or disorder of child organ due to pragnancy in traditional Chinese medicine.

General Nursing

1. The ward should be kept quiet, clean and ventilated and away from any factors inducing vomiting. It is appropriate for the patients to rest. The severe ones should be confined to bed.

2. Patients need emotional care and moral consolation to free their mind of misgivings so as to cooperate actively in recuperative medical care.

3. The patient should be given nutritious, light and bland semiliquid diet. Those with severe vomiting should be given multiple liquid meals with a little intake of food. If nececssary, intravenous transfusion should be given.

4. The patient should keep the oral cavity clean and rinse it out with clean water after each bout of vomiting in order to prevent aphthous stomatitis.

5. The patient should pass smooth stool. Those with consti-

pation may take honey three times a day in order to moisturize the stool.

6. Pay close attention to any changes of the patient's condition. The appearance of lumbo—abdominal pain, colporrhagia in small amount, threatened abortion, or vaginal bleedling during pregnacy and fetal abortion, etc. caused by severe vomiting, must be reported to the doctor promptly.

7. If the severe symptoms of deficiency of both *Qi* and *Yin*, such as frequent vomiting, fever and thirst, oliguria and constipation, red tongue, weak slippery pulse appear, it is likely to be toxemia of pregnancy. The doctor must be informed immediately to carry out emergency treatment.

Nursing According to Syndrome Differentiation

1. Dificiency of the Spleen and Stomach

Clinical Manifestations

Nausea and vomiting of liquid, anorexia, aversion to the smell of food, lassitude and sleepiness, pale tongue with white coating, slippery and weak pulse during the first trimester of pregnancy.

Nursing

(1) The patient with frequent severe vomiting should be confined to bed.

(2) The patient should control her emotions and keep herself away from anger and in cheerful mood to cooperate with the doctor in treatment.

(3) A nutritious light and bland diet is suitable. The patient can choose food according to personal preference and be advised to drink rice water, soya—bean milk, lotus root starch, etc. Body

fluid should be restored to prevent dehydration.

(4) Herbs for strengthening the spleen and stomach and regulating and lowering the adverse flow of *Qi* should be taken. The selected prescription is *Xiangsha Liujunzi Tang* with modification (Modified Decoction of Cyperus and Amomum with Six Noble Ingredients). Several drops of ginger juice should be mixed with the decoction to strengthen the stomach and relieve vomiting. After taking it, the patient should be kept in bed quietly.

(5) The patient should be advised to take food and herbs for tonifying the spleen and stomach, and drink plenty of light saline solution or the decoction of Radix Ginseng, Rhizoma Atractylodis Macrocephalae and Pericarpium Citri Reticulatae can be drunk as tea in order to strengthen the spleen and lower the adverse flow of *Qi*. Several grains of amomum fruit may be chewed at ordinary times to regulate stomach–*Qi*, smooth chest disorder and relieve vomiting.

(6) Acupuncture therapy: The needles are inserted into Neiguan (PC6) (Luo–connecting Point) and retained for 20 minutes. The patient with dificient–cold type should be treated with moxibustion therapy on Zusanli (ST36) to clear away heat and relieve vomiting.

2. Disharmony Between the Spleen and the Stomach
Clinical Manifestations

In the early stage of gestation: vomiting of bitter fluid, frequent belching, epigastric fullness distending pain in the hypochondrium, vexation and dizziness, mental depression, pink tongue with light yellowish coating, wiry and slippery pulse.

Nursing

(1) The ward should be clean, tidy, nice and comfortable. It

should be ventilated at regular intervals and be free from noise interference.

(2) Nurse the patient's emotion well, give more mental comfort to her and keep her in a good and cheerful mood in order that she can cooperate in the treatment.

(3) Herbs for soothing the liver, strengthening the stomach, lowering the adverse flow of *Qi* and arresting vomiting should be taken. The selected prescription is *Suye Huanglian Tang* with modification (Modified Decoction of Perilla Leaves and Coptis). Several drops of ginger juice should be mixed with the decoction before taken.

(4) Flos Chrysanthemi, Caulis Bambusae in Taeniam and Radix Scutellariae may be decocted and drunk as tea to clear away heat, to regulate the flow of *Qi* and strengthen the stomach.

3. Accumulation of Blood Stasis Type

Clinical Manifestations

In the early stage of gestation: vomiting due to retention of phlegm, epigastric fullness and anorexia, palpitation, shortness of breath, white—freasy coating, slippery pulse.

Nursing

(1) Nurse the patient according to the methods of Disharmony Between the Spleen and the Stomach.

(2) Herbs for invigorating the spleen for removing dampness resolving phlegm and relieving vomiting should be selected. The prescription is *Xiaobanxia Fuling Tang* with modification (Modified Decoction of Pinellia Tuber and Poria).

5.9 Excessive Fetal Movement (vaginal bleeding during pregnancy fetal abortion, abortion, habitual abortion)

After pregnancy, vaginal bleeding refers to frequent colporrhagia in small amounts which bleeds intermittently or drips without soreness of loins and abdominal or weighing sensation in lower abdomen. If the fetal movement and bearing–down sensation appear and slight soreness of loins and abdominal distension follow or there is a little colporrhagia, it is called *Zhuitai*. If the fetus aborts without being formed within the first trimester of pregnancy, it is called *Xiaochan* (Labouring with incompletely developed fetus). Fetal abortion after three months of pregnancy is simply called abortion.

General Nursing

1. The ward should be kept quiet and free from any noises and harmful stimulation. The patient should be confined to bed until colporrhagia stops.

2. Give the patient emotional care and comfort and dispel any misgivings of her so that she will have a positive attitude to the treatment.

3. The patient should take light, bland, nutritious and easily digested food and plenty of fresh vegetables and fruits. Pungent, rich, greasy and fried food is prohibited.

4. The patient must keep the vulva clean and be given a perineum pad, which must be kept after being used for the doctor's inspection. Changes of bleeding from vagina and abdominal pain, etc. should be observed. If colporrhagia is in pro-

fuse and abdominal pain becomes severe, it must be reported to the doctor for treatment.

5. If the symptoms of paleness, sweating and clammy limbs appear, blood prostration due to profuse bleeding from vagina is indicated. It must be reported to the doctor at once and emergency treatment be prepared. Blood transfusion may be necessary.

Nursing According to Syndrome Differentiation

1. Deficiency of *Qi* and Blood Type

Clinical Manifestations

At the first trimester of pregnancy: fetal movement and bearing—down sensation, colporrhagia in small amount, soreness of loins and abdominal distension, listlessness and lassitude, pale complexion, palpitation and shortness of breath, light tongue with thin white coating, thin slippery and weak pulse.

Nursing

(1) The patient should be confined to bed. Tiredness and sexual life must be prohibited to prevent injury to the fetus.

(2) The patient should be kept as calm as possible with the mind at rest and free from fear.

(3) Herbs for invigorating *Qi*, replenishing blood, invigorating the spleen and preventing abortion should be selected. The prescription is *Taiyuan Yin* with modification.

(4) If deficiency of both *Qi* and blood and loss of nutrition to the fetus occur, special care should be given to the patient's diet. She should take nutritious and light food, such as old hen soup, fish, meat, eggs and viscus of animals, etc. , or gruel cooked with Colla Corii Asini, Radix Astragali, seu Hedysari and Oryza Glutinosae, which can regulate, nourish and invigorate *Qi* and

blood as well as preventing abortion. Pungent tasting food must be prohibited.

(5) The needles can be inserted into Zusanli (ST36), Neiting (ST44), and Yanglingquan (GB34) points, etc. in combination with the other treatment once daily.

2. Deficiency of the Kidney Type

Clinical Manifastations

Colporrhagia, soreness of loins, weighing sensation, dizziness and tinnitus, frequent micturition, pale tongue with white coating, deep and thready pulse with a history of spontaneous abortion.

Nursing

(1) Nursing according to the methods of deficiency of both *Qi* and blood type.

(2) The patient with a history of spontaneous abortion should take more food for invigorating the spleen, such as Colla Corii Asini, Juglandis Regiae and Fructus Lycii. It should be taken after menolipsis and continued to the fifth—sixth mouth of pregnancy.

(3) Herbs for reinforcing the kidney and preventing abortion should be taken. The prescription is *Shou Tai Wan* with modification. The decoction should be taken warm.

3. Blood—heat Type

Clinical Manifestations

Colporrhagia in brighted colour, dysphoria, hot sensation in palms and soles, dry mouth and throat, lower—abdominal pain, tidal fever, dry stools, red tongue with yellowish coating, slippery and rapid pulse.

Nursing

(1) Keep the ward quiet, comfortable, ventilated, cool and suitable for sleeping. Assist the patient in keeping a free mind and avoiding distraction, and to have plenty time for sleep.

(2) Dietetic nursing: Advise the patient to drink plenty of light saline solution, eat fresh vegetables and sour fruits and take nutritious and high—protein food. Pungent and fried food should be prohibited in order not to support heat and impair *Yin*.

(3) Herbs for clearing away heat and preventing abortion should be selected. The prescription is *Bao—yin Jian* with modification (Modified Decoction for Keeping *Yin*).

(4) The patient with dry mouth and throat should often take Radix Ophiopogonis, Herba Cistanchis, Semen Sterculiae Scaphigerae and Caulis Bambusae in Taeniam after being infused in hot water, or pear juice or lotus root which can nourish *Yin*, clear away heat and remove heat from the blood.

(5) Acupuncture therapy: Shenmen (HT7), Shaohai (HT3), Neiguan (PC6), Taichong (LR3), Yanglingquan (GB34) and Zusanli (ST36) points, etc. may be needled.

4. Trauma Type:

Clinical Manifestations

Injury during pregnancy, abdominal pain and distension, fetal movement and bearing—down sensation colporrhagia, weak and slippery pulse.

Nursing

(1) The patient must be confined to bed and every attempt should be made to put her mind at ease, dispel her misgivings in order to prevent possible abortion.

(2) Herbs for supplementing *Qi*, nourishing blood, reinforcing the kidney and preventing abortion should be selected.

The presription is *Shengyu Tang* with modification.

(3) Medicine for promoting blood. circulation to remove blood stasis and plaster for external usage on the abdomen and waist must be prohibited in order to prevent blood from being abnormally accelerated and moving the fetus. If the upper or lower limbs are damaged, massotherapy can be used on the local part to ease the pain.

(4) Pay close attention to the patient's condition. The case with abdominal pain and bearing–down sensation, profuse colporrhagia and premonitory symptoms of abortion should be reported to the doctor and everything should be prepared for abortion.

5.10   Eclampsia Gravidarum

At the third trimester of pregnancy or just at the movement of delivery or after it, the patient collapses because of a sudden dizziness, and loss of consciousness. The symptoms of tic of limbs, trismus, staring blankly and dribbling appear. After a short time, the patient falls asleep or remains unconscious. This is called eclampsia gravidarum in traditional Chinese medicine.

General Nursing

1. The ward should be kept quiet, tidy, well–ventilated, at a comfortable temperature and humidity and free from irritations of sound and light.

2. The patient needs emotional care. It is necessary to console her, dispel her misgivings and fear, and give her ease of mind to cooperate actively in the treatment.

3. The patient should be kept in a single room with a

bedfender set up in order to prevent her from falling out of bed and given intensive care. She must be kept under continuous observation of the development of her condition. Blood pressure and fetal heart sound should be measured every four to six hours and kept on record.

4. Irritations should be avoided as far as possible. Each diagnosis, exam and nursing operation should be carried out gently and under sedation. The patient with aphagia may be fed with nasal drips. The patient in coma should fast.

5. The clothes must be kept clean in the case of those with fecal and urinary incontinence. They must be changed whenever necessary and the patient's skin kept clean.Liquid leakage should be prevented for those with skin edema during intramuscular or intravenous drip. The local part must be sterilized strictly to avoid causing infection.

6. Observe closely and record the changes of convulsion, mentality, blood pressure, pulse condition, temperature, urine and edema, etc. . First—aid medicine and instruments should be prepared well. The emergency case must be reported to the doctor for emergency treatment as soon as it appears.

Nursing According to Syndrome Differentiation

1. Hyperactivity of Liver Due to *Yin* Deficiency
Clinical Manifestations
At the last trimester of pregnancy: light—headedness, palpitation, shortness of breath, chest distress, feverish sensation accompanied with restlessness, flushed face, constipation, oliguria and dark urine, red tongue with light—yellowish and dry coating, string—taut thready, slippery and rapid pulse.

Nursing

(1) The patient must be confined to bed, have plenty of time for sleep and avoid overfatigue and overtaxing her mind. Her clothes must not be too warm.

(2) Good emotional care is necessary. As the patient is highly prone to nervousness and fear. She should be gently consoled during nursing in order to set her mind at rest and give her confidence in the treatment.

(3) The patient should be given a light, bland, nourishing, high-heat and high-protein diet with plenty of fresh vegetables and fruits. Pork liver, pork heart and jellyfish are all suitable foods. Smoking and drinking must be forbidden, and rich and pungent food should be prohibited.

(4) The medicine for nourishing *Yin*, suppressing the excessive *Yang* calming the liver and nourishing the blood should be selected. The best prescription is *Lingyang Gouteng Tang* with modification (Modified Decoction of Antelope's Horn and Uncaria Stem). If necessary, two dosages a day may be taken for several days. The dosages may be divided into smaller amounts and taken more frequently.

(5) If the patient suddenly goes into convulsions, her head should be turned to one side and a tongue-spatula packed with gauze put between the upper and lower teeth to prevent the tongue from being titter red. Shuigou (DU26), Hegu(LI4), Chengshan (BL57), Jiache (ST6), Taichong (LR3), Yongquan (KI1) and Quchi (LI11) points, etc. may be needled or pressed with the finger. One pill of *Angong Niuhuang Wan* (Bezoar Bolus for Resurrection) may be taken after being infused in water or the patient may be fed with nasal drip. The case should be reported

to the doctor for treatment.

(6) To those with airway obstruction caused by sputum, Tiantu (RN22), Fenglong (ST40) Neiguan (PC6) and Feishu (BL13) points, etc. may be needled to eliminate phlegm for resuscitation, or the patient's back may be pounded to facilitate the discharge of sputum. 60 ml of *Zhuli* Water (Bamboo Juice) and several drops of ginger juice can be fed frequently or administered as nasal drip to resolve phlegm. A little hot gruel can be taken after discharging sputum in order to restore the stomach *Qi*.

(7) The intake of salt should be limited for those with edema in the lower limbs. The patient should take a plenty of water melon and waxgourd juice or waxgourd peel may be decocted and taken as a drink to promote urination. Honey water can be given to those with constipation in order to lubricate the intestine and relax the bowels.

2. Hyperactivity of Fire Due to the Spleen Deficiency

Clinical Manifestations

Edema of face and limbs, chest distress with a tendency to vomiting, dizziness, fullness of eyes, anorexia, loose stool, greasy coating on the tongue, feeble, wiry and slippery pulse.

Nursing

(1) *Baizhu San* with modification (Modified Powder of Bighead Atractylodes Rhizome) may be selected as the medicine for reinforcing the function of the spleen to remove dampness, and calming the liver.

(2) The other nursing methods are as the same as that for those with hyperactivity of fire due to *Yin* deficiency.

5.11 Heterotopic Pregnancy

Heterotopic pregnancy is caused by fertilized ovum's

nidation in the organs outside the uterine cavity, such as oviduct, ovary and abdominacy and exfetation.

General Nursing

1. The patient must be given gentle emotional care and comforting and encouraged to dispel her misgivings and cooperate actively in the treatment.

2. The patient must be confined to bed and avoid being moved in order to prevent any danger from changing posture and increasing abdominal pressure.

3. Note carefully any abdominal pain, distension, bleeding and secretion from vagina. Observe changes of the patient's expression, blood pressure and pulse condition and record them. The posterior formix puncture should be prepared well before the operation.

4. If severe abdominal pain, pale complexion, sweating due to debility, cold extremities, fall of blood pressure and very faint pulse appear, syncope is indicated. The doctor must be informed to carry out emergency treatment.

Nursing According to Syndrome Differentiation

1. Shock Type

Clinical Manifestations

Sudden severe abdominal pain, tenderness, pale complexion, clammy limbs, profuse cold sweating, nausea, vomiting, fall of blood pressure, vexation, very faint pulse.

Nursing

(1) The patient should be nursed intensively and lie on her back.

(2) *Dushen Tang* may be selected as the drug for supplementing *Qi*, recuperating depleted *Yang* and rescuing the patient from collapse. It can be decocted quickly, and concentrated. It may be taken in frequent small amounts after dripping several drops of ginger in it in order to prevent vomiting.

(3) Liquid food and rice water, etc. may be fed by means of nasal drip to supply nutrition.

(4) Those with lowered blood pressure, profuse sweating and clammy limbs should keep themselves warm. *Renshen Tang* (Ginseng Decoction) may be decocted quickly and taken or Shuigou (DU26), Neiguan (PC 6), Zusanli (ST36) and Yongquan (KI1), etc may be needled in combination with the decoction treatment. The otopoints of sympathetic for raising blood pressure, adrenal gland, etc. can be selected to recuperate depleted *Yang* and rescue the patient from collapse.

(5) Medicine for promoting blood circulation to remove blood stasis can be given after the relieving of shock symptoms. The selected prescription is *Gongwaiyun Tang I*, (Decoction for Treating Ectopic Pregnancy).

2. Instability Type

Clinical Manifestations

Abdominal pain and tenderness which gradually ease, irregular colporrhagia which drips, stable blood pressure, thready and slow pulse.

Nursing

(1) The patient should stay in bed after being hospitalized for 1—2 days, and gradually start exercising. Those with negative reaction in pregnancy test may leave the bed and do light exercises.

(2) Herbs for promoting blood circulation to remove blood stasis to stop pain should be taken. The prescription is *Gongwaiyun Tang* with modification.

(3) Observe the condition of abdominal pain, the quantity and colour of bleeding from the vagina and the secretion such as blood clot or tissue. If the abdominal pain becomes severe and is accompanied by sweating and clammy limbs and fall of blood pressure, it must be reported to the doctor. Nursing should be done according to shock type.

3. Mass Type

Clinical Manifestations

Hematoma mass forming after abortion or rupture of ectopic pregrancy, light distending pain or pressing pain in the lower abdomen, little colporrhagia, pink and dull tongue, deep wiry and thready pulse.

Nursing

(1) Herbs for promoting blood circulation to remove blood stasis and removing hardness and dispersing entanglement should be taken. The prescription is *Gong Waiyun* II with modification.

(2) Observe any changes after taking medicine and examine the patient's routine liver function and blood test at regular intervals. If there is any deterioration, the doctor must be informed and the measure of stopping taking medicine or adding herbs for invigorating *Qi* and nourishing the liver should be taken.

(3) *Xuejie San* (Powder of Dragon's Blood) can be applied topically on the lower abdomen of the patient who has superficial swelling and is too weak to take Chinese medicine orally. Physiotherapy, or adhesive plaster applied topically may be prescribed.

(4) The patient can get up and move about after the embryo's dying, look after herself and add exercises gradually.

(5) Birth control must be known widely. A longer interval between successive conceptions can reduce the morbidity. Strengthen physical training to build up the ability against disease.

5.12 Postpartum Fever

Postpartum fever is characterized by continuous or sudden high fever accompanied by other symptoms. In modern medicine the fever caused by puerperal infection is also considered as postpartum fever.

General Nursing

1. The ward must be kept well ventilated, but there should be no draughts.

2. The patient should remain in bed, and be free from mental upsets and irritations and have ease of mind.

3. The patient with persistent lochia should keep semireclining position so that blood stasis can be benefited to be removed.

4. The patient should keep the vulva clean, washing it at regular intervals every day, and use sterilized perineum pad. The patient with laceration should have a new, clean dressing every day.

5. Care should be taken of the patient's oral cavity and skin. She should rinse her mouth regularly to prevent bacterial infection. Those who sweat heavily should dry the body with a towel and change the under wear frequently.

6. The patient with hyperactivity of pathogenic heat should

adopt toweling with warm water according to her condition. She should be advised to drink more boiled water. If necessary, venous fluid infusion should be selected.

7. The patient with dry intestine and constipation should drink plenty of fruit juice, eat plenty of vegetables, as well as sesame oil, honey, black sesame seeds and walnuts, etc. to moisturize the intestine and relax the bowels.

8. Observe and record the changes in the conditions of heat, pulse and tongue, emotions, complexion, abdominal pain, urine and lochia, etc.. If the symptoms of coma and delirium, pale face, cold extremities, faint and rapid pulse and other conditions of excess of heat appear, the doctor should be informed and treatment measures should be adopted.

Nursing According to Syndrome Differentiation

1. Blood—deficiency Type
Clinical Manifestations
Profuse bleeding after delivery, slight fever and spontaneous perspiration, no aversion to cold, red face, dizziness, tinnitus, palpitation, dry mouth, anorexia, constipation, pink tongue with thin coating, thready and weak pulse.
Nursing
(1) The patients should have plenty of rest. Clothing should not be too warm. The development of the patient's temperature should be observed and she should be advised to keep out of direct draughts so as not to catch a cold.
(2) A diet should be arranged according to the conditions of her case. She should be advised to take plenty of nourishing and light food, such as soup of boiled chicken and fish, tremella and

milk, etc.. The patient should avoid eating raw, cold and pungent food.

(3) Herbs for invigorating blood to benefit *Qi* and nourshing *Yin* and clearing away heat should be taken. The prescription—*Bazhen Tang* with modification (Modification Decoction of Eight Precious Ingredients) should be selected.

(4) Avoid using physical regulation of body temperature and any other methods of abating heat which give first place to inducing diaphoresis. Profuse sweating should be prevented.

2. Exopathic Disease Type

Clinical Manifestations

Postpartum fever and aversion to cold, headache, anhidrosis, aching limbs, or cough, running nose, thin and white coating of the tongue, floating pulse.

Nursing

(1) The patient should stay in bed and be sure to avoid exposure to wind.

(2) Herbs for nourishing the blood to expel wind should be selected. The prescription is *Jingfang Siwu Tang* with modification (Modified Decoction of Four Ingredients Pluse Schizonepeta and Ledebouriella). The decoction should be taken hot. Slight sweating appears after taking the hot medicine. If there is no sweating, gruel or brown sugar and ginger infused in hot water can be taken to help induce diaphoresis.

(3) Observe the condition of sweating after taking the medicine. Diaphoresis should not be induced much. The patient should towel herself dry immediately after sweating, change her underwear wet with sweat and shut the door and windows so as not to catch cold.

3. Noxious Pathogenic Factors Type

Clinical Manifestations

Fever and aversion to cold, or chill, dysphoria, dry mouth, abdominal pain, foul and putrid smelling, lochia, scarty dark urine, dry stool, red tongue with yellowish coating, rapid and strong pulse.

Nursing

(1) The ward should be kept well ventilated. The clothes and bedclothe should not be too warm.

(2) The patient should have plenty to drink during the high fever period, a light and nutritious diet with plenty water melon and other fresh fruit juice to supply body fluid.

(3) Herbs for clearing away heat and removing pathogenic heat from the blood and toxic material from the body should be selected. The prescription is *Liangxue Jiedu Tang* with modification (Modified Decoction of Removing Pathogenic Heat from the Blood and Toxic Material from the Body).

(4) Ramulus Cinnamomi, Herba Asari, Cortex Cinnamami, Rhizoma Zingiberis Recens and Flos Carthami, etc. can be infused in 75% alcohol and warmed up, which the patient with steady high fever can use to rub herself with. This has the function of promoting the flow of *Qi* by warming the channels and lowering the temperature.

(5) In addition, needling Hegu (LI 4), Quchi (LI 11), Fengchi (GB 20) and Lieque (LU7), should be combined with reduction.

(6) Pay close attention to the changes of the patient's condition, If the symptoms of pale complexion, cold limbs, profuse sweating and faint, thin and weak pulse appear suddenly, this suggests asthenia of *Yang—Qi* and should be reported to the doc-

tor. *Shen Fu Tang* (Decoction of Ginseng and Prepared Aconite) should be decocted quickly and taken in small doses atshort interals. Or one pill of *Angong Niuhuang Wan* (Bezoar Bolus for Resurrection) should be taken to recuperate depleted *Yang* and rescue the patient from collapse.

4. Blood Stasis

Clinical Manifestations

Several days after childbirth: constant onset of chills and fever, unsmooth lochia, lower abdominal pain, dull purplish tongue with ecchymosis, deep and wiry pulse.

Nursing

1. Observe carefully the changes of the condition of lochia including quantity, colour and quality. The patient with unsmooth lochia and dark blood with stasis should be prescribed 20 ml of *Yi Mu Gao* (Extract of Herba Leonuri for Activating Blood Flow and Removing Blood Stasis), which should be taken following its infusion with warm boiled water three times daily.

2. Herbs for promoting blood circulation to remove blood stasis should be taken. The prescription −*Shenghua Tang* with modification (Modified Decoction for Postpartum Troubles) should be selected.

3. Hot compress and moxibustion can be used on the lower abdomen of the patient with abdominal pain.

5.13 Lochiorrhea (Persistent Lochia)

Small amount of dark red bloody fluid is discharged from the vagina within 2−3 weeks after the delivery. It is called lochia. All lochia should be discharged over in 20 days after the childbirth. If lochia is profuse and the bleeding is persistent, it is called lochiorrhea.

General Nursing

1. The ward should be well ventilated.

2. The patient should stay in bed, be sure to keep herself warm and change her underwear in time after sweating in order not to catch cold.

3. Observe the conditions of quantity, colour, blood clots, abdominal pain and heat, and keep a good record of them. If lochia is in great amount, the patient should lie in semireclining position so that it can be discharged.

4. If the symptoms of excessive of lochia, red blood stasis, abdominal pain, pale complexion, dizziness, sweating, palpitation and shortness of breath appear, residual placenta should be considered and reported to the doctor who can take treatment measures.

5. The patient should keep the vulva clean. The perineum pad should be sterilized and changed frequently. Sexual life and tub bath must be forbidden in order to prevent bacteria from invading.

Nursing According to Syndrome Differentiation

1. Deficiency of *Qi* Type

Clinical Manifestations

Persistent lochia in great amount and light colour with watery quality, feeling of tenesmus in the lower abdomen, lassitude, pale complexion, light tongue, slow and weak pulse.

Nursing

(1) The patient should try to control her emotions have ease

of mind, be in good spirits and cooperate actively in the treatment.

(2) The patient should be sure to keep out of the wind and keep herself warm to prevent exopathogens from taking advantage of a weak point to invade the body and vital—Qi from being consumed.

(3) The patient should be provided with good nutriment, such as soft—shelled turtle, boiled chicken soup and longan pulp soup. She should not eat raw, cold, pungent and indigestible food.

(4) To the patient with a feeling of tenesmus in the lower abdomen, the acupoints of Tianshu (ST25), Qihai(RN6), and Guilai (ST29), etc. can be given moxibustion.

(5) Herbs for treating hemostasis by invigorating the blood should be taken.The prescription——*Buzhong Yiqi Tang,* with modification (Modified Decoction for Reinforcing Middle—*Jiao* and Replenishing Qi) should be selected.

2. Blood Stasis Type

Clinical Manifestations

Profuse and incessant lochia in small amount and dull purplish colour with blood clots, lower abdominal pain and tenderness, dull purplish tongue with petechia on the sides, deep and wiry pulse.

Nursing

(1) Take care of the patient's emotion and help to give ease of mind and keep functional activities of Qi in order, so that lochia can be discharged smoothly.

(2) Herbs for promoting blood circulation to remove blood stasis should be taken. The prescription —*Shenghua Tang* with

modification (Modified Decoction for Postpartum Troubles) should be selected.

(3) The patient with lower abdominal pain and tenderness may be given a hot compress or the acupoints of Tianshu (ST25), Qihai (RN6), Gulai(ST29)and Sanyinjiao(SP6)can be treated with moxibustion in order to force the blood clots to pass down and relieve the abdominal pain.

(4) 20 ml of *Yimucao Gao* should be taken after being infused in warm boiled water, three times a day .

3. Blood—heat Type

Clinical Manifestations

Persistent lochia in great amount and fresh or dark red with thick quality and fetid smell, flushed face, dry mouth and tongue, red tongue with yellowish coating, slight and rapid pulse.

Nursing

(1) Carefully observe the changes of the quantity, colour and smell of lochia and the whole body condition.

(2) Avoid irritating the patient's feelings and keep her in optimistic mood to strengthen her faith in treament.

(3) Herbs for removing pathogenic heat from blood and nourishing *Yin* and stopping bleeding should be taken. The prescription—*Baoying Tang* with modification should be selected.

(4) For the patient with dry mouth and tongue, Flos Lonicerae and Radix Ophiopogonis should be infused in boiling water and then drunk as tea in order to nourish *Yin* to clear away the heat.

5.14   Pelvic Inflammation

Inflammatory lesion takes place in the pelvic organs of

woman including endometrial inflammation, salpingitis, ovaritis, pelvioperitonotis and inflammation of pelvic connective tissue. It is in the range of invasion of *Ying* blood by heat, gynecological disease and mass in the abdomen in traditional Chinese medicine.

General Nursing

1. Advise the patient to take plenty of rest, keep regular habits and stay in bed during the acute period.

2. Take care of the patient's emotion, encourage her to have faith in conquering illness and to cooperate actively in the treatment.

3. The patient should be provided with plenty of nutritious and digestible food. She should drink plenty of water and eat more fresh fruits during the high−fever period.

4. The patient should keep the vulva clean and abstain from tub baths and sexual life during intermenstrual period in order to prevent infection.

5. Point−injection to Zusanli (ST36) and Sanyinjiao (SP6), etc. may be used interchangeably with injections of Radix Salviae miltiorrhizae, Radix Sophorae Flavescentis and Flos Chrysanthemi 1 ml of fluid may be injected into one point once a day.

Nursing According to Syndrome Differentiation

1. Heat of Excess Type
Clinical Manifestations
In acute pelvic inflammation: fever and aversion to cold, dry mouth with thirst, lower abdominal pain and tenderness, soreness and tenesmus of waist, increased foul leukorrhea with watery

quality and in yellowish colour, scanty dark urine, red tongue with yellowish or greasy coating, full and rapid or slippery and rapid pulse.

Nursing

(1) Because fever can impair *Yin*, the patient should be given bland and easy—digestible food, drink plenty of light salt water and juice of pear and have water melon and other fruits to nourish *Yin*, in order to clear away heat. Fried, roasted, greasy, pungent, sweet and sticky food should not be eaten.

(2) Herbs for clearing away heat and toxic material and promoting blood circulation to remove blood stasis and dampness should be taken. The prescription——*Qingre Jiedu Huayu Tang* with modification (Modified Decoction for Heat—cleaning and Detoxifying to Remove Blood Stasis) should be selected. Two doses should be taken per day at six hour intervals.

(3) The patient with high fever can be nursed according to the methods of high—fever nursing (2.1).

(4) In traditional Chinese medicine the enema is still used. 60 g of Caulis Sargentodoxae can be decocted into 100ml of decoction. At a temperature of 38℃ , the decoction may be poured slowly into the colon. Advise the patient to lie in bed and rest for half an hour. The treatment should be done once a day and five to ten times make one course of treatment. It must not be done before and after intermenstrual period.

(5) 2 ml of injection of Herba Andrographitis and the same dosage of injection of Flos Lonicerae can be used for intramuscular injection once every two days.

2. The Type of *Qi* and Blood Stasis

Clinical Manifestations

Swelling pain in the lower abdomen, which is severe just before and after the menstrual period, swelling pain of the breast, at the end of the menstrual period a small quantity of blood with masses and pure and thin lecukorrhea, pale tongue with white and greasy coating, thready wiry pulse.

Nursing

(1) The herbs for activating vital energy and blood circulation, removing blood stasis and stopping pain and clearing away the heat—evil and promoting diuresis should be taken. The prescription—*Qingre Huayu Tang* with modification (Modified Decoction for Clearing Away Heat—evil and Removing Blood Stasis) should be selected.

(2) Nutritious food such as meat and eggs should be provided more. Raw, cold, pungent and irritating food should not be eaten.

(3) Be sure to keep the vulva clean and wash it once a day. Be sure not to exposure to the rain and water or catch cold during the menstrual period so as to prevent the disease from becoming severe.

3. The Type of Stagnation of Pathogenic Cold—wetness

Clinical Manifestations

Sensation of oppression in the chest, painful ribs, swelling pain in lower abdomen during or after menstrual, loose and thin stool, clear and voluminous urine, dark tongue with thin coating, deep—slow—or deep—rapid pulse.

Nursing

(1) The medicine for warming channels and promoting circulation of *Qi* and blood should be taken. The prescription, *Wenjing Tang* with modification (Modified Decoction for Warming

Channels) should be seleted.

(2) If there is a swelling pain in the lower abdomen, stir–fried salt or antithesis amomum fruit mixed with vinegar can be applied to the abdomen.

(3) Keep herself warm during the period of menses and avoid catching cold.

5.15 Prolapse of Uterus

Prolapse of uterus refers to descent of the uterus into the vagina or even out of the vulva. It is also called " descent of uterus"in modern medicine.

General Nursing

1. The ward should be kept clean and quiet. The patient should have adequate rest, avoid activities and tiredness.

2. Diet should contain rich nutrition and be digestible. Food for regulating and tonifying the spleen and kidney should be provided. Raw, cold and pungent food should not be eaten.

3. Free movement of the bowels should be maintained, light cathartic can be given during constipation and over–strain to counteract constipation should be avoided.

4. Observe the extent of hysteroptosis, the condition of swelling, bleeding and ulcerating on its surface. If ulceration appears and yellow liquid seeps, it should be cleaned up and treated with application *Qingdai San* (Powder of Indigo Naturalis) to the area.

5. Keep the vulva clean and the underclothes soft and clean, changing or washing them once a day.

6. Effective birth control should be maintained. If further

births are required, they should be as few as possible and well spaced. Heavy objects should not be carried after childbearing.

7. Do more physical exercises of chest, knee joint in lying position or exercise the levator to strengthen the function of pelvic cavity muscle.

Nursing According to Syndrome Differentiation

1. The Type of Deficiency of *Qi*

Clinical Manifestations

Drop of the uterus into the vagina or out of the vulva, which becomes more severe after tiredness, sinking sensation in the lower abdomen, weakness of extremities, shortness of breath and words, pale complexion, profuse, thin and white leukorrhea, frequent urinating pale tongue with thin coating, thin empty pulse.

Nursing

(1) The patient's diet should be carefully regulated. Supple nutrition and provide eggs, fish, lean neat, soft—shelled turtle and porridge cooked with Radix Scutellariae or Radix Codonopsis Pilosulae to regulate and tonify the spleen and kidney. Raw, cold and pungent food should not be taken.

(2) The medicine for tonifying *Qi* and lifting energy should te taken. The prescription should be *Buzhong Yiqi Tang* with modification (Modified Decoction for Reinforcing Middle—*Jiao* and Replenishing *Qi*).

(3) Accupuncture therapy should be taken tonifying in points Baihui (DU20), Qihai (RN6), Dahe (KI12), Zigong (EX—CA1), Sanyinjiao (SP6), Taichong (LR3) and Zhaohai (KI6) to prevent oxhaustion of *Qi*.

(4) If the prolapsed uterus becomes swelling and ulcerated

with yellow liquid, Fructus Auratii 60 g and Fructus Mume 60 g, and Fructus Cnidii 30 g are decocted in water and be used to fume and wash the infected area. The power of Cortex Phellodendri, calcined *Gajie* Powder, powder of cuttlefish bone and calamine powder in suitable amount with Indigo Naturalis or Bormeolum Syntheticum are mixed with sesame oil, made into ointment and applied to infected area once a day.

2. Kidney Deficiency Type

Clinical Manifestations

Prolapse of uterus, sore and weak low back and legs, bearing sensation in the lower abdomen, dizziness, frequent urine, pink tongue with deep weak pulse.

Nursing

(1) Refer to the nursing of *Qi* deficiency.

(2) The medicine for tonifying the kidney, nourishing the blood, warming *Yang* and replenishing *Qi* should be taken. The prescription should be *Dabuyuan Jian* with modification.

(3) Radix Aconiti Praeparata 9 g, Cortex Cinnamomi 6 g and baked ginger 6 g are decocted in water and then taken. The moxibustion may be applied to point Baihui (DU20) on which a slice of ginger is put twice a day.

6 Nursing for Paediatric Diseases

6.1 Nursing Characteristics of Paediatrics

Children have their own characteristics in physiology and pathology. Physiologically they are active and grow rapidly but have tender,delicate and undeveloped organs.Pathologically,they are susceptible to diseases which will change quickly,and are prone to suffer from cold or heat,deficient or excess syndrome.In short,they grow quickly,but haven't developed fully;their blood and energy tend to be deficient,their superficial resistance to many diseases poor and the symptoms are changeable.A further difficult respect is that they are not always able to state their disease condition more wholly and precisely and to take care of themselves,so the nursing work of paediatrics has its own special characteristics.

1. Nurses should have high sense of responsibility. They should take care of the sick children carefully and patiently in daily life. They should build up a nurturing relationship with the sick children in their work and try to ease any fears they may have on doctors and nurses and all operations for nursing should be careful and gentle in order that there may be active cooperation between medical staff and the sick children in treatment and nursing service.

2. The ward must be kept tidy and clean. The air in it must be fresh and circulating. The temperature should be maintained

at 18℃—20℃ and up to 26℃ or so in summer. Relative humidity should be 55%—65%. When the windows are open for good ventilation, the sick children should not be directly exposed to draughts lest they catch cold. When the wards are being cleaned, moist utensils should be used to prevent dust from being raised. Excreta of the sick child should be disposed of immediately. Noise should be avoided, so as to prevent the sick children from being frightened.

3. Extreme care should be taken of sterilization and isolation to prevent cross infection. The furniture and air in wards should be sterilized regularly according to the particular disease. The beds and small tables should be cleaned with disinfectant. The sick children should be arranged in different wards according to their respective diseases. The visitors must be limited strictly to prevent cross infection. The milk bottles and tableware should be sterilized each time after use. Toys and basins should be clean and sterilized regularly. The sick children should be taught to wash their hands before and after meal and develop behaviour appropriate for their health.

4. Sick children's clothes must be appropriate for the disease and weather. They should be comfortable, soft, light and loose fitting. The sick children should not be overdressed, as cexcessive sweating may lead to cold. The qnilt should neither be too thick nor too thin. The diapers should be of soft cotton cloth and hygroscopic and cleaned and soaked in hot water after use and exposed to the sun .Other things should be sterilized according to the particular requirements and conditions.

5. Psychological care should be taken. Children have rich and varied feelings. They are naive and active. Being remote from

parents, family and familiar things with which they have close relationship, they are likely to be unhappy and reluctant to be away from them, this may cause their morbid manifestations such as loss of appetite and abnormal spirit. Such conditions are unfavourable to their recovery from disease. Therefore, nurses should be aware of the children's psychological state in their nursing and encourage the elder children to have the confidence to conquer the diseases. Let them enjoy entertainment when possible so as to boost their morale.

Sick children should have adequate time for sleep. They may often feel tired and sleepy because of sweating after taking medicine or recovering from disease. While sleeping they should not be woken, provided their breathing and complexion are normal. They need sufficient rest and sleep, especially during the period of recovery.

6. Note nursing for Disease Condition. Medical staff can obtain information about change of the sick children's disease condition mainly by careful observation, such observations should be regular, patient, careful, exact and thorough. Appropriate nursing measures can then be taken.

7. Note nursing for administration of Medicine. Children are often unwilling to take medicine so the dosage of herbal medicine should be small. The decoction should be thick and taken in small amounts many times a day. When administering decoction, a nurse should hold the sick child in her arms and then put a spoon with the decoction onto his mouth corner, letting the decoction flow slowly to the root of his tongue and being swallowed naturally, or drip the decoction into his mouth with a dropper. Be sure not to pinch the child's nose while letting him take the decoction,

as this may cause the decoction to go into the trachea. Flavouring can be added into the decoction to make it more palatable to the child. Pills and tablets for young babies must be ground into fine powder or dissolved in warm water, milk, rice soup and honey, then taken as decoction. The elder children should be encouraged to take medicine by themselves put with the help of the nurses. However, less responsible children should be watched until all the medicine has been taken as they may otherwise forget or hide it.The regulations and contraindication of administration should be noted carefully and any harmful reaction after taking medicine must be watched. The dosage of medicine should be properly controlled. The mounting method, aerosol inhalation and laser acupuncture may also be used.

8. Note Diet Nursing. according to the differences of ages and disease, condition of patients, the principle to provide food for sick children must be noted. The diet should be liquid, vegetarian and in small quantity, gradually becoming more solid, meaty and in a little more quantity, Food should be rich in protein,low in fat and suitably sacchariferous. More vegetables and fruits should be taken. The time, quantity and quality of diet should be fixed. Dietary hygiene is essential and the hands should always be washed before meals. Sick children must not be permitted to play during the meal to prevent food from slipping into the trachea.Diet should be controlled during the period of recovery and after recovery.Overeating must be avoided as this may induce a relapse.

9. Note safety Nursing. Children's ignorance, curiosity and playfulness may lead to accidents such as falling out of bed, poisoning, electric shock, burning, entering of foreign body into the

trachea, trauma, etc. Nurses must take great care and give the children safe education to prevent such unexpected accidents.All metal toys with sharp points and glass utensils must be kept off. The temperature of hot water bags must be kept under 60℃. The cap must be screwed tightly and the bag must be covered with cloth to prevent scalding. Nurses should take special care to ensure that no child falls from bed.

6.2 Measles

Measles is within the range of "epidemic febrile disease" in traditional Chinese medicine. It is characterized by fever, cough, koplik's spots and red skin rashes on the whole body. It is often developed in spring and winter. One attack confers permanent immunity. It belongs in epidemic febrile disease of TCM.

General Nursing

1. Refer to the characteristics of paediatric nursing (6.1) .

2. The isolation of respiratory tract should be taken until 5 days after the complete eruption of rashes, it can last until 10 days after the rashes have erupted if the sick has complications.

3. The environment should be quiet. The temperature in room should be a little higher in winter, 20℃ — 22℃ being suitable. The relative humidity should be 60% which is helpful for the complete eruption of rashes. The air in wards must be sterilized and kept fresh, so as to avoid cross infection. Dark colored curtains should be equipped and lamp—light should be controlled so as to keep the light gentle to avoid irritating eyes.

4. The sick children should stay in bed and not walk until the temperature becomes normal. They cannot go out until the rashes

have disappeared.

5. The patient's mouth and nasal cavity should be kept clean. The mouth should be rinsed with liquid made of Flos Lonicerae or saline solution. If lips become dry or broken, the ointment can be applied for xerocheilia. If there are sores in the mouth, the *Bingpeng San, Xilei San* and *Zhuhuang San* can be applied for aphtha.If the nasal cavities become dry and some scabs remain in them, paraffin oil can be used to moisten them, then the scabs are eliminated, so that the sick children won't scratch their nasal cavities with fingers. This can avoid injuring their nasal mucosa or causing bleeding.

6. The case of contact with the children suffering from measles should be quarantined and observed for 17 days and preventive measures must be taken .

Nursing According to Syndrome Differentiation

1.Initial Fever Stage   (Prodromal stage) (3—4 days)
Clinical Manifestations

Fever with aversion to wind and cold, cough and running nose, conjunctival congestion, photophobia, vomiting and diarrhea, koplik's spots on oral mucosa appearing after 2—3 days of fever, which is the evidence for early diagnosis of measles, thin and yellow tongue coating, floating and rapid pulse.

Nursing

(1) The nursing at this period is similar to that in common cold. The mouth must be examined twice a day since the second day of fever and watched whether the koplik's spots appear. Once the koplik's spots are found, corresponding nursing measures should be taken to promote and protect eruption. There are only

few cases whose mucosa of cheek has hyperaemia and no typical koplik's spots. The surface of mucosa is rough. Those who have been immunized by injection a short time before may have no typical symptoms. The koplik's spots may not appear, but nursing should not be neglected.

(2) Measles is a kind of eruptive disease. Once the rashes completely erupt, the toxin will be eliminated. If the rashes disappear, the toxin will not exist. In the early stage promoting the eruption of rashes is an important key in nursing of measles. The fresh reed rhizome 60 g or fresh Japanese raspberry root 60 g , can be decocted in water to be drunk instead of tea. Coriander 60 g can also be decocted to be taken in small doses at short intervals, in order to sweat slightly and promote the eruption of rashes. In order to avoid measles without adequate eruption resulting in a severe deteriorating case of measles, which is caused by blockage of skin striae due to catching cold, keeping warm is essential.

(3) Herbs for expelling the pathogenic factors from the surface of the body with drugs pungent flavour and cool in nature should be taken. A prescription of *Yingqiao San* with modification (Modified Powder of Lonicera and Forsythia) should be chosen. If the sick children have fever without perspiration, the tongue coating is thin and white, the pungent—warm herbs for relieving the exterior syndrome can be decocted for oral dose. The prescription of *Jingfang Baidu San* with modification (Modified Powder of Schizonepeta and Ledebouriella for Expelling Poison) can be used, too. The sick child should be covered with a quilt and kept in bed to let him have slight sweat, so as to promote eruption of rashes. Large sweating should be avoided to

prevent exhaustion of *Yin* fluid （a general term for various kinds of body fluid,such as blood, saliva, spermatic fluid） .

（4）Pay attention to protecting eyes. If gum in the eyes is too much or with dry scab it must be cleaned by warm water, or erythyomycin ointment can be used to eliminate it after eyes become moist. If eyes become red, swollen and filled with tears, Flos Lonicerae 9 g ,Flos Chrysanthemi 9 g, Rhizoma Coptidis 3 g are decocted in water and as an eyewash solution. Chinese goldthread water or antibiotic ointment may also be applied to the eyes.

（5）Food should be light. nutritious and easily digestible, liquid or semi—liquid food and porridge made of coriander can be provided to promote eruption of rashes thoroughly. Plenty of water should be given to the sick children.

2.Eruptive Stage （3—5 days）

Clinical Manifestations

High fever, cough, vexation, heavy breathing, severe conjunctival congestion, rashes behind ears and on neck, then spreading to forehead, cheeks, chest, back, limbs, hands and feet, finally to the underside of the arch of the foot. After complete eruption of rashes, appearance of bright red rashes, red tongue with yellow coating, full and rapid pulse.

Nursing

（1）This period is the time of complete eruption of rashes. Medicine should be taken for clearing away heat and removing toxic materials in order to make rashes erupt completely. The decoction for clearing away heat and expelling the superficial pathogens should be chosen. Observe carefully the order of appearance of rashes, their colour, density and the extent of complete eruption after taking the decoction. If any abnormal condition appears, the doctor should be immediately notified.

(2) Nursing of fever. Fever accompanying measles is a mechanism by which the body expels the toxin The sick child's temperature doesn't need to lower before the rashes have erupted thoroughly, provided he is not delirious, is sweating and the temperature is about 38℃ .If it exceeds over 39℃ , the temperature should be lowered, a warm and wet towel can be applied to the child's forehead or his face, neck, hands and feet may be washed in warm water to open striae of skin. Slight sweating should be induced to expel the toxin. In addition, CacumenTamaricis 120 g, coriander 30 g can be decocted in water and added to suitable amount of millet wine, with which the body is scrubbed to promote thorough eruption of rashes. Acupuncture can be applied to points Shenmen (HT7) , Shixuan (EX-UE11) and Fenglong (ST40) for the patient with hyperpyrexia and convulsion.

(3) Nursing of cough. The severity of cough is directly proportional to the severity of the measles. Medicine for stopping and relieving cough can be taken or the herbs for relieving cough and reducing phlegm are decocted for aerosol inhalation use, and done many times a day to relax irritated cough caused by dryness of respiratory tract.

(4) Maintain cleanliness of skin. If itching appears, the decoction of coriander,Schizonepeta (herba) and decoction of Perilla Frutescens can be used to wash and rub the irritated area to stop itch and promote the rashes to erupt thoroughly. The sick children's nails should be trimmed to avoid secondary infection due to scratching.

(5) Observe the condition of eruption, especially the condi-

tions of an improving case and a severe deteriorating case of measles. In the case of the former, rashes are bright red and the eruption of rashes is fairly well—distributed, the eruption and disappearance of rashes are regular. The rashes will disappear upon recovery. In the case of the latter, high fever is often seen. The spots of rashes are thick, purple and slow to erupt. The child may have lassitude. The rashes are less and their colour is slight. They will suddenly disappear without having erupted completely, or the child has difficulty in breathing, cyanosis, restlessness, convulsion, syncope and is prone to occurrence of complications such as pneumonia, throat inflammation, cardiac failure, encephalo—pathy, etc.. Observe carefully any changes of the condition.

(6) Eyes, nose and oral cavity should be given particular attention.

(7) Pay attention to regulation and nursing of diet and the light and vegetarian diet is suitable.

3. The Period of Recovery (5—7 days)

Clinical Manifestations

Rashes disappear from the upper to the lower part of the body after complete eruption, simulta neously followed by disappearance of fever, cough and conjunctival congestion. The spirit and appetite return to normal. Trace of brown spots and exuviation on the skin left along with disappearance of rashes disappear by themselves. Red tongue with pale coating, small and weaker pulse.

Nursing

(1) Medicine to nourish Yin, supplement Qi and regulate the stomach—energy should be administered. A suitable prescrip-

tion is *Shashen Maidong Tang* with modification (Modified Decoction of Root of Straight tadybell and Tuber of Dwarf Lilyturf), so as to support the sick body with deficiency of *Yin* and vital energy.

(2) During the period of recovery following the normalization of the function of the stomach and spleen, milk, eggs, lean meat and all kinds of vegetables, fruits and porridge with lotus seeds, Chinese yam can be eaten. Soup made of turnip or water chestnuts can also be drunk to expel the remaining toxic materials. Greasy, hard, sold, and irritating food should be forbidden and overeating should be avoided to prevent the stomach and spleen from damagement. Food hygiene is essential to prevent the patient from diarrhea and dysentery after the rashes have gone, and stool change should be noted.

(3) Take special care of the skin. As the rashes disappear, there will be scurf and some itchiness, *Lu Ganshi* (Calamina) liquid may be used to clean and scrub the skin in order to prevent infection due to scratching.

(4) Protect the patient from pathogenic wind—cold and any pathogenic factors which may lead to complications or cross infection during convalescence. Moderate physical activity may be permitted accompanied with plenty of rest.

6.3 Varicella

Varicella is an acute infectious viral disease with rashes. The clinical symptoms are characterized as fever, maculopapular, bleb and eruption with scabs on skin and mucosa in clusters. Generally the red maculopapular eruptions begin to erupt after about 24 hours of fever, then becoming bleb within a few hours, the centres becoming shrivelled and forming scabs 1—2 days later before drying out and dropping. The pigmentation will remain a few days. The characteristic varicella and rashes are distributed in the centripetal form more on the face and body than on the limbs. They will continuously appear in batches lasting 3— 5 days, so the rashes of different shapes and sizes in several periods can be seen. The disease is most common in winter and spring, rare in other seasons. The incidence is highest among children of one to six years old. One attack confers permanent immunity. Varicella is classified as one of the epidemic febrile diseases in tradition al Chinese medicine.

General Nursing

1. Refer to the characteristics of paediatrics nursing(6、1).

2. Since varicella is a serious infectious disease, the patients should be isolated from others to prevent touching or cross infection of respiratory tract until smallpox eruptions have become dry and formed scabs. All staff having contact with varicella patients should wear gauze mask and quarantine clothing.They should soak their hands in peracetic acid 1% solution after contact. The sick children's toys and eating utensils should be sterilized. Wards should be well ventilated. The air should also be sterilized.

3. The food should be light, easily digested and nutritious. Peppery and irritating food and sea food which can have a relapse should be avoided.

4. The beds should be kept clean and dry. Clothes and quilts should be soft, loose and comfortable to prevent the skin with varicella from being broken. The under— clothes should be

changed frequently and baths should be taken only in warm water. Neither showers nor cold baths should be taken as these may cause the small pox eruptions to ulcerate producing secondary infection.

5. The sick child's hands should be kept clean, the finger nails should be cut to prevent small—pox eruption from being scratched and broken causing secondary infection. When the skin itches, calamine washing solution or 5% solution of sodium bicarbanate can be applied externally to relieve itch. If the pox have been scratched, gentian violet 1% can be used to keep the eruption dry. *Chaqing San* (Powder of Chaqing) or *Qingdai San* (Powder of Indigo) can be applied to the skin.

6. The sick child should have bed rest, drinking plenty of boiled water, fruit juice, or gram soup to clear away heat, remove toxic material and lower the temperature.

7. The oral cavity, eyes and outer pudenda should be given special attention. If the smaupox eruption occurs in the eyes, erythromycin ointment may be applied or choloromyeatin liquid for eyes dripped to protect the eyes. If the oral cavity and the mucosa of outer pudenda ulcerate, *Bingpeng San* (Powder Made of Borneol and Sodium Borate) , *Xilei San* may be applied to the affected part, 2—3times a day.

8. The children who have contact with the sick children are easily infected with the disease.Quarantine should be observed for 21 days. They may be given an intramuscular injection with gamma globulin as a precaution.

9. Hormone treatment is contraindicated in case the virus spreads and the disease worsens.

Nursing According to Syndrome Differentiation

1.The Syndrome of Both *Wei* and *Qi* Systems　(the light type)

Clinical Manifestations

Slight fever, cough, rhinorrhea, thin distribtion of small—pox eruptions with clear liquid. itchiness, normal spirit and appetite, thin, white and yellow tongue coating, floating and rapid pulse.

Nursing

(1) During the period of pox eruptions of varicella, the patient should have complete bed rest, keeping their body warm. The patient should be protected from cold and wind, and sweat should be wiped off with a soft towel. Observe carefully the temperature, the density of eruption, its shape, colour distribution as well as the symptoms of whole body, keeping a note of all such conditions.

(2) Medicine should be administered to expel pathogenic wind and promote sweating to eliminate the exogenous pathogens from the body surface and clear away heat and damp. The appropriate prescription is *Yin qiao San* with modification (Modified Powder of Lonicera and Forsythia) . They should not be decocted in water for too long.

(3) If the patient has a slight fever, do not attempt to lower the temperature, but let him drink plenty of water, pear or orange juice.

(4) If the symptoms are not serious, Rhizoma Phragmitis 60 g , Flos chrysanthemi Indici 10 g, Flos Lonicerae 12 g, Radix Glycyrrhizae 3 g are decocted in water for oral dose and taken as

tea.

2. The Syndrome of *Qi* and *Ying* Systems (serious type)

Clinical Manifestations

High fever, vexation, or sleepiness small—pox eruption on the whole body, spreading to the hands and feet, big blisters with dim liquid, red ring around the blisters, or deep and purple colour, bleeding halo, yellow and greasy tongue coating, full and rapid pulse.

Nursing

(1) Administer medicine for clearing *Qi* and cooling *Ying*. The prescription chosen should be the decoction for clearing away the eruptions and expelling toxic materials. The decoction should be drunk cold.

(2) The sick child with high fever should have complete bed rest, drink plenty of water or a decoction made from Folium Bambusae 15 g, Rhizoma Phragmitis 30 g taken as tea to reduce fever. Observe carefully the change of temperature and the eruption condition. If the high fever does not lower, the poxes are very dense, the colour of poxes is bright red or dark purple and the liquid of bleb is dim, this indicates a syndrome caused by the toxic materials and heat stored in the body and blood. The Cornu Rhinoceri and Cornu Antelopis may be added to the decoction. If the patient has fainted due to emotional upset, refer to the nursing of the high fever 2.1.

(3) Take great care of the patients with small—pox eruptions to avoid secondary infection or more serious condition from developing. Special treatment should be given to those who have pox eruptions around the eyes, outer pudenda and ulcerated poxes. Refer to the general nursing for medicine for external use.

6.4　Epidemic Parotitis

Epidemic parotitis is an acute infectious disease in the respiratory tract which is characterized as fever, swelling and pain in the lower part of the ears—parotid. During the onset, the sick child has a fever and sore throat like the symptoms of a cold, but with one or both sides at the lower section of parotid becoming swollen 1—2 days later. Some patients have fever and parotid swelling simultaneously. The swelling develops slowly and has a feeling of pressing pain, but the affected area does not turn red and has no distinct boundary. Sometimes the submaxillary gland and sublingual gland become swollen early or later, the intrabuccal parotid duct may also become swollen. The course of the disease lasts about 1—2 weeks. It is termed "sudden swelling parotid", " *Hama Wen* " in TCM. This is a kind of epidemic febrile disease and occurs at any time during the year, but most frequently in spring and winter. It is common among of preschool—age and school—age children. The patients can be confered a permanent immunity after recovery.

General Nursing

1. Refer to the characteristic nursing of paediatrics

2. Strict isolation measures should be taken for the respiratory tract until the swelling of the parotid gland has disappeared. Eating utensils should be sterilized in boiling water.

3. The sick child should have complete bed rest until parotid swelling has disappeared. The patients with mild symptoms can walk around in the ward, but should avoid any possibility of developing complications.

4. Nutritious food, low in fat and salt is the most suitable. Sour and peppery food should be avoided as it will irritate the intrabuccal parotid duct causing pain. If the parotid gland becomes seriously swollen making opening of the mouth and chewing difficult, solid food should also be avoided.

5. Special care should be taken of the oral cavity. When the intrabuccal parotid duct is swollen, the oral cavity must be kept clean to prevent bacteria entering the parotid gland and causing suppurative inflammation. A decoction of Radix isatidis and light salt water can be used to rinse the mouth and clean the oral cavity for the sick baby.

6. Observe carefully the degree of pain or swelling of parotid gland, change of temperature, pulse condition, state of mind and condition of testicle to ascertain the extent of the disease and whether complications may develop. If symptoms such as high fever, vague mind, vomiting and stiff neck appear, it indicates complicated meningitis. If the symptoms of upper abdominal pain, vomiting and high fever appear, it indicates complicated pancreatitis. The complicated testitis and ovaritis will probably appear among children in late puberty The observation will continue for 3—4 weeks after illness.

7. External treatment: Medicinal paste may be applied to the swollen area of the parotid gland to reduce the swelling and relieve pain. The area of application should extend beyond the swollen area. It should be cleaned off and replaced once or twice daily. The local area must be kept clean. The medicines for external application and their uses are as follows:

(1) *Daqing Gao, Dahuang Gao, Furong Gao* can be used for external application.

(2) *Ruyi Jinhuang San* is mixed with warm water for external application.

(3) *Zijing Ding* or *Qingdai San* are ground and mixed with vinegar for external application.

(4) Mirabilitum and Indigo Naturalis in same amounts are mixed with vinegar into paste for external use.

(5) *Wanying Xiaohe Gao* may be used for external application after cleaning the affected part in warm water.

(6) Choose one of the following, Herba Portulacae, Herba Taraxaci or fresh cactus to crush into paste, add Borneolum Syntheticum 0.5 g each time and mix them together for external application.

(7) Fructus Evodiae 12 g should be ground into fine powder and flour 30 g added, then mixed with vinegar (which is decocted in clay pot) into paste and applied to the sole of the feet before sleep to lower the pathogenic fire from the upper part to lower part.

(8) The cupping method (a cup in which a partial vacuum is created over an acupoint for therapeutic purpose) may be used on one side over the swollen area, once a day. The disease can usually be cured with one or two applications of this treatment.

8. The child who has contact with the patient easily suffers from this disease. A decoction made from *Banlangen* (isatis root) 15—30 g may be taken or granules of the isatis root after being infused in boiled water can be taken, too for 3—5 days.

Nursing According to Syndrome Differentiation

1.The Syndrome of Stagnated Heat in Difensive System (slight type)

Clinical Manifestations

Lower fever, sore throat, nausea, vomiting, swelling parotid gland, a sense of sour and distension while masticating, the normality of mental disposition and appetite, gradual disappearance of swelling and recovering 3—5 days later, thin and white tongue coating, floating and rapid pulse.

Nursing

(1) Administer medicine for expelling wind pathogen, clearing away heat, dispersing swelling and the accumulation of pathogens. The prescription chosen should be *Yingqiao San* with modification (Modified Powder of Lonicera and Forsythia) .

(2) In the treatment the simple recipe should be used cooperatively with the proven prescription, For example, seven scorpions fried in sesame oil may be taken at a draught, once daily, continously for 3 days. The sick baby may take the powder made from fried scorpions which have been ground into fine powder with water.

(3) Semi—liquid and soft food such as eggs soup, porridge and noodles is better for the sick child.

(4) The sick child with low fever should drink much water, or water soaked from Flos Chrysanthemi 6 g, Spica Prunellae 10 g, may be taken as tea.

2. The Syndrome of Heat Stagnation in *Ying* and *Wei* Systems (serious type)

Clinic Manifestations

High fever, headache, lethargy, vexation, nausea, vomiting, swelling, pain or tenderness of parotid area, difficulty in opening mouth and masticating, swollen in lower jaw, dry stool, oliguria with reddish urine, or appearance of complications, thin, yellow and greasy tongue coating, smooth and rapid pulse.

Nursing

(1) This syndrome indicates the stagation of heat, so medicine for clearing away heat and removing toxic materials, dispersing the swelling and the accumulation of pathogens should be taken. The prescription chosen should be *Puji Xiaodu Yin* with modification (Modified Universal Relief Decoction for Disinfection) the decoction should be taken cool.

(2) External treatment refers to general nursing. The simple recipe and proven prescription are the same as for the syndrome of stagnated heat in *Wei* system.

(3) Liquid food, such as milk, egg soup, bean milk and lotus root starch, is more suitable.

(4) The patient with high fever, feels thirsty and tends to fidget as a result of inward transmission of the pathogenic heat. To counter serious heat pathogen and loss of body fluid, the patients should drink much water or cool beverage, such as *Juhua Lu, Banlangeng Ye* (liquid of dyers woad root Liquor Radicis Isatidis) or gram soup. Alternatively, acupuncture may be used on points Dazhui (DU14) , Quchi (LI11) and Hegu (LI4) to lower the temperature. If the temperature still does not lower, *Linyang Fen* (Powder of Antelope's Horn) or *Angong Niuhuang Wan* (Bezoar Bolus for Resurrection) can be taken.

(5) If vomiting occurs frequently, *Yushu Dan* may be taken in infusion. The oral cavity must be kept clean.

(6) If the patient suffers from constipation, senna leaves are soaked in water for drinking as tea. The patient should often eat bananas and even have an enteroclysis with glycerine if necessary.

(7) If the texticle becomes swollen and orchidoptosis causes

some pain, the testicle can be supported by a T—ban—dage to reduce the pain, the Herba Portulacae and Herba Taraxaci are decocted in water to fumigate or wash the scrotum. Acupuncture may be used on points Sanyinjiao (SP6) and Xuehai (SP10), once a day or Chinese medicine may be applied externally to the affected part. (Refer to the external treatment of general nursing)

6.5 Epidemic Encephalitis B

Epidemic Encephalitis B is a type of acute infectious disease char acterized by sudden attack, headache, high fever, coma and clonic convulsion. It is a vital infection carried by mosquitoes. It often occurs from July to September of summer and autumn. Children of 3—6 years old are easily affected. It is classified as an epidemic febrile disease in traditional Chinese medicine. It is known as " syncope due to summer heat" or " summer heat spasm". The sick child with mild symptoms will generally recover after 7— 10 days while those with more severe symptoms may take 2—3 weeks. During the emergency period, the complications of unconsciousness and collapse may occur and endanger life. The patient who has suffered from this disease for six months and still has symptoms, may retain sequelae.

General Nursing

1. Refer to the charateristics of paediatrics nursing.

2. The sick child should be isolated in a ward which has facilities to prevent the entry of mosquitoes nutil the temperature becomes normal. The sick child with severe symptoms should be placed in an emergency room. The ward temperature should be

kept between 24—26℃. The humidity should be regular and suit able.

3. High—protein food and sufficient water should be supplied to the patients, especially to those with continuous high fever, convulsion and profuse sweating. The food and water must be sufficient to promote the vital functions. Milk, thick bean milk, porridge cooked with mung bean powder and red bean powder with some sugar should be provided. Water should be supplied not only intravenously, but also in the form of juice of water melon, Bulbus Lilii and mung bean soup for drinking. Those who are unconscious and enable to eat should be given nasal feeding. Those who are conscious during the recovery period should be given semi—liquid and soft food.

4. Maintain oral hygiene. The sick child with a high fever can use Herba Agastachis water （Agastache Herba Agastachis 30 g decocted in water 200 ml） to clean the oral cavity, *Bingpeng You* （*Bingpeng San* 5 g, Sesame oil 10 g） is applied to keep the mucosa moist and prevent the oral cavity from infection. The patient who has high fever and loses consciousness should have oil applied to the nasal and lip area which are covered with wet gauze to keep the mouth, lip and respiratory tract moist.

5. Keep the respiratory tract clear. The child, who has convulsions, and becomes unconscious, easily produces obstruction of the respiratory tract, even suffocating due to cough, The obstacles to swallowing function, the accumulation of saliva and sputum should be cleared away so that respiration is unobstructed. The sick child should lie in a lateral recumbent position and turn over frequently . The back should be patted to promote the discharge of sputum and the blood circulation of the lungs. If the

sick child has ascaridis, it may manifest as nausea, vomiting cough due to irritation or convulsion as the ascarides are antiperistaltic in the esophagus oral cavity and trachea. Once this happens, the ascarides must be promptly removed. If the child has difficulty in breathing, oxygen should be supplied.

6. The child who is in bad condition or loses consciousness and becomes paralytic easily suffers from bed sores. It is essential that the bed should be flat, soft, tidy and dry. The skin must be kept clean to eliminate the bed sores. The paralytic limbs must be massaged to promote *Qi* and blood circulation and recovery of the organ's functions.

7. The sick child with unconsciousness and fecal and urinary incontinence must have his diapers changed frequently. The buttock should be kept clean and dry. If the urinary passage is blocked and the bladder is distended, the points Yinbao (LR9) and Jimen (SP11) should be massaged for 2—3 minutes, then the bladder from right to left.

8. Observe the disease condition. It develops very quickly at the acute period. Close attention must be paid to the sick child's mental state, consciousness, temperature, breathing, pulse, blood pressure and changes of pupil so that respiratory and heart failure, convulsion, bleeding, asphyxia and other complications can be found as soon as they develop.

Nursing According to Syndrome Differentiation

1. During the Acute Period
(1) Syndrome of Both *Wei* and *Qi* System
Clinical Manifestations
Sudden attack of fever with slight or no sweat, redness of

face and conjunctival congestion, headache, vomiting, lethargy, stiff—neck, oliguria with reddish urine, thin, white, yellowish and greasy tongue coating, floating and rapid pulse.

Nursing

a. Administer medicine for relieving exterior syndrome, clearing away and removing summer heat. The prescription chosen is based on *Yinqiao San* (Modified Powder of Lonicera and Forsythia) and *Baihu Tang* (White Tiger Decoction) with modification. They should be decocted in water for a short time.

b. The patient should rest in bed and drink plenty of water. A cold dressing may be put on the forehead. If palpitation due to fright and unrest or unconsciousness occurs, *Huichun Dan* 3—5 tablets or *Niuhuang Zhengjing Wan* (Bozoar Bolus for Relieving Convulsion) one pill may be taken in infusion to clear away heat, relieve convulsion and eliminate phlegm for resuscitation.

c. The patient who vomits constantly should lie in a lateral recumbent position, the head turned to the side to avoid vomitus entering the trachea causing obstruction to breathing. *Yushu Dan* may be taken to resolve turbid pathogen and stop vomiting. Acupuncture to stop vomiting may also be used on points: Zhongwan (RN12), Neiguan (PC6), Zusanli (ST36), Gongsun (SP4), or Hegu (LI4) is rubbed.

(2) The Syndrome of Intense Heat in Both *Qi* and *Yin* 9 systems

Clinical Manifestations

More severe condition, over 40℃ temperature after 3—4 days, higher fever, profuse sweating, thirst, restlessness, delirium, unconsciousness, stiff neck with repeated convulsions; yellow, thick and rough coating, bright red tongue, full rapid or wiry rapid pulse.

Nursing

a. This is the peak period of encephalitis B: high fever, convulsion and unconsciousness are the three main symptoms which are characterized as accumulation of interior heat, sputum, pathogenic wind combining together. The condition is dangerous and easily changable, so that the patient should be under intensive care. Watch carefully for changes of disease in order to handle the complex situation in cooperation with doctor's treatment.

b. Administer medicine for clearing *Qi*, cooling blood, nourishing *Yin*,clearing away heat, relieving convulsions and calming the endopathic wind. The selected prescription should be based on *Baihu Tang* (Modified White Tiger Decoction) and *Qingying Tang* (Decoction for Clearing Heat in the *Ying* System) with modification. The decoction should be cool and taken slowly.

c. The nursing of high fever (Refer to the nursing of high fever 2.1)

If the temperature is over 40℃ , measures for lowering the temperature must be taken to prevent the patient from convulsion and cerebral edema. The temperature in the room should be lowered and kept under 26℃ . The patient may be rubbed with a towel dipped in warm water or 30% warm alcohol to lower the temperature. Put an ice bag on the head and the main artery of the neck. The patient should have an enema with cold salt water if necessary. Acupuncture should be done on the points: Dazhui (DU14) , Quchi (LI11) , Hegu (LI4) and Fengfu (DU16) . If the patient continues to sweat heavily, the point Fuliu (KI7) may also be needled.

d. Nursing for convulsions. belts, cords and tight clothing must be removed to avoid restricting breathing. A board with gauze around it for pressing the tongue should be put between upper and lower teeth to prevent the tongue from being bitten. A protecting board should be placed round the bed to prevent the patient from falling down. Acupuncture should be also given to points: shuigou (DU26), Hegu (LI4), Taichong (LR3), Neiguan (RC6), An Mian and Yongquan (KI1). The propictary *Zixue Dan* 1—2 g, *Angong Niuhuang Wan* (Bezoar Bolus for Resurrection) 1／2—1 pill and *Zhibao Dan* 1／2—1 pill may be taken in infusion as well twice daily. In addition an intravenous injection with *Xingnao Jing* 6—10 ml can be made, twice a day to wake up the patient from unconsciousness by clearing away heat, stop convulsion and restore consciousness.

e. Nursing of unconsciousness (refer to the nursing of unconsciousness 2.2). If the phlegm in the throat makes a rumbling sound, *Xuanzhu Li* 10—50 ml may be taken at a draught to reduce the secretion in the throat or *Houzao Fen* 0.3 g may be taken in infusion to dissolve the phlegm, open the channel, disperse and promote the functional activities of *Qi*. The patient who has lost consciousness and with the abnormal eyes open should be rubbed around the eyes with cotton ball soaked in normal saline solution followed by an application of eye ointment. In addition a wet gauze soaked in saline solution may be placed over the eyes to prevent the cornea from dryness. If the patient's swallowing is obstructed, nasal administration of medicine may be done.

f. Attend carefully to any changes of the disease to avoid causing prostration syndrome.

(3) The Syndrome of Attack of *Ying* and Blood Systems by Heat.

Clinical Manifestations

Constant high fever, serious unconsciousness, constant convulsions or trembling of hands and feet, stiff—body, contracture, some spots on the skin, hematemesis, hematochezia, parched lip, thin tongue coating, small and rapid pulse.

Nursing

a. The syndrome of attack of *Ying* and blood is a dangerous and serious stage indicating the peak period of encephalitis B. It is the key stage which will determine whether or not there will be sequel. Combined treatment and nursing measures should be taken in order to save the patient from dangerous and emergent disease.

b. Administer medicine for cooling the blood, removing the toxic materials, clearing the heat, opening the channels, tranquilizing the mind and calming the endopathic wind. The prescription chosen should be *Shenxi Dan* with modification (Modified Miraculous Bolus of Rhinoceros Horn) . The decoction should be taken cool.

c. All measures for nursing of syndrome of intense heat in both *Qi* and *Ying* systems should be taken. The following measures should be added for the patient with constant high fever, clonic convulsion and unconsciousness according to the development of disease condition: *Linyang Fen* (Powder of Antelope's Horn) , *Xijiao Fen* (Powder of Rhinoceros Horn) 2 g may be taken in infusion for the patient with high temperature. At the same time the points *Shixuan* (EX—UE11) must be pricked for blood—letting. Point injection may be given to lower the temperature.

The patient with constant convulsions may take *Zhenjing San* (Powder of Relieving convulsion) 1.5—2 g or *Xiewei Fen* (Powder of Dry Scorpion Tail) 0.5—1 g with boiling water, twice a day. If the convulsions continue for a prolonged period, the patient should be given oxygen in high density to reduce the deficiency of oxygen in the brain.

If the patient has serious unconsciousness, red orpiment (Realgar) 1 g, Borneolum Syntheticum 0.3 g, powder of Spina Gleditsiae 0.3 g should be ground into fine powder and mixed with fresh grassleaves sweetflag rhizome juice to be taken 0.3—0.6 g each time, twice a day to resolve phlegm and restore consciousness.

d. The treatment of bleeding. Watch carefully for the position of any bleeding. If the nose is bleeding, a sterilized cotton ball or gauze can be applied to the nasal opening to stop the blood, The powder of Radix Pittospori, *Baibushuang* (plant soot), Lasiosphaera seu Calvatia and *Yunan Baiyao* (White medicinal powder for treating haemorrhage, wounds, bruises, etc) can be spread on the gauze which is wrapped to stuff the bleeding part. If the bleeding part is deep, gauze with vaseline can be used to stuff the bleeding part. At the same time a cold wet towel can be put on the forehead. The patient who spits blood or has hematochezia may take *Yunan Baiyao* 0.5—1.5 g, 3—4 times a day or *Daihuang Fen* (Pulvis Rhei), *Baiji Fen* (powder of bletilla tuber Pulvis Rhizoma Blettilae), Powder of cuttlebone (Pulvis os Sepiellae seu Sepiae) 1g each time and powder of root of noto—ginseng (Pulvis Radicis Notoginseng) 0.5 g dissolved in water and taken, three times a day. Observe carefully to ensure bleeding has stopped.

e. The prostration syndrome may be treated combining Chinese and western medical and nursing methods.

2. The Recovery Stage

The clinical manifestations at this stage differ markedly from person to person. The common symptoms are: lower fever, headache, mania, reticence, inactivity, dull expression, indistinct speaking, stiff—limbs, contracture, twitching of hands and feet and occasional epilepsy, etc.

Nursing

(1) The key of nursing at this stage is to relieve the symptoms and prevent any complications from developing. Apart from oral medicine, acupuncture, massage or injection at acupoints may be taken as the main therapy. The active and passive training of function with complex treatment and nursing can help the patient recover the ability of speaking, motion and coping with daily life.

(2) Highly nutritious food is needed to compensate for vital energy exhausted during the acute stage. Sea cucumber, chicken, fish should be cooked in soup and taken to tonify the kidney and strengthen the body resistance or restore normal functioning of the body to consolidate the constitution. The sick child who has difficulty in eating may need assistance and training. Nasal feeding may be given, if the child is unable to swallow. The unrse should train the sick child patiently to restore the swallowing function as soon as possible.

(3) The child who has paralysis and stiffness should be given careful skin protection to prevent the development of bed sores in addition to training his bodily functions. Keep the child warm, providing appropriate clothing according to the change of

climate, preventing him from external cold.

(4) If the child has difficulties in speaking, motion and coping with daily life or signs of development of insanity, close attention is essential to prevent possible accidents.

6.6   Scarlet Fever

Scarlet fever is an acute infectious eruptive disease, characterized by fever , laryngeal swelling,pain and ulcer,bright red diffuse rashes on whole body,desquamation in pieces after disappearance of rashes. The onset is abrupt. The skin rashes will appear in 1—2 days. They spread quickly from the neck, chest,back to the whole body. The characteristic of scarlet fever is that paleness round the mouth and strawberry—like tongue will appear. The desquamation in pieces will occur after the disappearance of rash, especially on the hands and feet. It is known in traditional Chinese medicine as " rash with decayed throat," " red rash" and "throat infections". It is regarded as being within the range of epidemic febrile diseases and often attacks in spring and winter. Children of 2—8 years old are particularly prone to it.

General Nursing

1. Refer to the characteristics of paediatric nursing (6.1) .

2. The patient must be strictly isolated to prevent secondary infection of the respiratory tract. The isolation should continue for 6—7 days from the onset to the disappearance of the disease. The clothes, quilts, eating utensils, toys and necessities of the sick child should be sterilized carefully.

3. The ward must be well ventilated and maintained at a

suitable temperature. The child should remain in bed during the eruption of rashes. Close attention must be paid to any heart complications. The activity of the sick child should be carefully controlled during the recovery period. Urine should be examined at regular intervals 1—2 weeks after the onset of the disease for the possible development of nephritis.

4. Hygiene of the oral cavity must be maintained. Wash it, using *Shuanghua Shui* (Decoction of honeysuckle flower) or warm salt water after meal or before sleep. The older sick child may gargle frequently to reduce pharyngeal swelling, remove the toxic materials and clean up the discharges from nose and throat.

5. Keep the skin clean. If the skin is itchy at the period of eruption, it may be relieved with a decoction of Radix Ledebouriellae, Cortex Dictamni Radicis and Fructus Cnidii applied to the skin or oil can be used to it, if there is dryness. Soapy water should not be used to wash the skin.At the period of desquamation calamine lotion may be applied and rubbed on the skin or the sick child may take a bath in the above mentioned decoction to relieve itch. If the skin has the phenominon of desquamation in large pieces, they may be cut with a pair of sterilized scissors. They should not be torn or peeled off by hand. The fingernails of the sick child should be kept short to prevent secondary infection from scratching the skin. The bed and quilt must be kept clean.

6. The food should be liquid or semi—liquid, nourishing, bland, neither too salty, nor too sweet. If pharyngitis develops, the pharynx will be irritated and hence made more painful by eating sour food, but sufficient water should be provided to the sick child.

Nursing According to Syndrome Differentiation

1. The syndrome of the pathogenic factor in the lung— *Wei* system (mild type)

Clinical Manifestations

Sudden attack of fever, chill, sore throat, red swelling and ulcer, little eruption of scarlet rashes, white or white and greasy tongue coating, floating and rapid pulse.

Nursing

(1) Administer the medicine for clearing away the heat and relieving sore—throat. The prescription should be *Yingqiao Mabo Shegan Tang* with modification (Modified decoction made of Lonicera, Forsythia, puff—ball and blackberry lily). Profuse Perspiration must be avoided.

(2) If the throat is painful and swollen, *Houzheng Wan* (pill for relieving sore throat) can be taken. Threat insufflation of *Qingdai San* (Powder of Indigo) and *Zhu Huang San* can be used 3—4 times daily, or *Qing Yang Wu Hua Ye* (Aerosol) can be used for clearing the throat with spraying inhalation, once or twice a day.

(3) Food which is swallowed easily, such as thin porridge, cooked wheaten food, egg soup and milk should be provided. The patient should drink plenty of fruit juice or decoction of fresh reed rhizome as tea.

2. Syndrome of Intense Heat in Both *Qi* and *Ying* Systems (serious type)

Clinical Manifestations

High fever, red cheeks, swollen, ulcerative and painful pharyngeal portion, scarlet rash spreading over the whole body, being more serious on back and chest, itching, thirst, dry stool,red strawberry—like tongue with small sticking, full and rapid pulse.

Nursing

(1) Administer medicine for removing toxic materials and relieving feverish rash. The prescription chosen should be *Qingwen Baidu Yin* with modification （Modified Antipyretic and Antitoxic Decoction）.The decoction is best taken cool.

(2) The treatment for the partial pharyngeal portion is the same as for the syndrome of pathogenic factor in lung—*Wei* system.

(3) Observe any change of temperature carefully.High fever of 39—40℃ during the period of eruption is common. The temperature will come down when the rash has erupted throughout the body. Watch carefully for any change of pulse rate or development of arrhythmia, convulsion and coma.

(4) Liquid food should be provided for the sick child. Water must be compensated timely for impairment of body fluids due to high fever. Drinks sweet in flavor, cool in nature and promoting the production of body fluids may be given, such as pear juice, water chestnut juice, lotus root juice or decoction of fresh reed rhizome （Rhizoma Phragmitis）, taken as tea.

6.7 Whooping Cough

Whooping cough is characterized as paroxysmal, spastic cough companied with laryngeal stridor during inhalation in clinical manifestation. This disease may occur in any season, but is more common in spring and winter. Infants from new—born up to the age of 5 years old are particularly prone. The younger the child is, the more serious the disease. Many complications tend to develop. Whooping cough may be spread through epidemic. Traditional Chinese Medicine calls it "paroxysmal cough", "Infectious cough" and cough due to renal deficiency.

General Nursing

1. Refer to the characteristics of paediatrics nursing.

2. The patient should be strictly isolated to prevent secondary infection of the respiratory tract. Isolation should continue from the onset of the disease for 40 days or from the onset of spasms and cough for 30 days. The clothes, quilts and necessities must be exposed to the sun or ultraviolet rays or may only be reused after boiling sterilization. Clothes and quilts must be often exposed to the sun and kept thoroughly clean.

3. The air in ward should be well ventilated, clear and completely free from smoke and the ward should be kept quiet. Dust and any kind of irritating smell should be avoided, so as not to evoke spastic cough.

4. The child must have thorough rest and sufficient sleep. If he coughs severely at night and is unable to sleep, powder of Chinese date kernel may be taken in infusion. Auricular—plaster therapy (According to the result of auricular diagnosis, a bean or seed of vaccaria segetalis is taped tightly to a particular ear acupuncture point and pressed as to stimulate the point for therapeutic purpose) can be taken in ear point of Shenmen (HT7) to help sleep. A sedative tranquilizer can be used if necessary.

5. The food should contain sufficient quantity of heat, rich nutrition. It should be easily digestive, liquid or semi—liquid.

Too sweet, salty, cold and hot food should be avoided. Food should be eaten slowly to avoid evoking cough. Pungent and irritating food or other food with unpleasant smell should be avoided.

6. The child needs gentle, psychological care as he suffers from the torment and pain due to spastic cough and has nervous emotion, he must be kindly and patiently cared for and comforted. He should not be made to laugh or cry loudly. Organize the older sick children to play nonvigorous games such as telling stories and reading picture books. Try best to make them quiet and divert their attention to reduce the attack of cough.

7. Pay attention to the nursing of oral cavity. Since the sick child may have spastic cough and vomiting for a long time, the absorption of vitamin B is influenced, tunica mucosa oris and tongue body, especially the frenulum of tongue may have erosion or ulceration, so the oral cavity should be paid special attention to keep clean. (Refer to the nursing of measles)

8. When the child suffers from the attack of spastic cough, he should lie in lateral recumbent position or in sitting position to avoid vomitus entering the trachea, Pat the sick child's back and change his lying position to promote his breath and reduce cough. If the phlegm is thick and ropy, aerosol medicine for removing heat from sick child's lungs can be used as aerosol inhalation to make the phlegm become thin and easily expectorated. If the spastic cough is serious, medicine for expelling phlegm can be taken, but medicine for relieving cough should not be taken to avoid the obstruction of lung *Qi*. A belt can be bound around the abdomen to avoid urinary and fecal incontinence, proctoptosis and hernia.

9. Observe the prolonged time of paroxysmal cough, the degree of severity of cough, the colour, the nature and quantity of phlegm, breath, complexion and consciousness. Observe the condition of sweat, vomiting, nosebleed, the bleeding spot on the skin and convulsion

10. The cupping method (applying a cup in which a partial vacuum is created over an acupoint for therapeutic purpose and massage therapy) may be used as an auxiliary therapy for removing the heat from the lungs, sending down adversely ascending Qi, relieving cough and resolving phlegm.

(1) Cupping should be done at points Feishu (BL13) and Dazhui (DU14), once a day, alternating between the two points day by day. The time of cupping should be 5—15 minutes each time. If it is too long, blisters will appear on the skin.

(2) Massage therapy may be frequently used to clear the lung channel of hand Taiyin. Knead the point Xiao Tianxin press and knead Tiantu (RN 22), push and press Danzhong (RN 17), palm—rub the rib area press and knead Feishu (BL 13) and Geshu (BL17).

11. Any child in the age group prone to this disease who has close contact with the sick child should be kept under quarantine observation for 23 days. An intramuscular injection of gamma globulin may be given as a precautionary measure. All babies upon reaching the age of two months should be inoculated with the triple vaccine "ria—pertussis—stetanus". The child should be given three injections during the course of the treatment, then more injections regularly to promote long lasting immunity.

Nursing According to Syndrome Differentiation

1. The Primary Stage of Cough

Clinical Manifestations

The primary stage of cough refers to the time from the onset of the disease to the development of spastic cough, generally for 7 —10 days at first attack of cough, rhinorrhea and slight fever. 1— 2 days later relieving of fever and cold caused by exopathogenic factor, but appearance of more serious cough, thin, white or yellowish tongue coating,floating and rapid pulse.

Nursing

(1) At this stage, the risk of infection is very high, isolation should be carefully carried out.Visiting should be strictly control- led so as to prevent cross infection. The air in wards should be thoroughly sterilized. Advise the patient to wear a mask before his diagosis is confirmed. He should not go out and contact with othet children.

(2) Administer medicine for stopping cough and venti- lating the lungs, relieving exterior syndrome and resolving phlegm, The prescription chosen should be *Sangju Yin* with modi- fication (Modified Decoction of Mulberry leaf and Chrysan themum) .

2. The Stage of Spastic Cough

Clinical Manifestations

From spastic cough to gradual weak symptoms, the period generally lasting for 2—6 weeks or about 2 months, paroxysmal cough, frequent and constant cough, noisy rhinorrhea with run- ning tears, laryngeal stridor during inhalation and vomiting, mild symptoms in the day time becoming worse at night, puffy face with eyes and nose bleeding, hemorrhagic spots on the face, especially round the eyeball socket, white and yellow tongue coating and strong pulse.

Nursing

(1) Administer medicine for relieving sputum and stopping cough. The prescription chosen should be *Suting Guntang Wan* with modification (Modified Suting Pills for Resolving Phlegm). The medicine Centipede Scolopendra and Radix Glycyrrhiza in the same amount are ground into fine powder 1—2 g of which is mixed with honey water for oral dose to be taken, three times daily. In addition a fresh gall bladder of chicken with sugar in suitable amount can be taken by the sick child 1—2 years old, half a bladder taken each time, twice daily. A whole bladder may be taken by the sick child over 2 years old, 1—2 times daily.

(2) The sick child should remain in bed and avoid unnecessary irritation. The examination, treatment and nursing should be done together to prevent the sick child from evoking spastic cough unnecessarily.

(3) Careful nursing is needed while eating. Fearing that eating may cause cough and vomiting, the sick child sometimes refuses to take food, the nurse should encourage the sick child to eat willingly or should patiently and carefully feed him. The sick child must stop eating while coughing so as to prevent the food entering the trachea and causing asphyxia. If the sick child vomits after eating, the food should be compensated for nutritional purposes. Carrot,pear and water chestnut juice may be drunk to resolve phlegm, nourish the lung,stop cough and promote the production of body fluid.

(4) When the sick baby is constantly attacked by spastic cough, he should be put under intensive care to ensure that

vomitus does not enter the trachea. The baby sometimes can not expectorate the ropy sputum which will block the trachea and may feel suffocated, leading to asphyxia or tic.The nurse should draw the sputum out and provide oxygen therapy and artificial respiration as emergency measures under the doctor' s supervision.

(5) Observe carefully any change of disease conditions and be prepared to deal with any complications. If high fever, asthma and nares flaring occur or the patient becomes unconscious, or develops convulsions due to high fever. the heat— blockage of lungs, brain and the complications of pnuemonia and cerebritis are indicated and emergency measures must be taken.

3. The Recovery Stage

Clinical Manifestations

About 2—3 weeks at the recovery stage, weakening and disappearance of paroxysmal spastic cough, tiredness, dull expression, low spirit, profuse sweating, white and thin coating on the tongue, slight and weak pulse.

Nursing

(1) At the later stage of spastic cough, the patient should take medicine for invigorating *Qi,* and nourishing *Yin,* moistening the lung and invigorating the spleen, because both the pathogenic factor and body resistance are weakened. the prescription should be *Renshen Wuweizi Tang* with modification (Modified Ginseng and Schisandra Fruit Decoction) .

(2) Dietetic nursing. As recovery progresses, more nutritious food should be gradually eaten to restore or reinforce the lungs and spleen. Milk, eggs, chicken soup and lean meat are suitable. Fresh vegetables, fruits, cool drinks and porridge cooked

with Radix Ginseng, Radix Astragali seu Hedysari, Bulbus Lilii and Radix Adenophorae Strictae or porridge cooked with tremella and Semen Phaseali should also be eaten to nourish the spleen, stomach, lungs and promote the production of body fluid. Food should be bland and the greasy food should fast to avoid producing sputum. Food should be varied so as to promote the appetite.

(3) The sick child easily catches cold because of his weakness and heavy sweating. After catching cold, the spastic cough will reappear, so sweat should be cleaned off with a towel to circumvent the possiblity of cold. The sick child should be encouraged to increase his activities to become fitter and have frequent exposure to the sun.

6.8 Paediatric Pneumonia

Pneumonia is a disease with inflammation in the respiratory tract. It is characterized as fever, cough and asthma, It occurs in all four seasons, but more often in spring and winter. The younger the age group, the higher the disease incidence and the more serious the condition is. Pneumonia may be a primary condition, but may also be a secondary condition arising from other diseases, such as coriza, measles, whooping cough and it may develop in the course of certain serious or long—standing diseases. In traditional Chinese medicine it is within the range of epidemic febrile disease known as"cough "and "syndrome of asthma".

General Nursing

1. Refer to the characteristics of paediatric nursing.
2. The isolation of the patient should be taken seriously.

Medical workers and visitors in contact with the sick child should wear masks to prevent cross infection.

3. The ward should be well ventilated with moist and sterilized air. The temperature should be suitable. The ward should be irradiated with ultraviolet ray once a day as a sterilization measure.

4. The sick children should be confined to bed, keep quiet to reduce the quantity of oxygen consumed and prevent possible heart failure. The sick children should be disturbed as little as possible, so examination, treatment and nursing should be coordinated to minimize disruption to their sleeping and rest. Their lying position should be changed regularly and their backs should be patted lightly to reduce the stasis of blood in lungs and phlegm obstructing the trachea.

5. Food should be bland, easily digestible, liquid and semiliquid. The sick children should drink much water. Greasy, pungent and irritative food should be avoided.

6. The oral cavity should be frequently cleaned with decoction of Cortex Magnoliae Officinalis and light salty water.

7. Ensure that the respiratory tract is kept clean, The patient with excessive secretions in the nasal and oral cavity should clean them out thoroughly. If too much phlegm is in the oral cavity, the nurse should encourage the patient to expectorate it, help him turn round and pat his back to ease expectoration or it may be drawn out with an aspirator if necessary. If the phlegm is too ropy and thick and not easily expectorated, ultrasonic nebulizative inhalation may be done to remove heat from the patient's lungs and make the phlegm dilute for easy discharge and promoting breathing. Examine the nasal catheter giving oxygen therapy carefully for any blockage.

8. Watch carefully for the sick child's complexion, temperature, respiration pulse, heart rate, and any change in liver size, the degree of severity of cough or asthma due to phlegm obstruction, changes in mental behaviour and the development of convulsions, etc. to find any complications at the early stage which may lead to heart failure and cerebritis.

Nursing According to Syndrome Differentiation

1. The Syndrome of Attack of Wind on the Lungs

The early stage of pneumonia may be divided into attack of wind—cold and wind—heat on lungs according to the different degree of pathogens.

(1) Attack of Wind—cold on the Lung

Clinical Manifestations

Fever, no sweat, cough, shortness of breath, white and thin phlegm, lack of thirst, white and thin tongue coating, normal tongue body, floating and tense pulse. This syndrome often occurs in the cold season.

Nursing

a. Ensure that the patient is kept warm. The clothes and ward temperature should be regulated according to the weather condition.

b. Administer medicine pungent in flavor and warm in nature for promoting the dispersing function of the lung. The prescription chosen should be *Hua kai San* with modification (Modified Powder for Relieving Bronchitis and Asthma) .it should be taken hot. After taking the decoction hot drinks and porridge may be taken. Cover the sick child with clothes and quilt to encourage some sweating. Observe the condition of sweating carefully.

c. Acupuncture should be given to Dazhui (DU14) , Quchi (LI11) , Hegu (LI4) while a high fever develops. Physical cooling therapy must be used carefully to avoid effection of the pathogenic agent dispelled from superficies.

d. Moxa roll moxibustion may be used to points Feishu (UB13) and Dazhui (DU14) to warm the lung and expel cold.

e. Cool food such as fruit and melon should not be given.

(2) Attack of Wind—heat on Lungs

Clinical Manifestations

Fever, sweating thirst, cough, ropy and yellow phlegm, shortness of breath and nares flaring, flushing complexion and lip, constipation or companied with mucous, red tongue body with yellow coating, floating and rapid pulse.

Nursing

a. The ward should be well ventilated. Clothes should be suitable, not too warm.

b. Administer medicine cool in nature for expelling fever, promoting the dispersing function of the lung and resolving phlegm. The prescription chosen should be *Maxin Shigan Tang* with modification (Modified Decoction of Ephedra, Apricot, Kernel, Gypeum and Licorice) . After taking the medicine, the sick child will sweat slightly.

c. If the symptoms of high fever and thirst appear, pear and water chestnut juice may be drunk and acupuncture may be used to lower the temperature at the same time. (The acupoint is the same as attack of wind—cold on lungs) .

d. If the expectorated phlegm is yellow and ropy, the decoction made of Flos Bambusae and Rhizoma Phragmitis may be drunk as tea or pear （one pear without peel）, the powder of Bulbus Fritillarial Cirrhosae 6 g and a little honey, which are mixed well, should be cooked and taken the juice frequently.

e. The sick child suffering from constipation should take *Dahuang pian* （rhubard tablets） or drink water with soaked pickled senna leaf as tea.

2. Accumulation of Phlegm and Heat in the Lung

Clinical Manifestations

High fever, vexation, yellow and ropy phlegm, difficult expectoration, flushing complexion, thirst, shortness of breath, flaring of nares, asthma due to raising shoulder and abdomen, purple round mouth, constipation or sometimes dilute and odorous, scanty urine, red tongue body with yellow coating, full and rapid pulse. This may easily develop to heart failure and encephalopathy. It is the advanced stage of pneumonia.

Nursing

（1） Administer medicine for clearing out the lung—heat and relieving asthma and cough. The prescription chosen should be *Qingfei Yin* with modification （Modified Decoction for Cleaning Away the Lung—heat）. The decoction is better taken cool.

（2） Food should be bland, liquid and semi—liquid. Too sweet food and cool drinks should not be taken to avoid promoting wetness and the production of phlegm. Orange, loquats, pears, water melons and fruit juice are beneficial in removing heat from lungs, nourishing *Yin* and resolving phlegm.

（3） The sick child whose temperature is over 39℃ should be confined to bed, drink much water. have the body rubbed with warm water or 30% warm alcohol or have a cold compress done on his forehead or be treated with acupuncture to lower the temperature on the same points as for wind—cold syndrome of lungs stroke. If the sick child has convulsions, *Wuli Huichun Dan* 3—5 pills may be taken once melted in water or the *Zixue Dan* 0.5—2 g can be taken once in infusion.

(4) If cough and a slight black ring round the mouth appear, continuous oxygen inhalation therapy should be given. If severe asthma, flaring of nares, purple complexion and hard breathing appear, the supplementory oxygen should be given continuously. The sick child must take a semisupination, his pillow must be higher to reduce the possibility of choking and to promote breathing.

(5) The sick child has a cough due to lung—heat or the phlegm is yellow and ropy but can not expectorate it easily, measures to eliminate phlegm should be taken. He should drink fresh bamboo juice, take *Chuanke San* (Powder for Relieving Asthma) or apply the *Chuanke San* (Powder for Relieving Asthma and Cough) mixed with vinegar to the acupoints Yongquan (KI1), Dachangshu (BL25) and he may also frequently drink decoction of green radish cut into slivers and taken with honey.

(6) In case of abdominal distension due to the disturbance of visceral function of intestine, the *Daihuang Fen* (Powder of Rhubarb) mixed with honey can be applied externally to the abdomen. Turpentine oil may be applied to the abdomen or an enema may be used to reduce abdominal distension and to assist regular breathing.

(7) The seriously sick child should be kept under observation at all times and watched for the appearance of dangerous

disease such as insufficiency of the heart— *Yang*, pathogenic factors lingering in pericardium, loss of consciousness and collapse. If the sick child has difficulty in breathing, pale and purple complexion, feels agitated and listless, has sweat and cool limbs, small and rapid pulse, the heart rate is faster than 160—200 times per minute and the liver becomes enlarged, complication of insufficiency and weakness of heart— *Yang* is indicated. Medical and nursing measures should be taken immediately and cooperatively. The sick child should immediately be given *Shenfu Longmu Jiuni Tang* or *Shenmai San* (Pulse—activating Powder). He should be kept warm and moxibustion applied to points Qihai (RN6), Guanyuan (RN4) and Shenjue (RN8) to make wetness nourish heart— *Yang* and give emergency treatment for collapse. The *Shenmai* (Palse activating) injection 10—20 ml, Jiski (fruit of citron) injection 5—10 ml and glucose injection 5 —10% diluted should be given as intravenous injection or drip. Cardiac stimulant should also be used without delay.

3. The Syndrome of Lingering Pathogens Due to Difficient Vital Energy

Clinical Manifestations

Long—term cough, phlegm —dyspnea, exacerbating due to the affection by exopathogens, lassitude, yellow complexion, poor appetite, cough with much sputum, sweating, low fever, red tongue body with white coating, small and rapid pulse, which are often seen during recovery stage of pneumonia.

Nursing

(1) At the recovery stage food for the sick child should be rich in nutrition. Food and dishes should be varied in order to stimulate the child's appetite. He should have plenty of fruits,

vegetables, dairy food, eggs, fish and lean meat to strengthen the spleen and replenish vital essence. If the *Yin* is deficient, the *Baihe Hongzao Tang* (Decoction of Lily Bulb and Chinese Date) should be taken. Litchis, loquats, pears and oranges are effective for nourishing lungs, promoting the production of body fluid and stopping cough.

(2) Administer medicine for replenishing *Qi,* nourishing *Yin,* clearing away the heat from lungs and removing phlegm. The prescription chosen should be *Buzhong Yiqi Tang* With modification (Modified Decoction for Reniforcing Middle— *Jiao* and Replenishing *Qi*) and *Shasheng Maidong Tang* (Modified Decoction of Glehnia and Ophiopogon)

(3) The sick child may have suitable physical activities to regulate the *Qi* and blood circulation, remove phlegm, reinforce the spleen and strengthen the health, but the time of actitivities must be limited. If the weather is suitable, the activities should be done outside with exposure to the sun. Take good precautions against cold and cross infection.

(4) Chronic persistent pneumonia: If persistent raucous sound remains in lungs, and the focus can still be seen through x —ray, physical therapy should be used, such as cupping therapy, mustard paste applied to the chest, ultrashort wave and ultraviolet ray therapy to promote the absorption of pathologic change.

6.9 Infantile Bronchial Asthma

Bronchial Asthma is a disease of the respiratory tract characterized by repeated onset of dypsnea. long expiration with wheeze. This disease may occur among new—born babies, but is most often seen among the children over 4—5 years of age. It is within the range of "syndrome of asthma" in TCM.

General Nursing

1. Refer to the characteristics of paediatric (6.1) .

2. Keep the ward quiet, the temperature and humidity suitable and stable. Facilities should be simple. Smoking must be forbidden and flowers and medicine with irritating smells should be kept out.

3. The patient must be kept warm to prevent catching cold, putting on more clothes promptly when the weather becomes clod. Especially the neck areas such as Tiantu (RN22) and Feishu (BL13) should be warm.

4. Food should be bland. Eating should not be excessive, The cool, raw, too sweet and salty food should not be eaten while the disease is attacking. At remission stage the sick child should eat easily digestible and absorbable food with rich nutrition and avoid eating anything which may evoke the attack of asthma such as milk, eggs, fish and shrimp. Greasy, pungent and irritating food should be contraindicated.

5. While the asthma is attacking, the sick child should remain in bed, taking a semireclining position or given a higher pillow to keep a comfortable position. The nurse should comfort the sick child and dispel his feelings of fear to avoid crying and making the disease more severe. At remission stage the sick child may be permitted to be have suitable exercises.

6. When the child has difficulty in breathing, oxygen therapy may be used at intervals, or Flos Daturae may be used as aerosal inhalation to ease the spasms of bronchus. The respiratory tract must be clear. Maintain hygiene of the oral cavity.

7. If asthma attack becomes serious and prostration of vital energy, shortness of breath and sweating appear, complexion, lip and fingernail are purple and livid, the limbs feel cold and pulse becomes small, the oxygen inhalation and *Shenfu Tang* (Decoction of Ginseng and Prepared Aconite) should be taken immediately to rescue from prostrating, the doctor should be reported and emergency treatment be prepared well.

8. Observe the disease condition.

(1) Note the time of attack, the seriousness or lightness of asthma, the condition of expectoration, the property of phlegm and the change of complexion and sweating.

(2) Watch for signs of impending attack, for example, the oppressed sensation of the chest, respiratory block, throat itch and dry cough, The prompt medical measures and early treatment can relieve, control and remit the symptoms. If asthma becomes regular, the patient should take medicine every 1—2 hours before the attack, which is beneficial to relieve and remit the symptoms.

(3) Observe the factors that evoke asthma, such as depressed emotion, sudden changeable climate, inhalation of dust, contact of pollen, fine hair, coal gas and paint. Look for the sensitinogen to avoid evoking asthma.

9. Asthma vaccine: Sanlian asthma vaccine made in China generally may be inoculated once a week or the long— acting preparation may be used once every 3—4 weeks until the attacks cease.

Nursing According to Syndrome Differentiation

1. The Stage of Attack

Some patients have some premonitory, symptoms appearing suddenly, for example. sudden nasal obstruction, sneezing, laryngeal itch and chest oppressed feelings and then the onset of asthma appears, some have no premonitory symptoms. They may have a sudden cough, short gasp, difficulty in breathing and are unable to lie on their back and have wheeziness in the larynx at the time of expiration, Asthma is classified into two kinds: cold and hot.

(1) The Syndrome of Cold Asthma

Clinical Manifestations

Sudden attack, grey and yellow complexion, cough, short gasp, wheeze in the larynx, nasal obstruction, speaking in low and deep voice, white, thin and foamy phlegm, no thirst, but preference for hot drinking, anhidrosis, white slippery tongue coating and floating, tense pulse.

Nursing

a. Cold asthma often occurs in spring and autumn. The pathogenic factor comes from wind—cold. The asthma will become heavier when the patient feels cold. The patient should be kept warm and avoid catching cold. The room should be warm and air must be circulated but the patient should not be directly exposed to draughts.

b. Administer medicine for promoting the dispersing function of the lung, dispelling cold, stopping cough and relieving asthma. The prescription chosen should be *Xiaoqinglong Tang* with modification (Modified Minor Decoction of Green Dragon). The decoction should be taken hot and *Dilong Fen* (Powder of Dilong) may be taken orally before meals at the same time, 1—3 g each time, three times a day to tranquilize the mind and relieve asthma.

c. The patient should avoid eating anything raw or cold.

d. At the attack stage of asthma, acupuncture, moxibustion, the auricular— plaster on ear points and cupping may be combined to control the symptoms. The points Dingchuan (EX–B1) , Jiechuan （Special asthma pt） , Tiantu （RN22) and Dazhui （DU14） should be needled, once a day.

If the patient has a serious asthma, the moxa roll moxibustion and cupping may be used cooperatively to Feishu (BL13) and Dazhui (DU14) .

Cupping therapy: First the needle is inserted into the point Pingchuan, followed by cupping therapy, with which the different sides of the body should be treated alternatly, once a day, ten minutes each time. The time of cupping should not be too long to avoid blistering the skin.

Auricular— plaster therapy on ear points: The points of asthma, endocrine and Pingchuan can be selected to treat various types of asthma.

The above therapies may be used singly at random or used alternately.

e. If the child coughs, having thin, clear white phlegm with foam after an attack of asthma, *Lengxiao Wan* （Pills for Relieving Asthma of Cold Type） may be taken for warming the lungs and resolving phlegm to relieve the symptoms and bring about a radical cure.

· (2) Syndrome of Asthma of Heat Type （asthma due to stagnation of hectic phlegm)

Clinical Manifestations

Sudden attack of asthma, flushing complexion, cough,

dyspnea, phlegm wheeze in larynx, rapid moving chest, heavy breath, vexation and uneasiness, thick, yellow and ropy phlegm, difficult expectoration, thirst, desire for drinking, sweating, greasy and yellow coating on the tongue, slippery and rapid pulse.

Nursing

a. The temperature in the room should be in the low side. Clean up the sweat immediately and change the wet clothes in time to prevent cold.

b. Administer medicine for clearing the heat, resolving phlegm, stopping cough and relieving asthma. The prescription chosen should be *Dingchuan Tang* with modification (Modified Asthma—Relieving Decocion), and decoction made from Semen Ginkgo 10g can be taken simultaneously, three times a day to nourish lungs, tonify the kidney and help inhalation.

c. If the phlegm is yellow, thick and can not be expectorated smoothly, pat the sick child's back lightly and allow him to drink *Shedan Chuanbei Ye* (Liquid made of Snake Gallbladder and Sichuan Fritillary Bulb) and *Xianzhuli Shui* (Fresh Bamboo Juice) to resolve phlegm and stop cough.

d. At the stage of attack, Borneolum Syntheticum 3 g can be mixed with vaseline 50 g to apply to the point Danzhong (RN17) . Acupunture, auricular—plaster and cupping therapy can be used in the same way as for the syndrome of asthma of cold type (1) .

2. The Remission Stage

As soon as the symptoms of repeated attack disappear, the remission stage will begin. The length of time of this stage has direct relation with the vital energy,deficiency and excess of body, the balance and coordination of three organs (lungs, spleen, kedney), and the changes of weather.

Clinical Manifestations

Emociation, cough with profuse sputum, shortness of breath on expertion, dyspnea, poor appetite, anorexia, tiredness, intolerance of cold, loose stool, feverish sensation over the palm and sole of the feet, night sweat, pale tongue, little tongue coating, deep and small pulse.

Nursing

(1) Herbs for tonifying the kidney, lungs and in vigorating the spleen should be taken. The selected prescription is based on *Jingui Shenqi Wan* (Bolus for Tonifying the Kidney—*Qi* of the Golden Chamber) and *Yupingfeng San* (Jadescreen Powder) with modification. If the child has feverish sensation over the palm and he sole of feet, night sweat due to deficiency of *Yin,* the prescription is based on *Liuwei Dihuang Wan* (Bolus of six Drugs Including Rehmannia) and *Yupingfeng San* (Jadescreen Powder) with modification and *Ziheche Wan* (Tablets made of Japasese Ardisia) should be taken together.

(2) Application method: Semen Sinapis Alba 3 g, Herba Asari 0.6 g pepper 1 g and Rhizoma Typhonii 1 g are ground into fine powder and mixed with ginger juice to be applied to the acupoint Feishu (BL13) before sleeping every night and removed in the next morning. If there is serious allergic reaction, the topical application of drug should be removed 1—2 hours later. It should be carried out once one or two days and there are seven days in one course of treatment.

(3) Keeping suitable temperature and striking a proper balance between activity and rest are important. The patient should

do suitable physical training out of doors, respire more in fresh air and be exposed to the sun in order to keep fit and reduce the chance of attack.

6.10 Stomatitis

Stomatitis is an oral disease characterized as hyperenia of mucous membrane, tongue and gingiva or oral herpes, erosion, ulceration, necrosis or the growing scab membrane due to pathologic change. It is generally a primary disease, but can develop into secondary disease. In traditional Chinese medicine it can be classified into "oral sore", " aphthae in children" and "acute ulcerative aphthae".

General Nursing

1. Oral hygiene is essential. The oral cavity should be rinsed with fresh saline solution, 3—4 times a day. If the mucous membrane has erosion and ulceration, the oral cavity should be cleaned with Folium Perillae, Cortex Magnoliae Officinalis decocted with water.

2. Prevent cross infection. The utensils for nursing the oral cavity must be sterilized. Seperate nursing utensils should be used for each patient. Hands should be washed before and after nursing. The milk bottle, breast — pump and tableware must be cleaned and sterilized after every use. If the child is breast—fed, the mother should be advised to maintain breast hygiene. She should wash the hands and clean the nipple with a cotton ball soaked in alcohol before breast —feeding. The sick child should be given water frequently rather than cleaning the oral cavity.

3. Food should be bland, not too acid,salty or irritative in order to relieve the difficulty of eating.If the sick child is breast — fed,the mother should not eat pungent and irritating food or drink alcohol. As the sick children often refuse to eat food because of pain, the nurse should feed them patiently.

Nursing Accoding to Syndrome Differentiation

1. Stagnated Heat in the Heart and Spleen
Clinical Manifestations
Bright red mouth and tongue, sore in oral cavity due to ulceration,ozostomia and pain, slobbering,anorexia, crying, restlessness, dry stool, oliguria with reddish urine, red tongue body, yellow, greasy and thick tongue coating, slippery and rapid pulse.

Nursing
(1) Heat— cleaning and fire — purging drug should be taken.

The prescription chosen should be *Qingre Xiepi San* with modification (Modified Powder for Clearing Away Heat and Purging the Spleen of Pathogenic Fire) . The decoction should be taken cool.

(2) The method for external treatment:

If the mouth and tongue become red and sores develop in the oral cavity due to ulceration, *Bingpeng San* can be mixed with honey to apply to the affected area for the mild symptoms, and *Xilei San,* (*Powder of Xilei*) *Zhuhuang San* and *Qingdai San* (Powder of Indigo) can be applied to the oral cavity for more serious symptoms. Fructus Evodiae 15 g can be ground into fine powder and mixed with vinegar to apply to the sole of feet for cooperative use, then removed 12 hours later. watch for the position of pathologic change carefully while applying the dressing. Observe carefully whether the original surface of the sores is healing, or whether new pathologic developments have appeared. No food or water should be taken within half an hour after applying the herbs to the oral cavity.

(3) If the sick child has dry stool, he should drink much fresh saline solution and have bananas and honey to loosen the bowel.

2. Flaring—up of Fire of Deficiency Type

Clinical Manifestations

Sores in mouth or on tongue, hyperemia on the surface of the sores, light persistent pain and ozostomia with long—standing case, long term repeated attack, vexation, thirst, flushing of zygomatic region, night sweat, feverish sensation over the palms and soles, red tongue, little coating on tongue and small, rapid pulse.

Nursing

The nursiag is basicly similar to the nursing of stomatitis.

(1) Medicine should be taken for nourishing *Yin,* clearing away heat, circulating blood, promoting tissue regeneration and astringing the wound. The prescription chosen should be *Zhibai Dihuang Tang* with modification (Modified Decoction of Anemarrhena, Phellodendron and Rehmannia) .

(2) The external treatment is same as that for stagnated heat in the heart and spleen. The powder of Radix Aconiti Praeparata 3—5 g is mixed up with vinegar, making a paste to apply to the sole of a foot, so as to conduct the fire back to its origin.

(3) Give close attention to the child with acute febrile disease, long—term disease and long—term diarrhea, constantly examining the oral cavity. If there is ulceration, *Liangxin San* (Powder for Removing Heat from Heart) should be applied immediately. Preventive action must be taken to protect the spread of disease through the whole body and build up the constitution.

3. Thrush

Clinical Manifestations

White scurf like grumose milk on mucous membrane of mouth or tongue, difficult cleaning of the mixing scurf, appearance of the hectic, unpainful and rough surface of mucosa after cleaning the scurf off, flush around the white scurf, fewer other accompaning symptoms.

Nursing

The nursing method is basically same as for aphtha.

(1) Borax water as for external use can also be used to wash the oral cavity followed by an application of Mirabilitum and powder of Cortex Magnoliae Officinalis, 3—4 times a day.

(2) This symptom can spread to the esophagus, trachea and affect swallowing and respiration. If it spreads to the intestinal tract, it will cause diarrhea. Observe carefully the sick child's respiration, stool and the way in which he takes milk.

(3) This disease is changeable and may continue f r a prolonged period so eating utensils and articles for daily use must be strictly sterilized.

6.11 Infantile Diarrhea

Infantile diarrhea is a disease of the digestive tract mainly fanifested as a frequent number of bowel movements and loose and watery stool. It may occure in any season, but is most common in summer and autumn, which is known as "diarrhea" in TCM. The spleen and stomach function of infants is much weaker than that of adult's, so the incidence of diarrhea infants is higher. The younger they are, the higher the incidence is, and the faster the disease condition develops. They are prone to deterioration of the case leading to impairment of *Yin* and *Yang*.

General Nursing

1. Refer to the characteristics of paediatric nursing (6.1) .

2. Take care with dietetic nursing. It is necessary for the sick child with light symptoms to control the diet, reduce the quantity of food and prolong the breast—feeding time. But it is necessary for those who have serious symptoms and frequent vomiting to eat nothing for the first 8—12 hours. During the fasting they can be given small but frequent amounts of water and thin rice water. After the fasting they can be given small amounts of milk and easily digestible food such as thick rice porridge. The food should be gradually increased from small amounts to more, from liquid to semi—liquid. According to the development or easing of disease condition, the food provided should be from liquid to solid, from a little to much, from vegetable dishes to meat dishes, and greasy, raw, cold and less digestible food should be avoided. The sick child with diarrhea of different types should drink plenty of water, millet gruel, hawthorn water and, dark plum water or take oral infusion of saline solution. The ingredients of the solution are NaCl 3.5 g, $NaHCo_3$ 2.5 g, KCl 1.5 g, glucose 20 g dissolved in rice water 1000 ml, or water to tonify the *Yin* fluid.

3. The beds for sick children must be isolated. The nurse should be sure to wash the hands after nursing. Eating utensils and diapers must be sterilized.

4. Keep the oral cavity clean and moist to prevent the development of aphthae and thrush. Water of Honeysuckle flower (Aqua Flores Lonicerae) or light saline solution can be used to wash the oral cavity followed by an application of sterilized vegetable oil or *Bingpeng* oil. The child with impairment of *Yin*, dehydration and tendency to open the mouth while sleeping, should have his mouth and nose covered with wet double—layer gauze, which should be changed frequently to maintain the moistness of the mucosa in oral and nasal cavities.

5. The buttocks should be kept dry and clean. Diapers should be changed frequently. The buttocks should be washed with warm water after bowel movements and wiped with a piece of soft cloth and oil can be applied to it to protect the skin. If the buttocks has become eczematous, it should be washed with antiseptics for astringing the wound and eliminating dampness such as *Huanglian Shui* (Coptis Decoction). After the buttocks is wipied drily, the powder of Pollen Pini and Calamina should be applied externally for the light case, Olium Radicis Arnebiae seu Lithospermi and yolk oil for the serious or the buttocks is exposed to the sun or the eczematous skin is treated by infrared ray to dry the eczema to promote tissue regeneration and astringe the wound.

6. The vomitive child should lie on one side or in semireclining position in order to avoid vomitus entering the trachea and causing asphyxia.The child who vomits frequently should take *Yushu Dan* and ginger juice orally and be given acupuncture and

massage therapy on points Neiguan (PC6) and Hegu (LI4) in order to relieve vomiting.

7. If the child has abdominal pain, acupuncture may be applied to points Zusanli (ST36) , Zhongwan (RN12) , Tianshu (ST25) and Changqiang (DU1) . Massage and chiropractic therapy (by kneading or massaging the muscles along the spine) may be used for sick babies. *Weian Gao* (Ointment for Regulating the Stomach) or put *Retong Ling* (Ointment for Clearing Away Heat and Stopping pain) on the abdomen. Observe carefully the reaction of the skin to the medicine and remove the medicine immediately if there is any scalding.

8. Observe the disease condition. Observe the times, quantity, smell and property of vomiting and diarrhea. Observe the condition of abdominal distension, pain and appetite. Note whether there is syndrom of impairment of *Yin* and *Yang*.

Nursing According to Syndrome Differentiation

1. Damp—heat Diarrhea

Clinical Manifestations

Frequent diarrhea, yellow and brown stool, loose, mucosy stools like paste and egg soup, a great quantity each time with foul smell, having a feeling of fever and pain after moving the bowels, redness of skin round anus, oliguria with reddish urine, vomiting, abdominal distension and pain, thirst, strong desire for drinking, fever, yellow and greasy tongue coating, slippery rapid pulse.

Nursing

(1) The patient should take medicine for clearing away heat, promoting diuresis, regulating the stomach and flow of *Qi*.

A suitable prescription *Gegeng Qinlian Tang* with modification (Modified Decoction of Pueraria, Scutellaria and Coptis.) The herbs must be decocted in water into concentrated decoction. The decoction should be given in small quantities but frequently to prevent vomiting.

(2) The diet should be supplied according to the rule of general nursing.

(3) Damp—heat diarrhea may easily cause areola of the skin round the anus. Care should be taken to protect the area.

(4) The sick child with serious diarrhea and distension (toxic enteroparalysis) may take mirabilite 30g, Pulvis Radicis et Rhizomae Rhei and honey to apply to the umbilical region. Be careful to compensate for potassium loss.

(5) Babies feet may be soaked in decoction Humulus Scandens 30—60 g, 2—3 times a day, 15—20 minutes each time.

(6) Massage therapy may be used for clearing away heat from the spleen, stomach, large and small intestine, reducing the heat in the six hollow organs, kneading the points Tianshu (ST25) and Guwei to clear away heat, promote diuresis, regulate middle—warmer energy and stop diarrnea.

2. Cold—damp Diarrhea

Clinical Manifestations

Yellowish, light brown or thin stool with light foul smell and much foam, obvious abdominal distension and pain, thirst, without desire for drinking, accompanied by both fever and aversion to cold.

Nursing

(1) Administer medicine for warming the middle—*Jiao* to dispel cold, regulating the flow of *Qi* and stopping pain. A suita-

ble prescription is *Heqi Yin* with modification （Modified the Decoction for Regulating the Flow of *Qi*）.The decoction should be taken hot. The sick child should lie in bed after taking the medicine and be covered with bed clothes.

（2）If the child has exterior syndrome caused by exopathic disease such as fever, aversion to cold, cough and running nose, he should remain in bed and to kept warm carefully, or be given moxibustion at points Dazhui （DU14）and Shenque （RN8）and take medicine for expelling cold and relieving exterior syndrome.

（3）The child who has abdominal distension and pain should be treated by warming the channels, expelling cold, regulating the flow of *Qi* and stopping pain. External treatments can be used such as a warm compress can be placed on the stomach, salt compress （refer to the nursing of acute appendicitis 4.8）, and paste ground from onion and ginger to the navel; or massage the point Shenque （RN8）in a clockwise direction or use moxa roll to heat the points Zusanli （ST36）, Zhongwan （RN12）, Qihai （RN6）, Sanyinjiao （SP6）. Salt can be placed in the navel and then ginger moxibustion is given to the navel but scald burn must be avoided.

（4）In addition that diet should be regulated according to general nursing, warm—pungent and warm—heat food should be provided to the child in order to help warm the middle—*Jiao* and expel cold, such as warm water with ginger and brown sugar, thin lotus root starch juice mixed with boiled water.

（5）Massage therapy: Apply acupressure to the point San Guan to tonify the spleen and channel, knead Wai Lao, knead navel, push the cervical vertabra, knead the point Guiwei, press the point Zusanli (ST36) to tonify the large intestine.

3. Diarrhea due to Improper Diet

Clinical Manifestations

Yellow, brown and rough stool with undigested food, acid and foul smell; eructation and vomit with acid and foul smell, paroxysmal abdominal pain, distension and urge to vomit, gradually weakened abdominal pain after vomiting and diarrhea. Anorexia, having history of improper diet, yellow, greasy and dirty coating on the tongue, slippery and rapid pulse.

Nursing

(1) Diet temperateness and regulation of the stomach function is essential in nursing. The patient may take *Baohe Wan* (Lenitive Pill) for promoting digestion and regulating the stomach to promote digestion of retained food and stop diarrhea. The diarrhea can not be brought under control if the retained food is not digested, so the sick child with food retained in the stomach should not take the medicine for inducing astringency and stopping diarrhea. If the undigested food is retained in the stomach, a tongue—spatula can be used for emesis.

(2) The sick child should fast for 4—8 hours after the onset, then be provided with thin, soft, liquid and easily digestive food. Greasy, raw and cold food should be avoided. Hawthorn juice, malt, millet bud soup and porridge water cooked with polished glutinous rice will assist digestion.

(3) Fructus Evodiae 30 g, Flos Syzygii Aromatici 2 g and pepper 30 grains are ground into fine powder. 1. 5g of powder per time is mixed with vinegar into a paste to apply to the umbilical region.

(4) Massage therapy: Knead the point Ban Men, to tonify

the spleen— channels and clear the bowels. Stroke Zhongwan (RN12) , abdomen, Tianshu (ST25) and Guiwei to activate the internal *Bagua* (eight combinations of three whole or broken lines formerly used in divination) , or chiropractic can be used to regulate the function of spleen and stomach.

4. Diarrhea due to Deficiency of Spleen

Clinical Manifestations

Long—term or repeated attacks of diarrhea, yellow, green or thin and rough stool without form, yellow complexion, cool limbs and relaxed skin, half— openning eyes during sleeping, bowel movement immediately after meals with rough stool, light tongue body, thin and white coating on the tongue, sunken and weak pulse.

Nursing

(1) Food should be provided for invigorating the spleen and replenishing *Qi* besides the necessary food according to general nursing. Porridge cooked with lotus seed, Chinese yam (rhizome) , coix seed, Chinese date or hyacinth bean can be eaten. The sick child should have meals regularly, the time and quantity should be fixed and over fullness, sweet and cold food should be avoided.

(2) Administer medicine for warming the middle— *Jiao,* strengthening the spleen, replenishing *Qi* and stopping diarrhea. The prescription chosen should be *Shenling Baizhu San* with modification (Modified Powder of Ginseng, Poria and Bighead Atractylodes)

(3) The child with long—term diarrhea and cold limbs due to insufficiency of *Yang* should maintain body warmth carefully, especially the lower limbs. The salt Sal, or Rhizoma Typhonii

should be pounded and mixed with the powder of Pulvis Corticis Cinnamomi and Pulvis Fructis Evodiae and flour mixed well to apply to the palm and the sole for warming *Yang* and stopping diarrhea.

(4) Massage therapy:Apply pressure to the points three passes, stroke the abdomen, knead navel, press upper seventh segment of spine, knead the point Gui—Wei and massage back for invigorating the spleen—channels and large intestine.

5. Impairment of *Yin* and *Yang*:diarrhea can cause impairment of *Yin* and *Yang,* generally sudden diarrhea causes impairment of *Yin,* but long— term diarrhea mainly causes impairment of *Yang.* However *Yin* and *Yang* have the same source, relying on each other. If impairment of *Yang* occurs, so does impairment of *Yin.* The symptoms of both impairments always exist simultaneously or in crossed state, though possibly one may be more serious than the other.

(1) Syndrome of lmpairment of *Yin*

Clinical Manifestations

Sunken sockets of eyeballs and dry fontanel skin without elasticity, vexation, thirst, oliguria. Crying without tears due to serious illness, anuria, cherry —like red lips and mouth, fast and deep breathing or sigh—like breathing, occassional clonic convulsion, dry tongue coating, sunken and small pulse.

(2) Syndrome of Impairment of *Yang*

Low spirits, pale complexion, half—open eyes and lassitude which are the early manifestation of impairment of *Yin* and *Yang* due to diarrhea; apathetic facial expression, cool limds, skin with different figures and exterior shallow and cool syndrome during breathing which are prostration syndrome of *Yang.*

Clinically, both impairment of *Yin* and *Yang* generally exist simultaneously, the difference lies only in the different extent of each.

Nursing

a. If the sick child has the impairment of *Yin* as the dominant syndrome, Fructus Mume, Herba Dendrobii, Radix Ophiopogonis, Radix Asparagi, Fructus Schisandrae, Radix Ginseng should be added to the prescription used in the original syndrome. If the child has the impairment of *Yang* as the dominant syndrome, Radix Ginseng, Radix Aconiti Praeparata, Fructus Schisandrae, Radix Ophiopogonis should be added to the original prescription. The child who has *Yin* and *Yang* exhausion simultaneously should be treated with the combination of traditional Chinese medicine and western medicine to achieve emergency treatment of collapse.

b. If the child has clonic convulsion, treatment should be given for calming the endopathic wind and relieving convulsion. Acupuncture can be used to points shuigou (DU26), Shixuan (EX−UE11), Yongquan (KI1). If the sick child can swallow. *Xiewei Fen* (Powder of Dry Scorpion Tail) should be taken orally to relieve spasm.

c. If his temperature doesn't rise, the child should be kept warm and given ginger moxibustion to Qihai (RN6).

6.12 Dystrophia

Dystrophia is a syndrome of deficiency and impairment of spleen and stomach mainly manifested as sallow complexion, emaciation, thin and withered hair, unnormal appetite and lassitude. It is involved in infantile malnutrition of TCM.

General Nursing

1. Refer to the characteristics of paediatrics nursing (6.1) .

2. Intensive care to daily life is needed. Putting on more or less clothes and regulation of the room temperature should be done according to the season and air temperature to prevent cross infection due to climatic conditions and seasonal pathogens in excess.

3. The diet should be monitored according to the sick child's age and disease condition. In case mother has no milk or deficient milk, cows milk, goats milk, bean milk, fermented drink made from ground beans or other drink which can substitute for milk should be provided for the sick child. There must be a regular quantity, quality and time for the feeding. If supplementary food must be added, it should be offered according to the following rules: At first liquid and little food should be given to the child and according to the relevent improvement of the digestive ability, solid and more food can be followed with the increasing in quantity and frequency of eating. The bad habit of food preference of sick child should be corrected. Patience is required in feeding the child without appetite. The cause of appetite loss should be found and corrected promptly. The child should be encouraged to have more time to become physically active in accordance with his state of recovery to improve the appetite.

4. Find out the cause leading to dystrophia. Massage or chiropractic therapy may be given according to the cause of disease. If the sick child is malnourished in any way, the corresponding supplement of nutrition should be provided.

5. The weight should be checked twice each week and recorded. changes in weight should be compared to help analyse

disease condition.

6. Nurses should familiarize themselves with the sick child's psychological state and try to resolve any bad influence on appetite due to mental factors.

7. Care should be taken of the oral cavity and eyes. The oral cavity should be rinsed with light saline solution and water made from Folii Perillae to prevent stomatitis. If the gingivae have bled and ulcerated and sores have manifested in mouth or on the tongue, *Xilei San* (Powder of Xilei) and *Zhuhuang San* (Powder of Zhuhuang) may be applied. The normal saline solution can be used with a cotton ball to clean eyes. Be sure to prevent the sick child from complications and deficiency of vitamine.

8. Organize some outdoor activities for the child, giving him frequent exposure to the sun to build up health. The limbs should be frequently massaged and given a rubbing bath in warm and fresh sulfur water.

9. Any complications should be frequently noticed. Children with dystrophia are prone to suffer from one or many kinds of deficiency of nutrients due to dystrophia and may cause exopathogenic problems due to weak resistence. Such complications should be found and corrected immediately.

10. The parents should be advised about the dietary requirements and supplementary feeding of their children and guided in training their children to develop good eating habits

Nursing According to Syndrome Differentiation

1. Weakness of the Spleen *Qi* Type
Clinical Manifestations
Yellow complexion, thin hair, emaciated physique, anorexia,

feelings of distension and fullness in the epigastric region and abdomen, feverish sensation over palms and soles, dysphoria, thin and white coating on the tongue, sunken and slippery pulse.

Nursing

(1) Administer medicine for strengthening the spleen and replenishing *Qi*, removing stagnation of *Qi* and regulating the stomach. The prescription chosen should be *Shenling Baishu San* with modification (Modified Powder of Ginseng, Poria and Big head Atractylodes).

(2) The recuperative diet should include food for strengthening the spleen, regulating *Qi* and promoting digestion, such as Chinese yam porridge, milk veteh porridge and lotus seeds porridge. In addition, sufficient protein, carbohydrate and vitamine should be provided to the sick child. Food such as milk, eggs, poultry and fish are good sources of protein. Food like cereal is a good source of carbohydrate.

(3) If the sick child has gastric and abdominal distension and fullness, keading the abdomen and chiropractic can be used to regulate the function of the intestine and stomach, remove the stagnation and regulate the flow of *Qi*, soothe the intestines and promote the movement of bowel.

2. Deficiency of *Qi* and Blood Type

Clinical Manifestations

Yellow complexion, emaciated physique, thin and withered hair, large head but thin neck, sunken abdomen, uncommunicative, dull expression, hypoevolutism or developmental arrest, bland tongue body, thin and greasy coating on the tongue, sunken and slight pulse.

Nursing

(1) Ensure that the diet is suitable. Apart from feeding according to deficiency of spleen and *Qi,* concentrated chicken, fish and soft—shelled turtle soup and ginseng and edible bird's nest porridge may be given to the child in order to replenish vital essence. The condition of the child suffering from this disease tends to be highly complicated. The child is prone to stubborn anorexia, so should be fed patiently. As the child's digestive ability is weak, food should be given frequently, but in small amounts. Observe the stool carefully and be familiar with the state of the digestive function.

(2) This disease may bring about rather serious conditions and both *Qi* and blood become deficient.Medicine for invigorating *Qi,* nourishing the blood, strengthening the spleen and stomach are required. The prescription chosen should be *Renshen Yangrong Tang* with modification (Modified Ginseng Decoction for Nourishing Body Fluid) .

(3) Nurses should be careful and gentle while working, especially for the child with serious dystrophia to prevent him from sudden heart failure and collapse.

6.13 Nephrotic Syndrome

Nephrotic Syndrome is characterized as anasarca, a great quantity of proteinuria, hypoproteinemia and hyperchotesterolemia in clinic. It is frequently seen among children 3—8 years old. It belongs to the scope of disease" *Yin* edema"in traditional Chinese medicine.

General Nursing

1. Refer to the characteristics of paediatric nursing.

2. The child at the edema stage should remain in bed, the serious patient must not leave the bed. If the child has hydrothorax and ascitis fluid which result in chest distress and short breath, he should take semire—clining position. As soon as the edema has relieved, the patient may take mild exercise, but too much may lead to relapse of the disease due to overstrain.

3. Diet: A high— protein, high calorie, low— fat, rich vitamin, easily digestible and bland diet should be provided. At the stage of edema, sodium salt and water intake should be limited. Salt— free diet should be qiven to those with edema and oliguria. When urine has become more voluminous and edema has disappeared, a low—salt diet may be offered, but a completely salt—free diet should not be adhered for a prolonged period, as this will cause anorexia and adversely affect the sick child's development due to hyponatremia leading to more serious edema. The diet may be supplemented with lean meat , eggs and milk to compensate for the albumen lost in urine. Porridge cooked with hindu lotus seed, tuckahoe Poria and Chinese yam rhizome may be provided to boost nutrition. In addition, a carp about 250 g, red bean (seed) 50 g and amomum fruit 10 g can also be boiled for eating. The decoction has the function of bringing about diuresis and promoting digestion of albumen.

4.Prevent infection and relapse.The sick child's resistance against exopathogen becomes weak and the Qi and blood become deficient because of the expulsion of a large quantity of albumen from urine. Infection of the upper respiratory tract and skin and other infectious disease easily occur. These may increase the seriousness of the disease and cause relapse. Essential precautionary and isolation measures must be taken. The infectious focus must be treated thoroughly.

5. Take particular care of the skin. The skin should be rubbed with water decocted from Herba Schizonepetae or alcohol 30% to maintain cleanliness and circulate the blood and *Qi*, promote dissipation of blood stasis and subsidence of swelling. The clothes should be light, soft, wide and loose and bedclothes should be kept clean, dry and soft. Intramuscular injections should be avoided as serious edema may cause malabsorption of the injection fluid. A patient who is spending a prolonged period in bed should be regularly turned over to prevent hydropneumatic edema and bed sores.

6. Maintain cleanliness of the oral cavity, rub and rinse out the mouth with Aqua Cortii Magnoliae Officinalis Eliminate infectious focus in throat, teeth and gums.

7. Record the food—intake and excretory quantity each day, especially during the edema and diuresis. Some urine should be retained for routine testing. Measure the weight, circumference of abdomen and blood pressure 3—4 times per week.

Nursing According to Syndrome Differentiation

1. Wetness and Heat Type

Clinical Manifestations

Fever, swollen throat, sores and ulcer on skin, anasarca, thirst, but no desire for drinking, scanty, yellow urine, thick and yellow coating on the tongue, slippery and rapid pulse.

Nursing

(1) Administer medicine for clearing away heat, removing the toxic materials and promoting diuresis. The prescription chosen should be *Wuwei Xiaodu Yin* with modification (Modi-

fied Antiphlogistic Decoction of Five Drugs) . If the edema is obvious, the fresh maize spike 60—120 g may also be decocted in water to take as a supplement. Water melon and wax gourd are beneficial to diuresis and elimination of swelling.

(2) The patient should have bed rest and limited activities.The first priority is to relieve the load of the kidney. Observe changes of temperature, blood pressure and urine. If the blood pressure is high, attemps should be made to lower it.

(3) At the early stage the key link of treating and nursing is to eliminate focus. If the throat is swollen and painful, the *Xilei San* and *Zhuhuang San* may be used to blow into the throat partially or aerosol fluid for clearing the throat may be used as spray inhalation to reduce the swelling, disperse accumulation of pathogen and ease pain. Alternatively Flos Lonicerae, Radix Platycodi and Radix Ophiopogonis are soaked in boiled water to be taken as tea for normalizing the throat. If the skin is ulcerated, the surgical treating and nursing for furuncle may be referred to 4. 1.

2. Deficiency of Both the Spleen and Kidney Type

Clinical Manifestations

Pale complexion, edema of whole body, especially the lower limbs, indentation remains in the skin after pressing, weakness and tiredness, gastric and abdominal distension, discomfort, loose and thin stools, white coating on the tongue, deep and small pulse.

Nursing

(1) Medicine for warming *Yang* and promoting diuressis should be administered.The prescription chosen should be *Shipi Yin* with modification (Modified Decoction for Reinforcing the Spleen) and *Wuling San* (Modified Powder of Five Drugs with

Poria) for taking in combination to promote diuresis.

(2) The child with serious edema should remain in bed at all times. The red bean (seed) 30 g, black soybean 30 g, may be boiled to eat for promoting diuresis. If the lower limbs have serious edema, the child can prop up the legs in a higher position to assist relief of the edema. If the edema is serious, the legs and buttocks should be raised with a soft pillow. The scrotum must be supported with a triangular bandage to avoid chafing the skin and aggravating the edema of the lower limbs. If the plasma protein is too low, plasma or plasma protein should be transfused intravenously. High quality protein food should be provided such as chicken soup, soft—shelled turtle soup and milk to increase plasma protein.

(3) If the gastric cavity and abdomen become distended, food intake should be reduced, but the frequency of meals should be increased. The hot compress may be placed on the abdomen. The sick child should take semireclining position.

3. Deficiency of Liver—*Yin* and Kidney—*Yin* Type

Clinical Manifestations

Edema, oliguria, headache, dizziness, vexation, insomnia, soreness of the Loins and weakness of the kness, little, thin and white tongue coating, wiry and small pulse.

Nursing

(1) Administer medicine for nourishing *Yin* and suppressing hyperactive *Yang*. The prescription chosen should be *Qiju Dihuang Tang* with modification (Modified Decoction Made from Bolus of Six Drugs, Rehmannia, with Wolfberry and Chrysanthemum) .

(2) Light, easily absorbed food should be chosen for pro-

moting diuresis to benefit treatment. The sick child can eat porridge cooked with Radix Astragali seu Hedysari and Semen Coicis to promote diuresis and eliminate dampness. Black edible fungus, softshelled turtle and animal's liver can be eaten for nourishing the deficiency of *Yin* fluid.

(3) For those who have vexation and restlessness, acupuncture can be used to points Anmian and Shenmen (HT7) . Drinking a suitable amount of milk before sleeping at night may help the child sleep better.

(4) Changes of blood pressure must be noted. If the blood pressure remains high or rises, the blood pressure should be tested twice daily. If the sick child suffers from dizziness, he should take *Naoliqing* (Pills for Clearing Away Dizziness) , often eat celery and Chinese hawthorn to lower the blood pressure. The diet should be low in salt. Auricular—plaster therapy (a small bean or seed of Vaccaria Segetalis is taped tightly to a particular ear acupuncture point and pressed to stimulate the point for therapeutic purpose) is used on points Shenmen (HT7) and Sympothetic.

6.14 Enuresis

Enuresis is a common disease among children over 3 years old. It often occurs in a dream, but the child is aware of it only after waking, it is also called" bed— wetting" . the light sufferer passes water only once in a night, but the more serious case may pass water many times in a night or just after falling asleep. It may occur to a patient when having a nap. The child under 3 years old may have enursis, but it is not considered pathological, because at this age the function of organs, linguistic ability and self—control, etc. are hypoplastic.

General Nursing

1. The sick child should lie in a lateral recumbent position while sleeping. This position will loosen the abdominal muscle so that the pressure on the bladder is relieved. The thickness of bed coverings should be suitable. The feet should not be kept too warm or pressed too heavily.

2. Pyschological nursing should be given to elder children. It is necessary to teach and guide them patiently, eliminate their nervousness and sense of shame, and encourage their confidence to conquer the disease.

3. The clothes and bedclothes should be changed promptly after enuresis. The skin should be kept dry, clean and warm.

4. The decoction should be taken only at day time. Solid food is suitable for supper. The quantity of drinking must be controlled after meals. The child should be encouraged to urinate before sleeping.

5. Become familiar with the time of the child's nocturnal urination and wake him up on time and urge him to urinate.

6. The child should develop regular urination habits. In the day time his playing should not be overstimulating, overexciting, and overtiring so as to avoid excessively long sleeping and enuresis due to tiredness or losing the balance of self—controlled ability.

7. The laser transmitter of helium or neon can be used to stimulate the points Shenshu(BL23) Zhongji (RN 3) , and Yeniao (handneedling) . Auricular—plaster therapy may be applied to the points Shenshu(BL23) , Urinary Bladder and

Subcortex.

8. Note the general condition, eliminate the disease of nervous, endocrine and urinary systems and find out which are the symptoms of primary or secondary enuresis.

Nursing According to Syndrome Differentiation

1. The Syndrome of Deficiency and Cold in the lower—*Jiao*.

Clinical Manifestations

Frequent enuresis, long— term disease course, heavy sleep and uneasiness on being awoken, cool hands and feet, inactivity, clear and voluminous urine, white and thin coating on the tongue, deep and slow pulse.

Nursing

(1) Administer medicine for warming the kidney and reducing volume of urine. The prescription chosen should be *Gongti Wan* with modification. The decoction should be taken hot.

(2) Porridge cooked with Chinese red dates, lotus seed and gordon euryale or dog meat 250 g and black soybean 10 g are cooked in soup for eating to warm and reinforce *Qi* of kidney.

(3) Acupuncture: needle the points Baihui (DU20) ,
Zhongji (RN3) , Sanyinjiao (SP6) and use moxibustion to Guanyuan (RN4) .

(4) Proved Prescription:

Ingredients:

chicken intestine	one section	(grilled)
Concha Ostreae	16 g	
Poria	16 g	
Oötheca Mantidis	16 g	
Cortex Cinnamomi	8 g	

Os Draconis   8 g

Administration:The ingredients are ground into fine powder, 3— 4 g taken each time, 2— 3 times a day to nourish the kidney—*Qi,* reduce secretion and assist urine retention. Alternatively sulphur powder 10 g and some bulbs of onion are pounded into paste to which vegetable oil is added to apply to the umbilical region, using it every 3—5 days.

2. Deficiency and Cold of the Spleen and Lungs Syndrome

Clinical Manifestations

Enuresis, yellow complexion, shortness of breath, spontaneous perspiration, poor appetite, watery and loose stool or bowel movements immediately after meals, having frequent cold and micturition during the day time, thin and white coating on the tongue, sunken and weak pulse.

Nursing

(1) Administer medicine for strengthening the spleen, replenishing *Qi* and arresting discharges. The prescription chosen should be *Buzhong Yiqi Tang* with modification （Modified Decoction for Reinforcing Middle—*Jiao* and Replenishing *Qi*）. The decoction should be taken hot.

(2) Porridge with howthorns, Chinese dates and Chinese yam rhizome should frequently be eaten. Alternatively pig's bladder and Radix Astragali seu Hedysari 60 g are boiled until tender and eaten frequently to strengthen the function of the bladder's storage.

(3) If the stool is loose and thin, ginger and red sugar may be decocted in water for oral dose to warm the spleen and expel cold.

(4) Applicating method:Galla Chinensis 3 g and Radix

Polygoni Multiflori 3 g are ground into fine powder and mixed with vinegar to apply to the umbilical region and covered with gauze. This method can be used consecutively 3—5 times, once every night. Pay attention to the response of skin to stimulating.

(5) If the child has frequent micturition, Yeniao point （in the horizontal lines of small finger's and the second finger's joint on palm) or the points Yinlingquan （SP9) Sanyinjiao （SP6) , Guanyuan （RN4) , Zhongji （RN3) and Shenshu （BL23) can be needled. Moxibustion therapy may be added for the weaker patients.

(6) The child should be protected from cold and have physical exercises, but should not be overfatigued.

3. The Syndrome due to Stagnated Heat in the Liver and Kidney

Clinical Manifestations

Enuresis occuring many times each night, urinating in small quantities each time or intermittent dripping of urine, impatience, sleep—walking, fever and sweating palms and soles or accompanied by night sweat, thin, white and yellow coating on the tongue, small and rapid pulse.

Nursing

(1) Administer medicine for nourishing *Yin* to purge pathogenic fire. The prescription chosen should be *Zhi Bai Dihuang Wan* with modification （Modified Pill of Anemarrhena, Phellodendron and Rehmannia) .

(2) Wash external pudenda before sleeping each night and apply talcum powder to it after drying to reduce the stimulation of external pudenda. Underpants should be changed frequently to avoid the stimulation due to rubbing.

(3) If the child urinates in a small amounts and has dripping urine, the points Zhongji (RN3) , Henggu (KI11) , Sanyinjiao (SP6) and Taichong (LR3) can be needled.

(4) Oötheca Mantidis 15 g, Fructus Alpiniae Oxyphyllae 15 g, Fructus Rosae Laevigatae 15 g and Fructus Psoraleae 15 g are decocted in water for oral use to reinforce the kidney and control urination.

(5) Point application with Chinese herbs.

Ingredients:

Moschus	3 g
Venenum Bufonis	2 g
Ramulus Cinnamomi	5 g
Herba Ephedrae	5 g
Realgar	5 g
Commiphora Myrrha	5 g
Boswelliae Carterii	5 g

These herbs should be ground into fine powder and put into a bottle for storage. Before application, some powder of the herbs should be mixed with a suitable amount of alcohol into paste and applied to the points Qihai (RN6) , Zhongji (RN3) and Sanyinjiao (SP6) . The mixed powder should be changed once 3—4 days.

20

护　　理

序

　　《英汉实用中医药大全》即将问世，吾为之高兴。

　　歧黄之道，历经沧桑，永盛不衰。吾中华民族之强盛，由之。世界医学之丰富和发展，亦由之。然而，世界民族之差异，国别之不同，语言之障碍，使中医中药的传播和交流受到了严重束缚。当前，世界各国人民学习、研究、运用中医药的热潮方兴未艾。为使吾中华民族优秀文化遗产之一的歧黄之道走向世界，光大其业，为世界人民造福，徐象才君集省内外精英于一堂，主持编译了《英汉实用中医药大全》。是书之问世将使海内外同道欢呼雀跃。

　　世界医学发展之日，当是歧黄之道光大之时。

　　吾欣然序之。

中华人民共和国卫生部副部长
兼国家中医药管理局局长
世界针灸学会联合会主席
中国科学技术协会委员
中华全国中医学会副会长
中国针灸学会会长

胡熙明
1989 年 12 月

序

中华民族有同疾病长期作斗争的光辉历程，故而有自己的传统医学——中国医药学。中国医药学有一套完整的从理论到实践的独特科学体系。几千年来，它不但被完好地保存下来，而且得到了发扬光大。它具有疗效显著、副作用小等优点，是人们防病治病，强身健体的有效工具。

任何一个国家在医学进步中所取得的成就，都是人类共同的财富，是没有国界的。医学成果的交流比任何其他科学成果的交流都应进行得更及时，更准确。我从事中医工作30多年来，一直盼望着有朝一日中国医药学能全面走向世界，为全人类解除病痛疾苦做出其应有的贡献。但由于用外语表达中医难度较大，中国医药学对外传播的速度一直不能令人满意。

山东中医学院的徐象才老师发起并主持了大型系列丛书《英汉实用中医药大全》的编译工作。这个工作是一项巨大工程，是一种大型科研活动，是一个大胆的尝试，是一件新事物。对徐象才老师及与其合作的全体编译者夜以继日地长期工作所付出的艰苦劳动，克服重重困难所表现出的坚韧不拔的毅力，以及因此而取得的重大成绩，我甚为敬佩。作为一个中医界的领导者，对他们的工作给予全力支持是我应尽的责任。

我相信《英汉实用中医药大全》无疑会在中国医学史和世界科学技术史上找到它应有的位置。

中华全国中医学会常务理事
山东省卫生厅副厅长

张奇文
1990年3月

出 版 前 言

    中国医药学是我中华民族优秀文化遗产之一，建国以来由于党和国家对待中医药采取了正确的政策，使中医药理论宝库不断得到了发掘整理，取得了巨大的成绩。当前，世界各国人民对中国医药学的学习和研究热潮日益高涨，为促进这一热潮更加蓬勃的发展，为使中国医药学能更好地为全人类解除病痛服务，就必须促进中医中药在世界范围内的传播和交流，而要使这一传播和交流进行得更及时、更准确，就必须首先排除语言障碍。因此，编译一套英汉对照的中医药基本知识的书籍，供国内外学习、研究中医药时使用，已成为国内外医药学界和医药学教育界许多人士的迫切需要。

    多年来，在卫生部门的号召下，在"中医英语表达研究"方面，已经作出了一些可喜的成绩。本书《英汉实用中医药大全》的编辑出版就是在调查上述研究工作的历史和现状的基础上，继续对中医药英语表达作较系统、较全面的研究，以适应中国医药学对外传播交流的需要。

    这部"大全"的版本为英汉对照，共有 21 个分册，一个分册介绍论述中国医药学的一个分科。在编著上注意了中医药汉文稿的编写特色，在内容上注意了科学性、实用性、全面性和简明易读。汉文稿的执笔撰写者主要是有 20 年以上实践经验的教授、副教授、主任医师和副主任医师。各分册汉文稿撰写成后，均经各学科专家逐一审订。各分册英文主译、主审主要是国内既懂中医又懂英语的权威人士，还有许多中医院校的英语教师及医药卫生部门的专业翻译人员。英译稿脱稿后，经过了复审、终审，有些译稿还召开全国 22 所院校和单位人员参加的英译稿统稿定稿研讨会，对英译稿进行细致的研讨和推敲，对如何较全面、较系统、较准确地用英语表达中国医药学进行了探讨，从而推动整个译文达到较高水平，因此，这部"大全"可供中医院校高年级学生作为泛读教材使用。

这部"大全"的编纂得到了国家教育委员会、国家中医药管理局、山东省教育委员会、山东省卫生厅等各部门有关领导的支持。在国家教委高等教育司的指导下，成立了《英汉实用中医药大全》编译领导委员会。还得到了全国许多中医院校和中药生产厂家领导的支持。

希望这部"大全"的出版，对中医院校加强中医英语教学，对国内卫生界培养外向型中医药人才，以及在推动世界各国人民对中医药的学习和研究方面，都将产生良好的影响。

高等教育出版社

1990 年 3 月

前　言

　　《英汉实用中医药大全》是一部以中医基本理论为基础，以中医临床为重点，较为全面系统、简明扼要、易读实用的中级英汉学术性著作。它的主要读者是：中医药院校高年级学生和中青年教师，中医院的中青年医生和中医药科研单位的科研人员，从事中医对外函授工作的人员和出国讲学或行医的中医人员，西学中人员，来华学习中医的外国留学生和各类进修人员。

　　由于中国医药学为我中华民族之独有，因此，英译便成了本《大全》编译工作的重点。为确保译文能准确表达中医的确切含义，我们邀集熟悉中医的英语人员、医学专业翻译人员、懂英语的中医药人员乃至医古文人员于一堂，共同翻译、共同对译文进行研讨推敲的集体翻译法，这样，就把众人之长融进了译文质量之中。然而，即使这样，也难确保译文都能尽如人意。汉文稿虽反映了中国医药学的精髓和概貌，但也难能十全十美。我衷心地盼望读者能提出批评和建议，以便《大全》再版时修改。

　　参加本《大全》编、译、审工作的人员达 200 余名，他们来自全国 28 个单位，其中有山东、北京、上海、天津、南京、浙江、安徽、河南、湖北、广西、贵阳、甘肃、成都、山西、长春等 15 所中医学院，还有中国中医研究院，山东省中医药研究所等中医药科研单位。

　　山东省教育委员会把本《大全》的编译列入了科研计划并拨发了科研经费，山东省卫生厅和一些中药生产厂家也给了很大支持，济南中药厂的资助为编译工作的开端提供了条件。

　　本《大全》的编译成功是全体编译审者集体劳动的结晶，是各有关单位主管领导支持的结果。在《大全》各分册即将陆续出版之际，我诚挚地感谢全体编译审者的真诚合作，感谢许多专家、教授、各级领导和生产厂家的热情支持。

愿本《大全》的出版能在培养通晓英语的中医人才和使中医早日全面走向世界方面起到我所期望的作用。

主编　徐象才

于山东中医学院

1990 年 3 月

目　录

说　明

　　护理是《英汉实用中医药大全》的第 20 分册。

　　本分册共分六章：第一章概论部分，阐述了中医护理的特点，中医精神护理，饮食护理和服用中药的护理等。第二章介绍了常见危重证的中医护理常规，辨证护理及应急措施。第三章至第六章介绍了内、外、妇、儿科常见病证的护理。各科首先介绍一般护理，然后根据不同症型进行辨证护理，体现了中医学说的人体通过经络系统与内脏体表各部组织器官之间构成一个有机的整体，与四时气候，地土方宜，周围环境，精神饮食息息相关的整体观念。本书以中医辨证理论为指导，结合中医传统治疗方法中的针灸、推拿及各种外治疗法等，并强调了未病先防的重要意义。

　　本分册汉文稿经北京中医医院护理部主任、副主任护师，中华护理学会中西医结合护理专业委员会副主任委员桂梅芬审阅。在山东泰安召开的《英汉实用中医药大全》英文稿统稿定稿会上，江启元教授，林晓琦女士，还有吴炜彤副教授帮助审阅了英文稿，在此表示感谢。

编　者

1 概论

1.1 中医护理发展简史

中医护理是随着中医学的发展而发展起来的，它的历史悠久，内容丰富。

古代医、护是合一的，如《史记·扁鹊仓公列传》中记载的，公元前 5—4 世纪的杰出医学家扁鹊通晓临床各科，应用针砭、火灸、汤液、热熨等多种疗法给人治病。扁鹊在为虢太子治病时，先使用针刺和汤剂；然后热熨两胁下，以使恢复体温。说明当时诊断、治疗和护理都由医生一人承担，没有设专人负责护理，也没有形成独立的学科，而大量的护理知识和经验均记载于历代文献和许多医家的临床经验，成为中医学的重要组成部分。

在我国最早的文化中就有各种泥湿敷、包扎、固定骨位以及"动作以避寒，阴居以避暑"等的记载，这实际就是中医护理的开端。

在成书于春秋战国时代（公元前 770~221 年）的我国最早的医学著作《内经》中，不仅概括总结了我们的祖先与疾病作斗争所积累起来的丰富经验，而且对人体的结构和功能以及疾病的病因、病理、诊断、治疗等，都作了系统的阐述；同时，也论述了中医护理学的各个方面，包括精神修养、生活起居、环境卫生、饮食调理与禁忌，服药方法和服药后的护理等。对中医护理事业的发展奠定了理论基础。

汉代张仲景著《伤寒论》和《金匮要略》中，对患者服药的辨证护理论述得十分具体，他还创造发明了猪胆汁灌肠方法，说明灌肠术早在我国汉代就已经应用了。另一位古代名医华佗，擅长外科技术，并首创了麻醉术，这给外科护理增加了新的内容。

他很重视体育锻炼，并模仿虎、鹿、猿、熊、鸟五种姿态动作，创造了五禽戏，对强身防病以及对慢性病的康复提供了新的治疗方法。

晋代（公元365～420年）葛洪著《肘后救卒方》中，记载了用狂犬脑敷贴狂犬咬伤创口的外科被动免疫疗法；皇甫谧所著《甲乙经》，发扬了针灸疗法，这些均给中医护理的发展增添了新的内容。

唐代陈士良著《食性本草》中，提出了食医方剂以及四时饮食与调养的方法，阐述了饮食护理与医疗的重要关系。孙思邈的《千金方》中记载了医务人员应有高尚的品德，如：对患者要不分亲疏、贫富、长幼、丑俊等，均应一视同仁，并要有高度的同情心和责任感。这种优良的传统至今仍然指导着临床工作。另外，他还擅长养生，主张"上医治未病之病"，《千金要方》和《千金翼方》中，记载了许多有关按摩、饮食、衣着及幼儿护理等方面的经验，强调食物宜熟后食，食后应漱口，饭后要散步，同时要求人们之间要和睦相处，可减少疾病的发生。在针灸方面，首创了阿是穴。他还发明了用细葱管导尿，说明我国唐代已有了导尿技术。王焘的《外台秘要》中，记载了各种外治疗法及新生儿护理方法，如：哺乳、包裹、沐浴等。

宋代（960～1279年）《本草衍义》中谈到关于食盐与疾病的关系，指出"水肿者宜全禁之"，即凡引起水肿的疾病，应食无盐或低盐的饮食。钱仲阳在《小儿药证直诀》中积极主张小儿有热病可用浴体法，即用温水擦浴降温，作辅助治疗。阎孝忠在《小儿方论》中，提出了小儿的喂养方法，在小儿出生半年后，可以米煮粥，取米汁喂之，十个月后可食稀粥烂饭，以助中气，则不易生病。还要求忌食生冷、油腻、甜食等。另外陈自明在《妇人大全良方》中，专门写有《食忌论》、《将护孕妇论》、《产后将护法》、《产后调理法》等，为中医妇科护理提供了极其宝贵的经验。

金元时期著名四大医学家刘完素、张子和、李东垣、朱丹溪，他们在医学上虽各持不同的学术观点，但对护理工作都是很重视的。在张子和著的《儒门事亲》中，他论述了很多护理内容，还发明了坐浴法治疗脱肛。他通过实践提出"恐胜喜，悲胜怒、怒胜思，……"的理论，强调以情胜情的心理治疗论点。李东垣认为脾胃为后天之本，强调注意后天的饮食调养，主张饮食宜清淡，少食膏粱厚味等。

明、清时代（1368～1840 年）护理内容有了新的发展，如明代胡正心说："凡患瘟疫之家，将初病人之衣，于甑上蒸过，则一家不得染"。这说明我国古代就开始对传染病患者用过的衣物使用蒸气消毒处理。清代叶天士对老年病的治疗与护理进行了较深的研究，强调老年人要学会养生，提出寒冷要保暖，饮食当薄味，戒酒肉厚味，心胸开阔，怡情悦志，戒怒等养身之道。另外，要勤劳，多锻炼，要早起早睡等防病抗老的经验。

由于中医的医疗与护理从来都是不可分割的，是相辅相成的，护理是医疗的组成部分，在整个医疗工作中占有十分重要的地位，经过历代的不断充实和发展。特别是针灸、刮痧、拔火罐、外治疗法、推拿按摩、气功、太极拳等的发明及应用，更丰富了中医护理的内容。

建国后，党的中医政策为中医护理事业的发展和提高创造了有利的条件。广大医务工作者和护理人员在临床工作中不断总结出大量有关中医护理和中西医结合护理的经验，并对中医学宝库中有关护理学理论进行发掘和整理，中医护理学的著作相继出版，并受到重视。中医的护理教育也在大力发展，全国已有十几所中等中医护理专科学校，有的中医学院还设有中医护理系，中医护理学已形成了一门独立的学科。特别是在全国各地大力振兴中医的大好形势下，中医护理人员正在根据中医护理的特点，结合临床实践，不断吸取现代护理学中的新技术，使中医护理进一步发展和提高，更好的为社会主义建设事业服务。

1.2 中医护理的特点

中医护理是遵循中医理论发展起来的，中医护理的基本特点，归纳起来可分为以下四部分。

1. 整体观念

中医认为，人体是一个以脏腑经络为核心的有机整体，人与自然界（包括气候、地理、社会环境等）一切事物都是对立统一的，而且人体各脏腑之间，内外环境之间，必须保持相对平衡，一旦失去平衡，就会发生疾病。因此在护理患者时，要创造一个良好的外界环境，在观察病情时，不仅要注意局部的病变，同时还要注意相关脏腑的变化，如：口舌生疮，因心开窍于舌，则为心火上炎所致；若伴有小便赤涩、刺痛，又因心与小肠相表里，心移热于小肠，小肠实热，而造成口舌生疮。所以在护理时，除口腔涂用冰硼散、锡类散或五枯散外，还应泻心火利小便，常用淡竹叶、白茅根煎汤频服之；另外宜多食绿豆汤、水果、蔬菜等清热泻火之品。忌食辛辣、炙煿、煎、炸、熏、烤助火之物。

中医较为重视四时气候、地理环境和患者体质对疾病的影响，因此在护理工作中必须周密考虑各方面的因素，对具体情况作具体分析，制定因时、因地、因人而异的护理方法。

(1) 因时制宜，即根据季节、气候的不同，采取不同的治疗和护理方法。如夏天气候炎热，阳气升发，人体腠理疏松开泄，感冒多为风热，服用解表药时，应指导患者不可出汗过多，以免耗伤阴液。冬天气候寒冷，腠理致密，感冒多为风寒，服用解表药时，应饮热稀粥或热开水，并盖被保暖取汗，以求邪从汗解。

(2) 因地制宜，即注意地理环境和气候条件的不同，如：南方湿热而多雨，北方干燥少雨，因此虽属同一种疾病，在护理措施也有所不同。

(3) 因人制宜，即应重视患者个体的差异。患者由于性别、年龄、体质强弱的不同，同一种疾病，其证候也不尽相同，故在护理时也应有所区别。

由于人体是一个有机的整体，精神情志正常与否，均和健康有很大关系，精神正常能使机体处于正常状态，适应周围环境和四时气候的变化，免受外邪侵袭；反之，情志异常，精神内伤，则可使气机升降失调，气血运行紊乱，五脏功能失职，从而引起各种疾病。如：狂喜则伤心，出现心悸、失眠、失神甚至发生狂乱等；大怒伤肝，致使肝气郁结，食欲减退，重者可出现面色苍白，四肢发抖，甚至昏厥；过思伤脾，脾伤运化失常，则出现腹胀便溏、头晕目眩、失眠多梦、健忘等；大惊伤肾，则会出现小便失禁等现象。因此护理人员要了解患者的精神状态，掌握情志的变化，做耐心细致的思想工作，消除不利于疾病的精神因素，使患者在情绪稳定，心情舒畅的条件下接受治疗。

另外，中医治病，除用药外，还非常重视饮食的调养作用。饮食调养也是中医护理的重要方面。中医传统的食疗原则，是以中医理论为基础，根据食物的四性（寒、热、温、凉），五味（酸、苦、甘、辛、咸）及其归经，再通过望、闻、问、切四诊的方法了解疾病发生的原因、病变部位、疾病性质及主要临床表现，进行辨证分析，然后选择和搭配食疗方剂。以胃脘痛为例，凡属初病、实证或病邪犯胃，治疗应以通为主的食疗方剂，除其病邪，通其气血；凡属久病、虚证或脏腑失调，食疗方剂应以补为主，调理脏腑。

2. 辨证护理

辨证是中医护理的主要依据，是在中医学理论指导下，运用四诊八纲，对患者的症状、体征进行综合分析，确定诊断属于何证，然后进行有效的治疗。这一理论也指导着中医护理工作的实践。以发热为例：同属发热患者，由于病因、病机、病证不同，其护理原则也不相同，如：发热伴有恶寒、无汗、苔白、不渴，则为病邪在表，治疗原则为解表，护理原则为避免风寒，以免再受外邪，要保暖，饮用开水或姜糖水，促使发汗；若壮热、大渴、大汗、苔黄，则为病邪入里化热，护理时应注意室内通风良好，多饮一些清淡饮料；气虚发热患者，在发热时尚伴有自汗、畏寒等症，则宜保暖，避免出汗等。由于疾病发展阶段的不同，护理也应随之而异，如湿温患者，早期为湿重热轻，室内温度不宜过凉，衣服不可过少，忌食生冷；后期湿蕴热炽，室内温度宜低，适量给予冷饮等。另外中医治病，谨守病机，即辨证时，强调疾病的动态、转归，所以护理时也应掌握各种疾病发展的规律，方可了解疾病发展的趋势。

3. 传统疗法

中医的传统疗法内容广泛，丰富多采，是中医的宝贵遗产。如：针灸、推拿按摩、拔火罐、刮痧、外治疗法（包括膏药疗法、热熨疗法、围敷疗法、熏洗疗法等），服药疗法，饮食疗法等。这些治疗方法不仅是中医治疗疾病的重要手段，也是中医护理技术操作的主要内容。由于这些疗法疗效显著，收效迅速，安全可靠，副作用少，易学易用，近几年来临床应用广泛，已突破了传统的治疗范围，有了进一步发展和提高。如针刺用于腹部手术后促进肠蠕动，减轻腹胀；推拿可解除手术后产生的尿潴留；耳针预防静脉输液、输血反应；用番泻叶泡水内服，代替清洁灌肠；麸熨疗法可协助治疗胃肠手术后早期发生的肠粘连等。

4. 治未病

《内经》中指出，"不治已病治未病"。这包括两个方面，首先强调未病先防。中医主张养生，要求人们平日做到饮食有节，起居有常，不妄劳作。注意锻炼身体，调摄精神，使身体正气充沛，阴阳平衡，就可以减少疾病的发生。因此应指导患者保持良好的生活习惯，稳定情绪，加强锻炼，如饭后散步，练气功，打太极拳等。另一方面强调对疾病应早期发现，早期治疗，防止疾病的发展与转变，因此要求护理人员应认真观察病情，早期发现疾病发生的先兆，及时采取相应的处理措施，控制疾病的发展。

1.3 精神护理

精神护理在临床上具有重要的意义，中医认为人是一个有机的整体，精神情志正常与否和健康有很大关系。精神正常，则阴阳平衡，正气内守，使机体处于正常状态，适应周围环境和四时变化，免受外邪侵袭。反之，情志过极，精神内伤，气机升降失调，气血运行紊乱，五脏功能失职，容易引起各种疾病。

不同的情志变化，会造成不同脏腑的病变，如：暴怒伤肝，狂喜伤心，久思伤脾，过悲伤肺，大恐伤肾等，在临床上确有实际意义。如暴怒会引起肝阳上亢，而出现头痛，眩晕，口干舌燥，两目干涩，失眠健忘等症状；思虑过度而伤脾，脾失健运，则易引起食欲不振，食后脘腹胀闷，倦怠无力等症状。

另外根据中医五行学说"恐胜喜，悲胜怒，怒胜思，喜胜悲，思胜恐"，就是以一种情绪平息另一种过极的情绪，即以情胜情的心理治疗方法。

中医十分重视精神护理，要求护理人员应掌握每个患者的各种心理状态及思想情况，调动患者的积极因素。首先应让患者知道精神因素对疾病的影响，发挥内因的作用，如肝病患者应戒怒，心病患者要防止过度兴奋或激动，肺病患者应保持乐观情绪等。而对其他危重患者，应适其意志，设法消除紧张、恐惧、忧虑、烦恼等不良精神刺激，做耐心细致的开导。安慰、解释工作，帮助患者树立战胜疾病的信心，更好的配合治疗，减轻患者的痛苦或早日康复。要做好精神护理工作，护理人员一方面应加强本身的修养，培养良好的医德和素质，具有踏踏实实、任劳任怨、认真负责的工作作风；对待患者应不论亲疏、贫富、长幼、丑俊、恩怨，均要一视同仁。另一方面要掌握一定的中医基础理论知识，运用于临床，结合患者疾病和思想动态，有的放矢的做好精神护理。

1.4 饮食护理

食物是治疗疾病，恢复健康的重要物质基础。《内经》指出"药以调之，食必随之"。所以中医在用药物治疗疾病的同时，还很注意饮食的调养作用。饮食调养也是中医护理的重要内容之一，因此护理人员应掌握饮食治疗的法则，以提高护理工作质量。

1. 食物宜忌

(1) 食物与疾病的关系：疾病有阴阳、寒热、虚实、表里之分，食物有寒、热、温、凉之性，辛、甘、酸、苦、咸之味，因此，食物的性味必须与疾病的属性相适应，否则会引起相反作用而影响治疗。在指导患者饮食时，应根据疾病的不同，选择不同性能的食物，以达到"虚则补之"、"实则泻之"、"寒者热之"、"热者寒之"的目的。例如：热证宜食凉性食物，忌食辛辣、醇酒、炙煿等热性食物；寒证宜食温性食物，忌食生冷，瓜果等凉性食物；阳虚者宜温补类食物，忌寒凉；阴虚者宜清补淡薄滋润类食物，忌温热；疔、痈为火毒之证，当忌食油腻、荤腥，以免助火生痰，增加病势；皮肤病一般忌鲜发鱼虾之类，避免生风透发更加作痒；痔疾忌食辛辣刺激之物，以免大便燥结，引起便血及便后疼痛。

(2) 食物与药物的关系：食物和药物同出一源，均来源于自然界中的植物和动物，药物所具有的性味、归经、特性，食物也同样具有。因此，药食的性能也有协同和相互克制的作用，协同者则可以增强疗效，如：当归加羊肉、生姜可增加温补生血作用；赤小豆炖鲤鱼可增强利水效应；黄芪加薏米可提高渗湿利水的功效。若药食性能相反，则会减低疗效甚至起副作用，如：萝卜与参类、地黄同用，则消食、耗气，致使参类、地黄失去补气作用；另外，荆芥忌鱼蟹；白术忌桃、李；蜂蜜忌葱；甘草忌鲢鱼，铁屑忌茶叶；黄连、桔梗、乌梅忌猪肉等。

（3）食物之间的关系：食物的性能各不相同，而在调配中也有相须、相使、相畏、相反的不同，如：羊肉、生姜同属温性，二者相互协同发挥作用，增强温补，可治疗虚寒性腹痛；蟹与生姜是一寒一温，以温祛寒，故可同食；而蟹与柿子，两者都属寒性，食后可导致胃寒，故不可同食。因此要掌握食物的性能及宜忌，才能做到食物间的合理调配，增强食物的协同作用，提高疗效。

（4）食物的烹调与疾病的关系：食物的烹调加工方法很多，同一种食物由于烹调方法不同，对疾病也有宜忌之别，所以在食物的烹调方面，要适应患者身体情况和疾病的需要。如肉类、鸡鸭等禽类，应文火煮烂，以利于消化吸收，才能适于胃肠疾患或久病气血双虚者食用，若这类食物用煎、炸、熏、烤等烹调方法，则可使食物性多燥热，食后伤耗胃阴，易发生内热病证；又如：蛋类，蒸蛋糕、煮蛋汤、冲蛋花，一般均不忌食；但煎、炒则碍胃，不易消化。因此食物合理的加工烹调，对配合治疗疾病，有着重要的意义。

2. 饮食护理的基本要求

（1）以中医理论为基础，指导饮食的辨证实施；要掌握每位患者的身体情况和不同病证选择适体疗疾的食物，食物的性能必须与疾病的属性相适应，如寒证应选用温热性食物，忌食寒凉；热证应选用寒凉性食物，忌食温热，否则会引起反作用。临床实践证明，某些疾病的发生，突然变化，恢复期延长，以及愈后复发等，大都与口腹不慎，恣意饮食有关。因此饮食护理是临床护理工作的重要环节。

（2）饮食有节：要注意四时饮食的调节，食量应节制，定时定量，不宜过饥、过饱；饮食冷热应相宜，硬软要适度，以保证脾胃运化功能正常，有利于疾病的恢复。反之，脾胃功能损伤，致使营血不和而加重病情。

（3）注意饮食卫生：食物宜清洁、新鲜；饭前应洗手，饭后要漱口，防止病从口入。饮食要有规律，应先饥而食，食勿过饱，不宜偏食、贪食，晚餐不宜多食，食后应散步，饱食不可即卧。另外食前应保持心情舒畅，做到怒后勿食，食后勿怒，以利于脾胃受纳，运化功能保持正常，促使身体早日康复。

3. 食物的分类

食物的种类繁多，不胜枚举，根据中医的传统分类，可归纳为谷类、蔬菜类、瓜果类、肉食类等。因食物的性味、性能的不同，可分为以下几类：

(1) 辛辣类：包括姜、葱、蒜、胡椒、辣椒、酒等属于热性动火类食物，适用于寒证疾病，热证患者忌用。

(2) 生冷类：包括瓜果、生冷拌菜、冷饭、冷菜和冷制食品等性凉多属寒性食物，适用于热证疾病，脾胃虚寒者宜少用或忌用。

(3) 膏粱厚味：主要是指禽、蛋、肉食、乳品等类以及经过煎、炒、炸、烤、爆、熏等烹调后的食物，性多燥热，易损耗胃阴，故热性病不宜食用。

(4) 补益类：各种食物均有一定的补养作用，但因性味不同，一般分为平补、清补、温补等。应根据病情的需要，体质的强弱和四时气候的变化等灵活运用。

4. 食物的性味

常用食物的性味主要是指四气，即寒、热、温、凉。一般把微寒归于凉，大温归于热，性温和的称为平性，因此临床上对食物的性味分为温热、寒凉、平性三类：

(1) 温热性的食物

①肉类：狗肉、牛肉、鸡肉、龟肉、羊肉、雀肉、虾肉、白花蛇肉、乌梢蛇肉等。

②菜类：黄豆、蚕豆、刀豆、淡菜、胡萝卜、葱、蒜、韭菜、芥菜、油菜、香菜、胡椒、辣椒等。

③其它：红糖、面粉、羊乳、江米等。

(2) 寒凉性的食物

①肉类: 鸭肉、鹅肉、兔肉、鳖肉、牡蛎肉、蟹肉等。

②菜类: 菠菜、白菜、芹菜、苋菜、竹笋、黄瓜、苦瓜、茄子、冬瓜、紫菜等。

③水果类: 梨、西瓜、柑、橙、柚等。

④其它: 大麦、绿豆、白糖、生蜂蜜等。

(3) 平性的食物

①肉类: 猪肉、鲤鱼肉、墨鱼肉等

②菜类: 赤小豆、黑豆、豇豆、四季豆、丝瓜、木耳、百合、莲子、大枣、土豆、黄花菜等。

③其它: 鸭蛋、山药、杏仁、葡萄、桃子、无花果等。

5. 常见食物的主要功效

(1) 有解表作用的: 辛温解表的有生姜、葱白、香菜等; 辛凉解表的有淡豆豉、茶叶、洋桃等。

(2) 有清热解毒作用的: 冬瓜、南瓜、黄瓜、西瓜、苦瓜、绿豆、扁豆、菠菜、田螺、鸭肉、梨、苋菜、西红柿等。

(3) 有清热解暑作用的: 绿豆、扁豆、西瓜、甜瓜、茶叶、柠檬等。

(4) 有清咽利喉作用的: 苦瓜、柿霜、荸荠、鸭蛋、黄瓜、芋头、薄荷等。

(5) 有祛湿利水作用的: 赤小豆、蚕豆、海带、紫菜、鲤鱼、黑鱼、西瓜、冬瓜、大白菜、芹菜等。

(6) 有镇咳、祛痰作用的: 萝卜、冰糖、梨、杏仁、白果、桔子等。

(7) 有健脾益胃作用的: 饴糖、大枣、莲子、山药、花生、生姜、葱、蒜、山楂、花椒、茴香等。

(8) 有补益作用的: 平补类的有猪肉、牛肉、鲤鱼、黑鱼、青鱼、葡萄、蛋类等; 清补类的有白果、百合、甲鱼、海参等; 温补类的有羊肉、狗肉、鸡肉、雀肉等。

（9）有预防感冒的：生姜、大蒜、葱、醋、豆豉等。

（10）有透疹作用的：香菜、香菇、荸荠、黄花鱼、鲜鲤鱼、鲜虾等。

（11）有解毒作用的：如生姜、醋可解鱼、蟹之毒；茶叶、白扁豆解药物中毒；山羊血、空心菜可解荤类中毒；蜂蜜解百毒；大蒜抑菌解毒。

（12）有润肠通便作用的：桑椹、蜂蜜、香蕉、核桃仁、芝麻油、松子、海带、猪肉等。

（13）有涩肠止泻作用的：莲子、炒山药、藕用于脾虚泄泻；大蒜、马齿苋适用于热性泄泻；山楂、焦麦芽、焦谷芽用于伤食泄泻等。

（14）有驱虫作用的：石榴、南瓜子、使君子、榧子、大蒜、椰子、胡萝卜等。

（15）有止血作用的：黄花菜、藕粉、木耳、刺菜、柿饼、香蕉、莴苣、韭菜等。

（16）有降血脂、血压、防止血管硬化作用的：海带、海蜇、紫菜、黑木耳、山楂、洋葱、香菇、大蒜、茶叶、芹菜、蜂蜜、豆类制品等。

（17）有通乳作用的：鲫鱼、猪蹄、莴苣、鲤鱼，产后气血不足而少乳宜用鲢鱼等。

（18）有治疗消渴作用的：糯米、猪肚、猪肉、桑椹、豆类、山药、洋葱、茭白等。

6. 常见病证饮食宜忌举例

呼吸系统疾病：包括急、慢性气管炎，哮喘、肺脓疡，肺结核，胸膜炎等疾病，常见症候如：咳嗽、咯痰、哮喘等。在急性发作期多为外邪所引起，故不宜过早滋腻补养，否则易于留邪，应清淡素食，多食水果，新鲜蔬菜，忌食辛辣、烟酒、油腻、甜粘食物。如果咳嗽痰黄，肺热盛者，宜选萝卜、桔子、梨、枇杷等或加粳米煮粥食之，以清热化痰；痰中夹血者，宜食藕片、藕汁，以清热止血；久病邪退，肺阴虚者，选用百合、银耳、甲鱼等滋阴补肺。

肝胆系统疾病：包括肝硬化，急、慢性肝炎，胆道系统感染及胆石症。饮食宜清淡，多进蔬菜及瘦肉、鸡、鱼类、忌食辛辣、烟酒刺激之品，少食动物脂肪。急性期应以素食为主，恢复期可稍进荤食。如肝脾肿大，可选食甲鱼、淡菜等。消腹水者可食鲫鱼、赤小豆汤，或常食黄芪、大枣粳米粥及动物肝，应低盐或无盐饮食。黄疸者可食鲤鱼、黄花菜、大枣、葡萄干、田螺等，以退黄疸。

1.5　服药护理

中药的剂型很多，药效各异，临床常用的有汤、膏、丹、丸、散、酒剂等。随着中药剂型的不断改革和发展，为解决汤剂服药困难及贮存携带方便，现已制成合剂、冲剂、片剂、针剂等。护理人员全面掌握药物的性能与各剂型的使用方法及其护理，将有利于提高疗效，促进患者早日康复。

1. 常用剂型

(1) 汤剂：常用多种药物配伍后加水煎煮去渣取汁而成，其特点：配方灵活，随症加减，奏效迅速，适用于急慢性疾病及复杂多变的症候。汤剂不仅内服也可外用，多用于熏洗疗法。

(2) 丸剂：即用多种药物配方后，共研细末，以水或蜂蜜调制成丸。丸剂吸收较缓慢，但药效持久，携带方便。适用于慢性疾病。

(3) 膏剂：是将药物反复煎煮去渣浓缩，掺入冰糖、饴糖、蜂蜜等调制成膏，如益母草膏、鹿胎膏等内服膏剂。另外，还有膏药或软膏可供外用。

(4) 散剂：即将一种或多种药物配方研碎成粉末状，可内服，也可外用。

(5) 酒剂：即将一种或多种药物浸泡于白酒中，使药物的有效成份溶于酒中，经过滤去渣而成。

(6) 丹剂：是使用盐、矾、硝、银等矿物质，在密闭条件下，经过加热升华或降华而制成的红、白等色结晶物，多做外用。有时也将某些具有特殊疗效，比较贵重的丸剂称为丹如：紫雪丹、小儿回春丹、至宝丹、避瘟丹等，多做内服。

(7) 冲剂：即把药物精选配方制成颗粒状，以开水冲后速溶成药液，即可内服，如：感冒冲剂、降压冲剂等。

(8) 片剂：即将一种或多种药物配方，研碎成粉末状，再加适当的辅料混合压制成片，如：犀羚解毒片，牛黄解毒片等。

2. 汤剂煎法

汤剂是临床上最常用的剂型，中药的煎煮方法对药效关系很大。

(1) 煎药容器：以砂锅、瓦罐为宜，现在也采用搪瓷器皿或铝锅。忌用铁锅，以免与药物发生化学反应而影响药效。

(2) 煎药前，先将药物加水浸泡1小时左右，有利于药物有效成份的煎出。加水量可因药物而异，如粉性大，含淀粉多的药物吸水性大，宜多加水；而贝壳类、矿物类可少加水；补养药宜久煎可多加水；解表药宜轻煎，少加水。

(3) 煎药的时间与火力，要根据药物的性能而定，如：解表药宜武火（急火）快煎，待药煮沸后5分钟左右即可，补益药应文火（小火）慢煎，煮沸后再煮约30～60分钟为宜。

(4) 煎药时应按药物不同的性质采用相应的方法，以保证药物的疗效。

①先煎：贝壳类、矿物类及某些果实、根茎类药物，如：磁石、代赭石、龙骨、牡蛎、龟板、瓦楞子、石决明、乌贼骨等，气味不易煎出者，均应先煎15～30分钟。生半夏、生附子、川乌、草乌等有毒药物，应先煎数小时，以减轻其毒性。

②后下：薄荷、藿香、钩藤、大黄等芳香辛散类药物，不宜久煎，应在其他药物基本煎好后再下，煎3～5分钟即可，以防

有效成分逸散。

③包煎：为防止绒毛类药物、小颗粒或有粘性的药物如旋覆花、车前子、青黛、赤石脂等，混入同煎浑腻难服，宜布包入煎。

④烊化：如阿胶、鹿角胶、饴糖之类，可放入煎好的汤药汁或水中徐徐加热，搅拌熔化后内服。

⑤泡服：如番泻叶、胖大海、双花、青果、寸冬、甘草等药可用沸水浸泡代茶饮。

⑥贵重药品的煎服：人参、西洋参、羚羊角片等贵重药物，宜单味煎煮，然后兑入汤药中同服。

3. 服药方法

根据疾病的轻重缓急、部位、性质及药物性能的不同，对服药的方法也有不同的要求。

(1) 按疾病的轻重：汤剂一般每日1剂，分两次服，两次间隔4～6小时为宜；重病者，每日两剂，每两小时1次；重危患者可少量多次频频喂服；神志不清或其他原因不能口服，可采用鼻饲法给药；呕吐者可将药汁浓缩后少量多次频服。

(2) 按病变部位分：病在下焦宜饭前服药，病在上焦和一般疾病均宜饭后服药。

(3) 按药物的性能：补养药宜空腹服；对胃肠道有刺激性的药物宜饭后服；安神药、润肠通便药宜睡前服；治疟药应在发作前两小时服；驱虫药宜在睡前及早晨空腹服；调经药应在行经前数日开始服用。

(4) 按疾病的性质分：一般疾病宜温服；寒证宜热服；热证宜冷服；对真热假寒或真寒假热证则可反佐，即寒药热服或热药冷服；发汗解表药宜趁热服，以助发汗。

(5) 其他剂型：散剂可用汤剂冲服或以蜂蜜调和用水送服，也可装入胶囊内吞服。丸剂：水丸可直接用水送服，蜜丸可分成小粒吞服，或用温水溶化后服用。膏剂宜用开水冲服。

4、服药的观察及护理

由于药物所具有的性能、气味、特性各不相同，因此服药后注意观察认真护理十分重要。

（1）服发汗药要掌握药量，服后应饮热稀粥或热开水，卧床盖被，以助药力，使其遍身微微出汗为宜，要防止大汗淋漓，汗出过量易耗伤津液，忌食生冷瓜果。

（2）服泻下药应观察大便次数、颜色及量，达到治疗目的后，即停止服药。

（3）服驱虫药后，注意观察有无药物毒性反应，检查大便有无寄生虫排出。

（4）服排石药后，应观察有无腹痛现象，检查大、小便，了解排石情况。

（5）服用酒剂应根据患者的酒量，切勿过量，防止引起头晕、头昏、呕吐、心悸等不良反应。

（6）呕吐患者在呕吐后应休息片刻，使胃气和降后再服药，服药前先食数滴姜汁或针刺内关穴以止呕。

（7）服用攻下药或峻下逐水药，对容易发生的不良反应要向患者说明，避免产生思想顾虑和紧张情绪。服药后应密切注意患者的反应，发现异常，及时处理。

2　危重证护理

2.1　高热护理

　　发热是临床常见的症状之一，可在许多疾病中出现。发热的原因可分为外感和内伤两个方面，内伤发热一般起病缓慢，病程较长，发热而不恶寒，或感到怯冷，但得到衣被则减。其热时作时止，或有定时，并感手足心热，伴有头晕神倦，自汗盗汗，脉弱无力等证候。外感发热，发病较急，病程较短，伴有恶寒，其寒虽得衣被亦不减，并有头痛，鼻塞，脉浮等证候。

　　1. 高热者应卧床休息。

　　2. 病室温、湿度适宜，光线不宜太强，空气新鲜，适当通风，但勿直接吹向患者。

　　3. 患者可因心情不畅，肝气不舒，气郁化火而加重身热，故应做好情志护理，尤其对内伤发热者，由于病程长，病情复杂，应鼓励患者减少思想负担，保持乐观主义精神，使疾病早日康复。

　　4. 饮食宜清淡，营养丰富，易于消化，根据发热轻重给予流汁或半流汁饮食。同时应辨证进食，禁食油腻、荤腥、辛辣食物。

　　5. 发热多损耗津液，临床表现口渴，小便短赤症状，应鼓励患者多饮水，可用麦冬、淡竹叶、灯芯草等泡水代茶饮，外感风热者多饮清凉饮料，如温开水，果子露、西瓜水等。外感风寒者多服热饮料，如热粥、热姜水等。忌食生冷。

　　6. 加强口腔护理，发热患者呼吸急促，加之汗出，耗伤津液，故表现口干舌燥，易发生口腔炎。可给双花、连翘、黄连、蒲公英水煎漱口，霉菌感染者涂大蒜注射液，或苦参注射液；口腔溃疡者可涂冰硼散，锡类散、柿霜、五枯散（五倍子 36 克加白糖 3 克，微火炒黄，加枯矾 25 克，共研细末，贮瓶备用）等，口唇干裂者可涂油剂。

7. 保持皮肤清洁，汗后用干毛巾擦拭，及时更换汗湿衣被，切勿受凉。对长期卧床患者注意皮肤护理，预防褥疮。

8. 注意观察体温变化，每 4 小时测量体温一次，必要时随时测量，并记录。高热者根据病情适当采取降温措施，注意不要影响热型的观察，以免延误诊断或导致虚脱。应首先辨明发热的原因，热在表者忌用物理降温，以免汗腺受冷的刺激而闭塞，致使热邪外达无出路，热不得解，因此应采取发汗解表法使热邪外达。壮热、口渴等里热证可采取物理降温。热甚便秘者，可给大黄粉 3 克或大黄片 5 片内服。

9. 针刺降温，可取曲池、大椎、风池，配印堂、太阳、合谷等穴，或用三棱针刺双太阳、印堂、十宣、尺泽等少量放血。耳针疗法取神门、皮质下、交感，中强刺激，捻转 5 分钟后，留针 30 分钟。

10. 热毒内陷心包患者出现高热，烦躁，神昏谵语，甚至痉厥者，即服紫雪丹 1.5～3 克，或安宫牛黄丸 1 丸，并报告医师，采取措施。

11. 体温骤降，汗出肢冷，面色苍白，表情淡漠或烦躁，脉象细数或脉微欲绝者，为虚脱征兆，应及时协助医生进行抢救。

12. 患者出现吐血、衄血，肌肤发斑、尿血、便血者，为热入营血，迫血妄行，应报告医生抢救。

13. 观察寒热，出汗，口渴，饮水，舌苔，脉象，神智，呼吸，面色，二便等变化，发现异常，及时处理。

14. 外感发热患者汤药宜热服，并多服热饮料，加盖衣被；内伤发热者汤药宜温服。注意观察服药后出汗情况，如出汗时间的长短，出汗部位、性质、气味等。若出汗过多，可停服中药，并向医生报告。

2.2 昏迷护理

昏迷的主要临床表现是患者神志不清，意识丧失，对各种刺激失去正常反应。引起昏迷的原因很多，如颅脑疾病，药物或化学药品中毒等，凡是昏迷均属危重症候。

1. 安置危重病室，病室环境宜安静，光线适宜，空气新鲜，备齐抢救用品、药品及安全护理物品。

2. 安排特护，制定护理计划，建立特别记录，注意观察体温，脉象，呼吸，血压，瞳仁的变化，做好记录，发现异常变化及时报告医生，以便采取治疗措施。

3. 密切观察病情变化

(1) 观察昏迷深、浅程度的变化，神志逐渐转清为病情好转，若昏迷程度继续加深，示病情加重，应协助医生，进行抢救。

(2) 若患者出现面色苍白，口开手撒，呼吸低微，四肢不温，汗出粘冷，血压下降，脉象细弱，示为闭转脱的危象，要配合医生，有效的进行抢救。

(3) 对昏迷原因尚未明确的患者，应严密观察有无高热，项强，头痛，抽搐，半身不遂，呕吐，黄疸等兼症出现，一旦发现，应及时报告医生，为诊断提供参考。

4. 保持呼吸道通畅，及时清除痰涎或呕吐物，一般适宜采取平卧位，头偏向一侧，取下假牙，舌后坠者应拉出，以免阻塞气道。若患者表现气息急促，面色青紫，肢体抽搐时，均应给氧，必要时行气管切开术。

5. 加强口腔护理，防止并发症发生。抽搐者用牙垫垫于牙齿咬合面，以免咬伤口舌。牙关紧闭者可用乌梅擦牙，或针刺下关、颊车、合谷等穴。张口呼吸者，可用一层湿纱布盖于口唇上，保持粘膜湿润。

6. 注意保护眼睛，昏迷患者，眼睑常有闭合不全，可定时滴眼药水，或用生理盐水湿纱布遮盖眼部等。可防止因角膜干燥而发生角膜溃疡和炎症。

7. 加强皮肤和肢体护理，二便失禁者，采取适当方法，以免刺激皮肤，并及时清洁臀部。瘫痪或偏瘫者，应做好肢体护理。

8. 预防泌尿系感染，记录尿量，如 6 小时以上无尿者，应辨清是尿潴留，还是尿少或尿闭，给予相应的处理。

9. 保持大便通畅，3 天无大便者，给予缓泻剂或灌肠等。

10. 昏迷初发患者 2～3 天内暂禁食，由静脉供给所需营养，2～3 天后仍未清醒者，应给鼻饲流汁饮食，原则为病初宜清淡，后期则需保证充足的营养，并应保持足够的水份。当病情好转，吞咽动作恢复时，及时停用鼻饲，通过口腔进食。

11. 遵照医嘱对闭证、脱证患者分别进行处理。

(1) 闭证：热闭患者鼻饲安宫牛黄丸、至宝丹、紫雪丹或静脉滴注清开灵注射液，亦可针刺人中、十宣、百会、合谷、涌泉等穴，或十宣放血；浊闭患者鼻饲苏合香丸；痰闭患者鼻饲竹沥水、生姜汁，或针刺天突、丰隆、内关等穴。

(2) 脱证：亡阳者给予参附汤，可灸气海、关元、百会、膻中、神阙穴（隔盐灸），针刺人中、合谷、足三里；亡阴者服生脉散或益心口服液。

2.3 厥证护理

厥证是以突然昏倒，不省人事，面色苍白，四肢厥冷为主要表现的一种病证。一般昏厥时间较短，清醒后无偏瘫失语，口眼㖞斜等后遗症。从现代医学观点来看，休克、昏厥、中暑、低血糖昏迷及精神性疾患等，均属厥证范畴。

因引起厥证的原因不同，临床又有气厥，血厥，痰厥，暑厥，食厥之分。

1. 立即使患者平卧或取头低位，呕吐及有痰者头偏向一侧，松解衣扣，注意保暖。

2. 保持病室环境安静，室内光线宜偏暗淡，使患者充分休息。

3. 厥逆时可喂糖水或开水，醒后可食清淡的流汁或半流汁饮食。

4. 观察神志、瞳仁、面色、体温、呼吸、脉象、血压及二便的变化，做好记录。发现异常及时报告医生，采取措施。

5. 注意询问病史及发病诱因，观察其全身情况，进行全面检查，分辨虚实，针对病因，进行原发病治疗与护理。

6. 因药物引起过敏反应而厥逆者，应立即皮下注射 0.1% 盐酸肾上腺素 1 毫升，给予氧气吸入，立即报告医生进行抢救。

7. 针灸治疗，实证可针刺人中、承浆、十宣、涌泉等穴，用强刺激，进针后每隔 3～5 分钟行针 1 次。虚证可配合灸法，取百会、气海等穴，至恢复正常为止。

8. 气厥患者常因精神刺激而诱发，应特别加强精神护理，劝慰患者及家属解除紧张、恐惧心理，避免不良刺激。

9. 血厥患者应及时测量血压，观察血压的变化，做好输血前的准备，虚证患者可服独参汤，根据病史做好原发病的治疗与护理。劝导患者加强休养，避免过度操劳，注意摄生，增强体质。

10. 痰厥患者应取侧卧位，痰不易咳出者可拍其背部，必要时用吸痰器吸痰，或即服竹沥水 30 毫升等，消除痰液，保持呼吸道通畅。

11. 暑厥患者，室内要通风凉爽，立即采取物理降温，急服清心开窍药物如：牛黄清心丸 1 丸，用凉开水调服，或服用十滴水、人丹等。多饮凉开水、绿豆汤、西瓜水等清凉饮料。

12. 食厥患者暂禁食，可用探吐法或中药催吐剂排出胃内容物，并服用和中消导药物，如保和丸、四消糖等。腹胀便秘者，可服缓泻剂如大黄片、番泻叶泡水代茶饮等。

13. 厥逆时间较长而导致昏迷患者，则参照昏迷护理。

14. 厥证缓解后，仍需严密观察病情变化，防止复发。

2.4 心悸护理

心悸是自觉心跳快并伴有心前区不适感，临床有生理性和病理性两种。中医学将心悸分为惊悸和怔忡两种。惊悸多由外因引起，其症状较轻，发作时间短，日久可发展为怔忡。怔忡以内因为主，其症较重，且时时发作。心悸的发生与精神因素，心血不足，心阳衰弱，水饮内停，瘀血阻络等有关。

1. 病室环境要安静，避免噪音，以防惊吓刺激引起心悸发作。

2. 心悸发作常与精神过度紧张、激动或思虑有关，故应加强精神护理，使患者心情舒畅，正确对待疾病，安心休养，积极配合治疗。

3. 重症患者或心悸发作时，应卧床休息，兼有喘息气促症状时，可取半卧位，并给于氧气吸入。轻症患者可适当活动，活动量应逐渐增加，以不加重症状为度，避免劳累和剧烈运动。

4. 饮食选用具有补养作用的食物，如山药、大枣、莲子、桂圆、甲鱼、猪心、海参等食品，应少量多餐，勿进食过饱，忌辛辣刺激性食物和烟、酒。痰多者忌食肥甘油腻食品。兼有水肿者控制钠盐的摄入。

5. 严密观察病情变化

(1) 注意心悸发作的情况，是经常性还是阵发性，与活动，精神，进食的关系，以协助诊断。

(2) 观察心悸伴随症状，若伴有咳嗽、胸痛、胸闷、呼吸困难、尿少、浮肿者多为心力衰竭；若伴有胸痛，出冷汗、血压下降，提示心肌梗塞；若伴有高热，全身中毒症状严重者，则应考虑中毒性心肌炎。发现以上情况，应报告医生及时处理。

(3) 观察心悸发作特点，持续时间和规律。

（4）注意观察血压，心率，心律的变化，发现异常报告医生及时处理。

（5）注意面色，舌象，脉象的变化。面部烘热，舌质红，脉细数者多属阴虚火旺；面色㿠白，舌质淡，脉细弱者多属阳气虚衰；面色不华，舌质偏紫，脉涩或结代为心血瘀阻；面浮肿，苔腻、脉迟滑者是痰湿或寒的表现。

6. 心悸发作时可针刺心俞、内关、神门、膻中等穴位。

7. 保持大便通畅，便秘者给予轻泻剂，如清宁丸3克，日服2次。

8. 患者心跳骤然停止，应立即采取胸外按摩、人工呼吸、心内注射等抢救措施。

9. 服用洋地黄类药物前，要测脉搏和心率，心率应测1分钟，若低于60次，则应考虑停药。注意观察有无服用洋地黄毒性反应，一旦出现，立即报告医生采取措施。

3 内科常见病证及护理

3.1 感冒

感冒是常见的外感疾病。以鼻塞，流涕，头痛，咳嗽，恶寒，发热等为特征。轻者称为伤风，重者称为重伤风，如在一个时期内广泛发病，证候多类似者，称为时行感冒，即流行性感冒。

一般护理

1. 保持室内空气新鲜，适当通风，勿吹向患者，以免复感加重病情，注意防寒保暖，随气候变化及时增减衣被。

2. 流行性感冒应按呼吸道隔离，病室空气消毒宜用食醋熏蒸法，每立方米用食醋 5～10 毫升，以 1～2 倍水稀释加热，每日 1 次或隔日 1 次。

3. 轻症患者勿须卧床休息，重症或发热者应卧床休息，热退后可起床，症状消失后恢复工作，但要注意劳逸结合，防止过劳。

4. 给予营养丰富，清淡易消化的食物，忌食油腻甜粘食物。轻症宜食半流汁饮食，重症宜食素流汁，宜多饮水。

5. 注意观察发热，恶寒，出汗，咳嗽，舌象，脉象的变化。

6. 汤药宜轻煎不可过煮，1 剂分 2 次服，如服头煎药后出汗较多，体温骤降者，应立即报告医生，并停服二煎药。出汗为病邪外达但不可太过，以微汗遍及全身为宜，出汗后尤应避风保暖，以防复感。若服药后仍无汗，热势继续上升，应报告医生。

7. 患者应注意锻炼身体，增强机体的抗病能力。

辨证护理

1. 风寒证

临床表现

恶寒重，发热轻，无汗，头痛身楚，鼻塞流涕，咳嗽痰喘，口不渴或喜热饮，舌苔薄白，脉浮紧。

护理

(1) 病室温度宜偏高。

(2) 禁食生冷食物，宜多服热饮料。

(3) 服用辛温解表宣肺散寒的药物，方选荆防败毒散加减。汤药宜热服。服后避风盖被取汗，同时多服些热饮料或食热粥、米汤之类，以助药力。

(4) 高热者不宜用物理降温，以防毛窍闭塞，邪达无出路。

(5) 针灸治疗以祛风散寒，解表宣肺为目的，取列缺、迎香、风池、合谷等穴位，头痛加印堂、太阳等穴位。

(6) 可给生姜3片、葱白5节、淡豆豉9克水煎服，或犀羚解毒片1日3次内服。

2. 风热证

临床表现

身热较著，微恶风寒，汗泄不畅，头痛目赤，流黄浊涕，咳嗽，痰粘或黄，咽喉肿痛，口渴欲饮，苔白微黄，脉象浮数。

护理

(1) 病室温度宜凉爽，适当通风。

(2) 多食水果如西瓜、洋桃等，多饮清凉饮料如绿豆汤。

(3) 服用辛凉解表，宣肺清热的药物，方选银翘散加减，汤药宜温服，衣被适中不可过暖，汗多衣湿时待汗止后更换湿衣，以免重感。

(4) 针灸治疗以疏散风热，清利肺气，取尺泽、鱼际、曲池、大椎、外关等穴位。咽喉肿痛加少商，用三棱针点刺放血，或服用喉症丸、六神丸等。

(5) 可给竹叶 12 克，薄荷 3 克、杏仁 3 克、连翘 3 克，用水煎服，桑菊感冒冲剂 1 袋，日服 3 次。

3. 暑湿证

临床表现

身热，微恶风，汗少，头重如裹，肢体酸重疼痛，咳嗽痰粘，鼻流浊涕，心烦口渴，渴不多饮，胸闷，脘痞，呕恶，甚则腹胀、便溏，舌苔厚腻或黄腻，脉象濡或濡数。

护理

(1) 胃肠道症状明显者，食清淡的流汁饮食。

(2) 服用清暑解表，芳香化浊的药物，新加香薷饮加减，药宜温服，胃肠道症状明显者，可少量多次服，也可加生姜汁服用。

(3) 针灸治疗以达清暑化湿，疏表和里，取中脘、合谷、足三里等穴位，热重加大椎、曲池，湿重加阴陵泉穴。

(4) 可用六一散 12 克、薄荷 6 克，开水泡服，或藿香正气丸 1～2 丸，日服 2 次。

3.2 痢疾

痢疾为夏秋季节常见的肠道传染病，以腹痛腹泻，里急后重，大便脓血为主症。

一般护理

1. 做好消化道隔离，防止交叉感染，对其排泄物、餐具、便具及所接触的物品，均应严格消毒。大便培养连续 3 次阴性后，方可解除隔离。

2. 病室应空气新鲜，温度适宜，急性患者应卧床休息，慢性患者可适当锻炼，增强体质。

3. 观察腹痛情况，大便次数、颜色及全身情况，若出现高热、昏迷、痉厥则为邪陷心营的危重症候，应报告医生，采取抢救措施。

4. 便后用软纸轻擦肛门，用温水洗净，必要时可外扑爽身粉，或涂少量油类。

辨证护理

1. 湿热痢
临床表现

发热恶寒，腹痛腹泻，大便带粘液或脓血，肛门灼热，里急后重，口干喜冷，苔黄腻，脉象滑数。

护理

(1) 食流质或半流质饮食，宜清淡，鼓励患者多饮温开水或淡盐水，以补充液体，防止伤津。

(2) 服用清利湿热、行气和血药物，方选芍药汤、葛根芩连汤加减，汤药宜温服。

(3) 针刺天枢、大肠俞、膈俞、足三里，血海等穴位。

2. 疫毒痢
临床表现

发病急骤，痢下脓血，腹痛剧烈，里急后重，高热面赤，口渴烦躁，甚至谵妄，昏迷痉厥，舌红绛苔黄，脉洪数。

护理

(1) 病情严重的患者可暂禁食6～8小时，病情稳定后食流质饮食，多饮水，保持水电解质平衡，恢复期患者逐渐恢复正常饮食，忌食油腻、煎炸等不易消化的食物。

(2) 注意观察体温的变化，高热者报告医生，采取治疗措施（参照2.1高热护理）。

(3) 注意观察病情，如患者出现神昏谵语、抽风痉厥，烦躁不安，面色苍白、脉象细弱等。应报告医生，采取治疗措施（参照2.3厥证护理）。如出现呼吸深浅，节律不齐，或叹息样呼吸，为呼吸衰竭危象，应及时报告医生，采取抢救措施。

(4) 服用清热凉血解毒药物，方选白头翁汤加减。可配合保留灌肠。

(5) 针刺大椎、内关、天枢、四缝、十宣等穴位。

3. 虚寒痢

临床表现

痢下稀薄紫暗，或夹有粘沫，久痢不复，腹痛里急，形寒肢冷，神疲纳呆，苔薄白，脉沉细。

护理

(1) 腹部注意保暖，腹痛时可用热水袋、炒盐或小茴香热敷。

(2) 给予易消化，营养丰富的食物，可食些大蒜、葱、姜之类的热性食物，少食粗纤维及油腻、生冷食物。

(3) 服用温补脾肾，涩肠固脱药物，方选养脏汤合四神丸加减，汤药应热服。

(4) 灸足三里、天枢、神阙、大肠俞等穴位。

4. 休息痢

临床表现

久病不愈，时发时止，痢则腹痛，里急后重，大便夹有粘液或少量脓血，苔薄白，脉细弱。

护理

(1) 注意调节饮食，体虚者应加强营养，常食健脾益气，化滞和胃药物，方选六君子汤加减，发作时加香连丸，汤药应温服。

(2) 针灸取足三里、中脘、脾俞等穴位。

3.3 支气管炎

支气管炎分急性、慢性两种，属中医学咳嗽的范围。急性支气管炎多属外感咳嗽；慢性支气管炎多属内伤咳嗽。以春冬气候多变的季节较为多见。小儿和年老体弱者易发病。临床以咳嗽、咯痰或喘促等为主症。

一般护理

1. 室内清洁，空气流通，保持适宜的温度和湿度，避免干燥，防止灰尘、烟雾和特殊气味刺激，以免诱发咳嗽或使咳嗽加重。

2. 发热者应卧床休息，年老体弱者可延长休息时间。

3. 饮食宜高热量，清淡易消化食物，宜多饮水。忌食辛辣刺激之物，戒烟、酒。

4. 注意观察发热、咳嗽、痰液的性质以及舌苔、脉象的变化。

辨证护理

1. 风寒外束，肺失宣降
临床表现
咳嗽，痰稀薄白，恶寒微热，鼻塞流涕，喉痒声重，舌苔薄白，脉浮。
护理
(1) 注意保暖，室内温度宜偏温，注意气候变化，外出时戴口罩，以防复感外邪，加重病情。
(2) 忌食生冷瓜果。
(3) 服用疏散风寒，宣肺止咳药物，方选杏苏散加减。药宜热服，并观察服药后的效果。
(4) 通宣理肺丸每次服1～2丸，每日2次。
(5) 针灸治疗，取列缺、合谷、肺俞、外关等穴位。

2. 风热犯表，肺失宣畅
临床表现
咳嗽痰稠，咳而不爽，口渴咽痛，身热。舌苔黄，脉浮数。

护理

(1) 室内空气宜清爽，避免直接吹风。

(2) 多食具有清热化痰作用的食物，如橘子、柚子、萝卜、牛肉等，多服清凉饮料。

(3) 服用疏风清热，宣肺止咳药物。方选桑菊饮加减，汤药宜温服。

(4) 痰稠咳而不爽的患者，取坐位或半卧位，可轻拍背部，或用双花、桔梗、远志各 3 克水煎药液，做雾化吸入，稀释痰液，以利排痰。

(5) 发热者按时测量体温，并报告医生（参照 2.1 高热护理）。

(6) 针灸治疗，取尺泽、肺俞、曲池、大椎等穴位。

(7) 桑菊片 3 片，日服 3 次，或桑叶 9 克、杏仁 9 克、生石膏 30 克、甘草 1 克，用水煎服。

(8) 注意口腔清洁，可用银芩汤（双花 9 克、蒲公英 9 克、黄连 9 克、黄芩 9 克，水煎 500 毫升）漱口。

3. 脾不健运，痰湿壅肺

临床表现

咳嗽痰多，痰白粘或稀，胸脘满闷，舌苔白腻，脉濡滑。

护理

(1) 饮食宜清淡，戒烟、酒，忌食肥脂肉类食品，以免助湿生痰。

(2) 服用健脾燥湿，化痰理肺药物，方选二陈汤加味。观察服药后的效果。

(3) 针灸治疗取中脘、丰隆、肺俞等穴位。

(4) 橘红丸每次服 1～2 丸，日服 2 次。或半夏 9 克、茯苓 12 克、陈皮 3 克、甘草 3 克，用水煎服。

4. 肝郁化火，火热扰肺

临床表现

气逆作咳，面红喉干，痰质浓稠，心烦口渴，舌苔薄黄，少津，脉弦数。

护理

(1) 加强情志护理，避免情绪激动，保持心情舒畅。

(2) 服用平肝泻火，清肺降逆药物，方选咳血方加味。

(3) 针灸治疗，取肺俞、肝俞、经渠、太冲等穴位。

(4) 桑白皮9克、黄芩9克、黛蛤散9克，水煎服。

3.4 支气管哮喘

哮证是一种发作性的痰鸣气喘疾患。喉中有痰鸣音，呼吸气促困难。喘是指呼吸困难而急促，甚则张口抬肩，鼻翼煽动，不能平卧。两者相兼名为哮喘。初发病多属实证，如反复发作则转为虚证。

一般护理

1. 室内设施简单，保持整洁，安静，空气流通，不要放置有刺激气味的花草和其它物品。

2. 哮喘发作时，需卧床休息，取半卧位或端坐位，并及时给氧。

3. 有吸烟习惯者，应劝其戒烟。

4. 饮食宜清淡，避免食用可能诱发哮喘发作的食物，如鸡蛋、牛奶、鱼、虾等。忌食生冷、过咸、甜的食物。

5. 加强精神护理，保持心情舒畅，避免因精神因素影响而发病。哮喘发作时，安慰患者消除紧张情绪。

6. 嘱患者尽量避免接触烟雾、灰尘和有刺激性气味，以免诱发哮喘发作。

7. 注意观察哮喘发作的先兆，如胸闷，呼吸不畅，鼻咽痒，喷嚏，流涕等，应尽早给以处理。

8. 密切观察哮喘发作的时间，轻重程度，持续时间，伴发症状，咯痰情况，体温，舌象，脉象等的变化。

9. 了解患者的生活环境，饮食习惯，家族过敏史等，以寻找诱发因素，并注意避免接触。

10. 痰不易咳吐的患者，可给予中药煎剂做雾化吸入或轻拍背部，以助排痰。

11. 平时注意锻炼身体，增强体质，如气功、呼吸操、太极拳等。

辨证护理

1. 实证

(1) 寒饮伏肺

临床表现

呼吸急促，喉中有哮鸣音，咳痰清稀，呈泡沫状，胸膈满闷，面色晦滞，口不渴，或渴喜热饮，或兼有头痛，发热，恶寒，无汗等。舌苔白滑，脉象浮紧。

护理

①注意保暖，避免受凉，外出时戴口罩。

②服用温肺散寒，豁痰利窍药物，方选射干麻黄汤加减。药宜热服。多服热饮料，忌食生冷。

③针灸治疗，取列缺、尺泽、风门、肺俞等穴。

④每晚睡前服哮喘丸3粒。将洋金花叶制成卷烟状，哮喘发作时点燃吸入，可缓解症状。

(2) 痰热遏肺

临床表现

咳喘气粗，痰黄质稠，面红发热，有汗，口渴，烦躁，咳引胸痛，舌苔黄腻，脉象滑数。

护理

①注意口腔清洁，可给银苓汤漱口。

②发热者，及时观察体温的变化。

③服用清热宣肺，化痰降逆药物，方选麻杏石甘汤加减，药宜温服，注意观察服药后的效果。

④针灸治疗，取合谷、大椎、丰隆、膻中等穴位。喘甚者加肺俞、云门等穴拔火罐。

⑤蛇胆川贝散每次服 1 支，日服 3 次。

2. 虚证

临床表现

起病较缓，病程较长，呼吸气短，语言无力，自汗恶风，动则气喘，口唇指甲青紫，四肢欠温，舌质隐紫，脉象细数。

护理

(1) 防止疲劳和情志刺激，以防诱发哮喘。

(2) 随气候变化，注意防寒保暖，严防受凉。

(3) 服用补肺益肾、降气化痰药物，方选平喘固本汤加减。汤药宜热服。

(4) 肺气虚者，可给黄芪膏，每次服 15 克，日服 3 次。

(5) 针灸治疗，取定喘、膏肓、肺俞、太渊等穴位。

3.5 肺脓疡

肺脓疡中医学称"肺痈"。是肺部生脓疡的病证。以发热，咳嗽，胸痛，咯吐大量腥臭脓血痰为特征。临床按病程先后的各个阶段，分为初期，成痈期，溃脓期和恢复期。

一般护理

1. 病室清洁，室内保持良好通风，空气新鲜。

2. 注意室温的调节，做好防寒保暖，避免重感，以防加重病情。

3. 急性期发热、吐脓痰及咳血时，应卧床休息。病情好转后，应下地活动，可促使脓痰排出。

4. 饮食宜清淡，多食蔬菜，不宜过咸，忌食辛辣油腻厚味，和海腥发物，如黄鱼、虾、螃蟹等。应多饮水。

5. 戒烟和酒。

6. 观察体温，呼吸，舌苔，脉象的变化，并做好记录。

7. 注意观察咳痰的情况，以及咯痰的色、质、量、味的变化。

辨证护理

1. 初期

临床表现

恶寒发热，咳嗽，咯白色粘沫痰，痰量由少渐多，呼吸不畅，口干鼻燥，舌苔薄黄或薄白，脉浮数而滑。

护理

(1) 注意观察患者咳嗽、胸痛及痰量的变化。

(2) 服用清肺解表的药物。方选银翘散加减。汤药不宜久煎，宜温服。注意观察服药后的效果。防止成痈。

2. 成痈期

临床表现

发热汗出，寒战，胸闷胸痛，烦燥不安。咳嗽气急，吐脓性痰，有腥臭味。舌苔黄腻，脉滑数。

护理

(1) 观察发热，胸痛，痰液量、色、气味的变化。患者出现壮热寒战，胸闷、咳嗽时，牵引胸部隐痛，吐腥臭痰，示肺痈已成。

(2) 服用清肺化瘀、消痈药物。方选苇茎汤加减。

(3) 大便秘结者，可给予缓泻剂，以保持大便通畅。

3. 溃脓期

临床表现

咳吐大量脓血痰，腥臭异常，胸中烦满而痛，喘不得卧，身热面赤，烦渴喜饮。舌质红或绛，苔黄腻，脉象滑数。

护理

（1）发热者给予半流质饮食，多吃水果，如：橘子、梨、枇杷、萝卜等，以润肺化痰。可食苡米粥，以助排痰。多服清凉饮料，取鲜芦根煎水代茶饮。

（2）加强对患者口腔护理，给予银芩汤，或用淡盐水漱口，保持口腔清洁。

（3）注意痰杯消毒，杯内应加入适量消毒液。

（4）服用排脓解毒药物，方选加味桔梗汤加减。

（5）痰稠不易咳出者，可用清热化痰药物，用水煎液，做雾化吸入，以利排痰。

（6）根据病灶的部位，安置患者适当的体位，以利体位引流排痰。

（7）注意观察病情，若发现大量咳血，咯血时，应警惕出现血块阻塞气道，或气随血脱的危象，一旦出现，应立即报告医生，采取抢救措施。

（8）取鲜薏苡仁适量，捣碎炖汤服，每日3次，以助排痰。或荷叶适量煎浓汁，加白蜜服之。

4. 恢复期

临床表现

身热渐退，咳嗽减轻，咯吐脓血渐少，臭味亦减，痰液转为清稀。或见胸胁隐痛，气短，自汗，盗汗，低烧，潮热，面色不华，形体消瘦，舌质红或淡红，脉细数无力。

护理

（1）鼓励患者下床活动，但不宜过劳。

（2）给予高热量、高蛋白饮食。食量逐增，不宜过量，以免损伤脾胃。

（3）因病程较长，患者思想负担较重，故应加强对患者的精神护理，保持心情舒畅，以利疾病恢复。

3.6 高血压病

高血压是以头痛，眩晕，时发时止，或头重脚轻，步履不稳，血压升高为特征，属中医学的头痛、眩晕病范畴。

一般护理

1. 病室光线不宜太强，环境安静、舒适，保证有充足的睡眠时间。

2. 早期高血压患者可参加工作，但不要过度疲劳。要坚持适当锻炼，如打太极拳、练气功等。

3. 给予热量较低和清淡的膳食。多吃蔬菜、水果、高维生素食物。饮食不要过量。少食盐，忌食辛辣、甘肥、油腻食物，避免饮酒。

4. 观察血压的变化。血压波动明显者，应报告医生，采取措施。

辨证护理

1. 肝郁化火，风阳上亢

临床表现

头痛眩晕，面赤目红，烦躁多怒，口苦咽干，小便黄少，舌质红，脉弦数有力。

护理

(1) 掌握患者心理，做好精神护理，劝导患者解除忧虑，恼怒，保持心情舒畅和乐观的态度。

(2) 服用清泻肝热，佐以养阴的药物，方选龙胆泻肝汤加减。

(3) 针灸治疗，取行间、水泉、印堂等穴位；耳穴压豆神门、降压沟等。

(4) 菊花60克，煎水代茶饮。龙胆泻肝丸每次服9克，每日服 2 次。

2. 肝肾阴虚，肝阳上亢

临床表现

眩晕耳鸣，失眠多梦，烦躁易怒，尿赤不畅，腰疼腿酸，甚则四肢麻木。脉弦细，舌质黯红。

护理

（1）注意观察病情变化，若发现有唇舌麻、肢体麻木，口眼㖞斜等中风征象，应立即让患者卧床休息，并及时报告医生，进行处理。

（2）本证每因劳累、或恼怒而发病，故患者应注意休息，做好精神护理。

（3）针灸治疗，取肝俞、肾俞、三阴交、足三里等穴位。

（4）脑立清每服 10～20 粒，每日服 2 次。

（5）服用育肝肾阴，潜镇肝阳药物，方选镇肝熄风汤加减。汤药宜温服。

3. 阴阳俱虚，虚阳上逆

临床表现

头痛，眩晕，目糊耳鸣，面微红，口干自汗出，失眠多梦，肢冷腰酸，筋惕肉瞤，行动气急，舌暗红苔少，脉象弦细。

护理

（1）加强饮食调补，多食红枣、黑芝麻、山药、核桃等。

（2）服用滋补肾阴，温肾助阳药物，方选肾气丸加减。

（3）针灸治疗，取气海、三阴交、足三里、脾俞等穴位，用补法。

（4）桂附地黄丸每次服 1 丸，每日服 2 次。

3.7　脑血管病

本病是以猝然昏仆，不省人事，伴口眼㖞斜，半身不遂，语言不利；或不经昏仆，而仅以㖞僻不遂为主症的一种疾病，中医学称中风。因外邪侵袭而发病者，称为外风，又称类中风或类中。本病的发生，病情有轻重缓急的差别，轻者仅限于血脉经络，重者常波及有关脏腑，所以临床将中风分为中经络、中脏腑两大类。中经络一般无神志改变而病轻；中脏腑常有神志不清而病重。

一般护理

1. 昏迷患者，参照 2.2 昏迷护理。

2. 病室环境宜安静、清洁，空气新鲜。

3. 急性期患者要绝对卧床休息，避免搬动。

4. 根据病情可食清淡的半流质或流质饮食，多饮水，昏迷者给予鼻饲。忌烟、酒、肥甘及刺激性食物。

5. 严密观察病情，如神志、瞳仁、血压、舌象、脉象、体温、呼吸、二便、语言、肢体等情况的变化，并做好记录。

6. 情志所伤，五志过极，是本病的主要发病因素之一，故应做好精神护理，使患者保持心情舒畅，安心养病，积极配合治疗。

辨证护理

1. 中经络

临床表现

头痛、头晕，突然口眼㖞斜，口角流涎，语言不清，肌肤不仁，手足麻木，或恶寒发热，肢体拘急，关节酸痛，甚则半身不遂，舌苔薄白，脉象浮数。

护理

(1) 疾病初起，应卧床休息，头部宜放平。待病情好转后，逐渐恢复活动。

(2) 服用平肝熄风、化痰通络药物，方选牵正散合导痰汤加减。

（3）注意观察病情，遇有变化及时处理，以免反复发作，使病情由轻转重，出现中脏腑之候。

（4）病情稳定后，进行按摩、推拿、针灸等治疗，并指导患者练气功、打太极拳，以利机体功能恢复。

（5）忌用止血剂，以免血液凝滞，影响疗效。

2. 中脏腑

（1）闭证

临床表现

突然昏倒，不省人事，牙关紧闭，面红、目赤、口眼㖞斜，肢体偏瘫或兼拘急，二便闭塞，舌红苔黄，脉滑数。

护理

①患者应绝对卧床休息，取头高侧卧位，尽量避免搬动，以防引起病情恶化。

②保持口腔清洁，做好口腔护理。

③保持呼吸道通畅，必要时给予吸痰。

④阳闭者喂服或用鼻饲法，服局方至宝丹或安宫牛黄丸；阴闭者急用苏合香丸，温水化开喂服或鼻饲。

⑤服用熄风清火、豁痰开窍药物，方选羚羊钩藤汤加减。

⑥两目闭合不全者，给予生理盐水纱布敷盖，以免角膜干燥受损，必要时可给氯霉素眼药水点眼。

⑦观察体温变化，体温在39℃以上者，头部可放置冰袋，或酒精擦浴，夏季室内可吹电风扇。

⑧严密观察患者的神志、瞳仁、呼吸、血压等变化，发现异常，及时报告医生进行抢救。

⑨保持二便通畅。便秘者，可服缓泻剂，如生大黄粉5克，或番泻叶9克，泡水代茶饮。也可用开塞露。尿潴留者，可推拿箕门穴，或针刺中极、三阴交，必要时可行导尿和灌肠。

⑩针灸治疗，取人中、十二井、太冲、丰隆、劳宫等穴位，以平肝熄风，豁痰开窍。牙关紧闭加地仓、颊车，吞咽困难加照

海、天突等穴位。

(2) 脱症

临床表现

昏沉不醒，目合、口张、手撒、遗尿、鼻鼾息微、四肢逆冷，脉细弱或微。

护理

①服用救阴回阳固脱药物，方选参附汤合生脉散加减。观察服药后的效果。

②观察呼吸、出汗、肢温、血压等变化，若出现冷汗如油，面赤如妆，脉微欲绝，或浮大无根，为危候，应报告医生，及时抢救。

③用艾柱灸关元穴。神阙穴隔盐灸，以回阳固脱。

(3) 后遗症

临床表现

半身不遂，口眼㖞斜，语言不利等。

护理

①做好精神护理，避免情志刺激，保持心情舒畅。

②起居有常，以防六淫之邪侵袭而加重病情。

③饮食有节，给予清淡易消化的食物，忌食肥甘及刺激性食物。

④病情稳定后，及时指导患者坚持肢体功能锻炼，循序渐进，可选择推拿、按摩、太极拳、散步等方法。

⑤半身不遂者给予针灸治疗，取合谷、手三里、曲池、肩井、环跳、血海、阳陵泉、足三里、昆仑等穴位。手足瘛疭不能握物，取申脉、臑会、腕骨、合谷、行间、阳陵泉等穴位。也可采取头针疗法，取运动区、足运感区、语言区。耳针取偏瘫相应的穴位。

⑥语言不利者，应早期进行语言训练，采取由简单到复杂的方法。

3.8 冠状动脉硬化性心脏病

以胸骨后、心前区出现发作性或持续性闷痛，疼痛常放射至颈、臂或上腹部，短气、喘息不得卧，有时伴有四肢厥冷、青紫。脉微细。属中医学，真心痛、胸~的范畴。

一般护理

1. 病情轻者可适当活动，短气、喘息不能平卧者，可取半卧位，病情重者应卧床休息。

2. 饮食有节，给予清淡饮食，多食水果、蔬菜，可少量多餐。勿过食肥甘、生冷食品，忌烟酒，避免饮食不当损伤脾胃，脾胃运化失常可导致发病，或加重病情。

3. 情志失调是本病发生和病情加重的主要因素，故应做好情志护理，使患者解除顾虑，避免紧张和激动，保持情绪稳定，积极配合治疗。

4. 严密观察患者疼痛的部位、性质、程度、持续时间、发作诱因、舌象、脉象、呼吸、心率、心律、血压和出汗等方面的情况变化，给予及时处理，并做好记录。

5. 保持大便通畅，让患者养成按时排便的习惯，大便时无努责，以免发生意外。便秘患者，应多食蔬菜、水果、蜂蜜等，必要时给予缓泻剂，如大黄片、番泻叶等。

6. 心前区疼痛突发、疼痛较甚者，要立即休息，可服冠心苏合香丸 1 粒，舌下含化硝酸甘油片 0.3~0.6 毫克。可采用针灸治疗，取膻中、内关、足三里、通里、曲池、神门、间使、郄门等穴位。

7. 胸闷气短，呼吸困难患者，应给予氧气吸入。

8. 病情稳定后，指导患者适当进行身体锻炼，如太极拳、气功等。避免劳累和剧烈的运动。

辨证护理

1. 胸阳不振，心脉闭阻
临床表现

胸闷憋气，阵发性心痛，心悸，气短，面色苍白，畏寒肢冷，或自汗出，夜寐不宁，食欲不振，小便清长，大便稀薄，舌苔白润或腻，脉沉缓或结代。

护理

(1) 室温适宜，注意保暖，以防感冒加重病情。

(2) 给予易消化的饮食，多食具有助阳作用的食物，如刀豆、对虾、核桃仁等，忌食生冷食物。

(3) 服用温助心阳，宣通脉络的药物，方选瓜蒌薤白桂枝汤加减，汤药宜热服。

(4) 针灸治疗，取心俞、厥阴俞、内关、通里等穴位，针后加灸，以达助阳散寒。

2. 气滞血瘀，心络受阻
临床表现

阵发性心胸刺痛，痛引肩背，胸闷气短，舌质暗，脉沉涩或结代。

护理

(1) 注意观察患者心胸疼痛的情况，及时给予处理。

(2) 服用行气活血，化瘀通络的药物，方选血府逐瘀汤加减。

(3) 针灸治疗，取膻中、巨阙、膈俞、心俞等穴位，针用泻法。

(4) 五灵脂 30 克、蒲黄 30 克，共研细末，每服 6 克，黄酒送服。

3. 脾虚聚痰，阻遏心络
临床表现

体多肥胖，嗜睡身倦，咳嗽痰稀，胸闷憋气作痛，头蒙如裹，心悸不宁，苔白或腻，脉滑或弦滑。

护理

(1) 节制饮食，不宜过饱，以减轻体重，降低心脏负担。饮食不宜过甜，忌食油腻，煎炸食品，以免助湿生痰。

(2) 服用健脾化痰、除湿养心的药物，方选导痰汤加减。

(3) 针灸治疗，取巨阙、膻中、郄门、太渊、丰隆等穴位，针用泻法，以通阳化浊。

4. 肝肾阴虚，心血瘀阻

临床表现

胸闷气憋，夜间胸痛，头昏耳鸣，口干目眩，夜寐不宁，盗汗，腰酸腿软等，舌质嫩红，脉细数或细涩。

护理

(1) 夜寐不宁的患者，可给予枣仁粉 10 克，睡前服，或耳穴压豆，取心、肾、神门等穴。

(2) 夜间盗汗患者，每晚睡前用五倍子粉适量，醋调外敷神阙穴。

(3) 心绞痛常在夜间发作，故夜间要加强护理，注意巡视，发现有发作先兆，及时给予处理。

(4) 服用滋补肝肾，活血化瘀药物，方选养阴通痹汤加减。

5. 阴阳两虚，气血不继

临床表现

胸闷心痛，夜间可以憋醒。心悸气短，头晕耳鸣，食少倦怠，恶风肢冷，或手心发热。舌质紫暗，苔白少津，脉细弱结代。

护理

(1) 若出现心痛持续，或突然出现四肢厥冷、青紫，脉微细，血压下降，是阳虚欲脱的危候，应急服四逆汤合生脉散，回阳救脱。并立即报告医生，进行抢救。

（2）服用调补阴阳，益气养血药物，方选炙甘草汤加减；或柏子养心丸 1 丸，日服 2 次。金匮肾气丸 1 丸，日服 2 次。

3.9 慢性肺源性心脏病

慢性肺源性心脏病，简称肺心病。是继发于支气管、肺或肺血管慢性疾患的一种心脏病。临床以咳嗽气促，心悸，胸闷腹满，不能平卧，肢体浮肿，面唇紫绀为主要特征，属中医学咳嗽、痰饮、心悸等范畴。

一般护理

1. 病室空气新鲜，定时进行空气消毒，工作人员及探视者，入病室要戴口罩，防止交叉感染。患者要注意保暖，尤其秋冬季节，气候变化时尤应注意，防止感冒。

2. 心肺功能代偿良好者，应适当活动，以增强体质，但勿过劳。心肺功能衰竭者，应绝对卧床休息，心悸气短，不能平卧的患者，可取半坐卧位，尽量减少活动。

3. 饮食宜清淡易消化，忌食辛辣、生冷、咸、甜食物，禁止吸烟。

4. 注意口腔清洁，防止霉菌感染，可用苦参煎剂，或银芩汤漱口，口腔溃疡，可涂锡类散，冰硼散等。

5. 清除痰液，保持呼吸道通畅。要鼓励患者咳嗽排痰，咳痰无力者，可适当更换体位，或轻拍背部，以利于排痰；咳痰不爽者，可做雾化吸入，使痰液变稀薄，易于咳出。

6. 咳嗽时可服竹沥水，莱阳梨止咳糖浆，或针刺取定喘、风门、肺俞、合谷等穴位。咳剧加尺泽、列缺等穴位。痰多加丰隆穴。

7. 观察呼吸次数、节律、深浅等情况，呼吸困难者，可采取低流量、低浓度持续吸氧法，用氧过程中注意观察患者神智、呼吸、发绀等变化。

8. 观察患者发热情况，若发热恶寒，咳痰黄少而粘稠，舌质红，苔黄腻，脉滑数，多为热邪蕴肺。年老体弱者，正气衰竭，无力抗邪，正邪交争之象可不显著，故咳嗽加剧，痰色变黄，舌质变红，亦要考虑有外邪存在。体温下降，面色青紫，四肢厥逆，大汗淋漓，脉微欲绝，示元阳欲绝，应报告医生，进行抢救。

9. 观察血压的变化：严重感染，心力衰竭，呼吸衰竭，消化道出血等情况，均可使血压下降，如发现异常，及时报告医生，采取治疗措施。

10. 观察咳痰量、色、气味以及排痰难易等情况，一般痰色白量少，示病邪较轻；痰量增多，色黄稠，示邪热较重。

11. 观察舌苔、脉象、神志的变化，如发现患者表情淡漠，嗜睡懒言，或兴奋躁动，言语不清，为肺性脑病，应报告医生，并按昏迷护理（参照2.2昏迷护理）。

12. 平时让患者服用一些扶正固本的食物和方药，以增强体质。

辨证护理

1. 风寒外束，水射心肺

临床表现

咳嗽喘促，痰白而稀，心悸，身体疼重，肢体浮肿，面部尤甚，发热恶寒，小便清长，舌苔薄白，脉浮紧。

护理

(1) 患者因肺虚，卫表不固，怕风易汗，故应注意保暖，汗后尤应注意防止感受风邪，加重病情。

(2) 因肺气虚弱，复加痰阻，则咳嗽、喘促，稍劳即著，故患者应卧床休息。

(3) 服用解表散寒、温里化饮药物，方选化饮解表汤加减，或用止咳定喘丸，每次服9克，日服2次。

2. 脾虚停饮，阻遏心肺

临床表现

喘息气短，心悸食少，大便溏薄，四肢浮肿，面色苍白，唇色青紫，舌质淡润，苔白腻，脉沉弦滑。

护理

(1) 因脾阳不振，则食少便溏，饮食宜用温肾健脾、固涩止泻的食物，如羊肉、刀豆、核桃仁、莲子、山药等。

(2) 浮肿严重者，应注意皮肤护理，观察记录尿量。

(3) 服用温阳健脾、散结化痰药物，方选苓桂术甘汤加减。

(4) 二陈丸每次服 9 克，日服 2 次。

3. 肾不纳气，冲气上逆。

临床表现

咳嗽喘促，呼多吸少，时而暴然喘促，咯痰不爽，心悸不安，胸闷痰多，精神不振，表情淡漠，嗜睡，昏迷，苔白腻或淡黄腻，舌质暗红或淡紫，脉细滑数。

护理

(1) 注意神智变化，患者表现神智淡漠，意识朦胧或嗜睡时，要积极改善患者的换气功能，清除呼吸道分泌物，给予氧气吸入。可针刺治疗，取人中、十宣、涌泉等穴位。可服安宫牛黄丸或至宝丹，以清心开窍。若出现躁动抽搐，针刺行间、中脘、肝俞、心俞等穴位。可给全蝎粉 3 克，蜈蚣粉 3 克，开水冲服。

(2) 皮肤粘膜出血，咯血，便血时，服用清热凉血止血药物，注意观察出血的情况。

(3) 肾不纳气者，可服金匮肾气丸 1～2 丸，日服 2 次。

3.10 急性胃肠炎

本病以恶心呕吐，腹痛腹泻，发热为特征。夏秋季节发病较多，属中医学呕吐、泄泻、霍乱的范围。

一般护理

1. 保持病室清洁，空气新鲜，经常通风，以免秽气刺激引起患者呕吐。

2. 发热、呕吐、腹泻严重的患者，应卧床休息，不宜过多翻动。呕吐后即用温开水漱口，排泄物要及时清除干净，污染的衣被及时更换。

3. 因饮食不节，进食过多，或过食生冷、油腻、不洁食物等，可导致伤胃滞脾而发病，故饮食护理十分重要，轻者可给流质饮食；重者或有剧烈呕吐者应禁食，待病情好转后，逐渐恢复饮食，初进流质、半流质、软饭，正常后改为普通饮食。饮食应清淡，软、烂宜消化，禁食肥甘、油腻和刺激食物。酌情多饮水。

4. 观察呕吐时间，呕吐物内容，量、颜色、气味，观察大便的形状、次数、颜色，必要时留取标本，化验检查。

5. 观察病情变化，若呕吐急暴，呈喷射状，兼有剧烈头痛，神智不清者，为邪陷心肝的重症；呕吐物中带有鲜血或呈咖啡色，为胃络损伤；头昏、烦躁、嗜睡、呼吸深快，为阴津耗竭；呕吐不止，面色苍白，出冷汗，四肢发凉，脉象细弱，为虚脱之象。发现以上情况应报告医生，采取治疗措施。

6. 中药煎剂宜少量多次分服，必要时可以浓缩，亦可加生姜汁3～5滴，或针刺内关穴，耳穴压豆取胃、神门穴。

7. 泄泻严重患者，便后用温水清洁肛门，外扑爽身粉。

8. 针灸治疗，取天枢、内关、足三里等穴位，泄泻严重加关元；呕吐重者加金津；发热加曲池。有寒加艾灸，阳气欲脱加灸神阙穴。

9. 耳针治疗，取小肠、交感、神门、胃、脾穴点。

10. 可采用刮痧疗法，或盐熨脐部。

辨证护理

1. 暑湿型

临床表现

吐泄频作，脘闷恶心，腹痛即泄，吐泄物皆秽臭，心烦口渴，或伴有发烧，舌苔黄腻，脉濡数。

护理

(1) 注意观察患者发热的情况，高热时采取降温措施（参照2.1 高热护理）。

(2) 服用清暑化湿，辟秽和中的药物，方选燃照汤合连朴饮加减。

(3) 针刺治疗，取足三里、内庭、天枢、曲池、十宣等穴位。

(4) 给予六一散 30 克、扁豆 9 克，水煎服。

2. 寒湿型

临床表现

恶心呕吐，泄吐清稀，脘腹胀鸣，身重体倦，头痛，肢冷，或兼恶寒，低热，舌苔白腻，脉濡缓。

护理

(1) 饮食宜热，清淡，易消化，注意补充盐类，忌食生冷。

(2) 服用散寒燥湿、芳香化浊药物，方选霍香正气散加减。汤药应热服。

(3) 针刺治疗，取足三里、天枢、大肠俞等穴位。

3. 虚寒型

临床表现

吐泄频繁，粪便及呕吐物清淡，腹疼喜按喜暖，面色苍白，四肢厥冷，苔白，脉沉迟或细微。

护理

(1) 注意保暖，勿受寒邪，以免加重病情。

(2) 饮食宜热，多服热饮料，忌食生冷。

(3) 针刺治疗，取足三里、大肠、百会、涌泉等穴位。用艾柱灸神阙穴。

(4) 腹痛时可用艾灸中脘，或腹部热敷。

4. 积滞型

临床表现

呕吐酸腐食物，嗳气饱胀，腹痛厌食，泄下酸臭，便后痛减，舌苔厚腻，脉弦滑。

护理

(1) 应使胃中所停滞的食物全部吐出，必要时可用探吐法，使胃中积滞物吐出。

(2) 服用消食化滞和中药物，方选保和丸加减。

(3) 根据食滞轻重控制饮食，必要时可禁食 24 小时。

(4) 腹胀患者可服木香顺气丸，每次服 9 克，每日服 2 次。

(5) 针灸治疗，取四缝穴、三焦俞、中脘、足三里等穴位。

3.11 溃疡病

溃疡病又称消化性溃疡。临床以慢性、节律性、周期性上腹部疼痛和特异性的并发症为特征。属中医学胃脘痛、肝胃气痛、心痛等范畴。

一般护理

1. 合理安排生活，避免过度疲劳，疼痛较重或伴有出血症状的患者，应卧床休息。

2. 做好精神护理，因精神紧张、受刺激和忧虑均是发病的诱因，要指导患者避免精神刺激，保持稳定情绪，对治疗树立信心。

3. 饮食适宜，对治疗和防止疾病发作，及并发症的发生，具有重要的意义。饮食要营养丰富，易消化，根据病情可食流质、半流质或软饭，饮食有节，冷热适宜，要少量多餐，勿暴饮暴食，避免生冷、油腻、辛辣刺激性食物。禁止吸烟和饮酒。

4. 观察胃痛的部位、性质、时间、规律和伴随症状，如突然上腹部剧烈疼痛，继而全腹痛，面色苍白，脉象细数，血压下降，则应报告医生，并协助医生进一步检查，以明确诊断，有穿孔或出血者应做好手术前的准备。

5. 观察呕吐物、大便的形状及伴随症状，如呕吐物为咖啡色或暗红色，大便色黑或柏油样便，伴有头晕、心悸、面色苍白、出汗等症状，应注意观察有无出血情况，做好记录，定时测量血压、脉象等，应报告医生，并做好抢救工作。

6. 病情较轻和稳定者，应适当锻炼，如太极拳、气功疗法等，以增强体质，但不宜剧烈活动。

辨证护理

1. 肝胃不和

临床表现

胃脘疼痛，双胁胀闷，嗳气泛酸，善怒而太息，情绪不稳，口酸苦，舌苔薄白，脉弦。

护理

(1) 服用疏肝理气，和胃止痛药物，方选柴胡疏肝散加减。

(2) 针灸治疗，取中脘、肝俞、内关、阳陵泉等穴位。

2. 肝胃郁热

临床表现

上腹疼痛，痛无定时，胃中灼热，反酸嘈杂，心烦易怒，口苦咽干，喝喜凉饮，或见呕血黑便，舌红苔黄，脉弦数。

护理

(1) 服用养阴柔肝、和胃泻热药物，方选一贯煎加减。

(2) 针刺中脘、梁丘、内庭、丘墟等穴位。

3. 脾胃虚寒

临床表现

胃痛久发，绵绵作痛，多在饭前或夜间痛，遇冷则加重，喜暖喜按，少食痛减，多食腹胀，面色萎黄，神疲乏力，四肢不温，舌质淡苔薄白，脉濡细。

护理

(1) 注意保暖，勿受寒凉，饮食宜热，禁食生冷。

(2) 胃痛时可腹部热敷。

(3) 服用健脾和胃、温中散寒药物，方选附子理中丸合黄芪建中汤加减。

(4) 针刺治疗，取足三里、中脘、脾俞等穴位。

4. 血瘀络伤

临床表现

上腹部疼痛较重而持久，痛处不移，食后痛甚，压按更痛，反复黑便或吐血，舌质紫暗有瘀斑。

护理

(1) 宜卧床休息。

(2) 服用化瘀止血，理气和胃药物，方选膈下逐瘀汤加减。

(3) 观察有无呕血、便血，一旦发现，及时报告医生，采取治疗措施。

3.12 泌尿系感染

临床以尿频，尿急，尿痛为主症。肾盂肾炎多伴有腰痛的症状。本病属中医学淋病、腰痛的范畴。

一般护理

1. 急性期的患者，应卧床休息，慢性期可适当活动，但勿过劳。

2. 注意观察尿的次数、尿量、颜色等。必要时留取标本送验。腰痛者肾区可给予热敷。

3. 饮食宜清淡，营养丰富，多食水果，多饮水或红小豆汤，以清热利尿。禁食辛辣刺激性食物。

4. 进行卫生方面的宣传教育，注意外阴部清洁和经期卫生。

辨证护理

1. 湿热蕴结型

临床表现

尿频，尿急，尿痛，小便浑浊或黄，尿道有烧灼感，下腹部坠胀，腰痛，恶寒发热。苔黄腻，脉滑数。

护理

(1) 观察发热的情况，做好记录。(参照 2.1 高热护理)。

(2) 尿急，尿频，尿痛的患者，可行中药坐浴，清洗阴部。可用双花、蒲公英、艾叶各 30 克，煎水熏洗。

(3) 服用清热利湿药物，方选八正散加减。汤药宜温服。

(4) 针刺治疗，取大椎、曲池、关元、三阴交等穴位。

2. 脾肾阳虚型

临床表现

面色㿠白，腰酸肢冷，乏力，口渴喜热饮，纳呆便溏。苔白，脉沉细。

护理

(1) 注意情志护理，以防惊恐或思虑过度伤及脾肾，加重病情。

(2) 服用健脾益肾，清湿热的药物，方选四君子汤加减。汤药应热服。

(3) 针灸治疗，取肾俞、足三里、中脘、阳关等穴位，配合艾灸。

(4) 注意保暖，勿受凉。多服热饮料。

3.13 肾炎

肾炎是以肾脏病变为主的变态反应性疾病，主要为双侧弥漫性肾小球炎症。主要临床表现有浮肿，血压增高，尿有改变，如尿少、血尿、蛋白尿。按临床表现与病理变化的不同，分为急性肾炎与慢性肾炎。属于中医学水肿范畴。

一般护理

1. 急性发作期应卧床休息，至症状全部消失，尿常规化验正常为止。若尿常规化验有明显异常，浮肿或高血压严重者，需卧床休息，严重水肿而致胸闷憋气者，取半卧位。轻型或恢复期患者，可适当活动，但不宜过度劳累。

2. 室温适宜，患者切勿受凉，预防感冒。

3. 限制水、盐摄入。急性期和有浮肿患者应严格限制钠盐摄入，水肿消退后改为低盐。每日饮水量或补液量视尿量而定，一般应比前一日总出量多 500 毫升为宜。

4. 做好口腔护理，可给银芩汤漱口。注意对卧床患者皮肤护理，防止褥疮和发生感染。

5. 每日记录出入量，腹水者按要求测量腹围，每周测体重1次，高血压者每日测血压 1～2 次，并做好记录。

6. 注意观察水肿发生的部位，程度，消长规律，尿的次数、尿量、颜色、体温、血压、舌象、脉象的变化。

7. 注意观察并发症的出现，如患者突然出现头痛、恶心、呕吐、嗜睡，甚则意识不清，惊厥等表现，为高血压脑病。如有心慌、气短、吐粉红色泡沫样痰，为左心室衰竭表现。以上均属病情危重，应即报告医生，采取抢救措施。

8. 服用逐水或攻下药物时，应观察其用药效果及反应。记录出入量。

辨证护理

1. 风水相搏

临床表现

水肿从眼睑开始，继则四肢，甚至全身皆肿，来势迅速，小便量少，兼有恶风，发热，身痛，苔薄白，脉浮紧。

护理

(1) 注意保暖，勿受凉，预防上呼吸道感染。

(2) 外感症状明显者可食半流质饮食，一般给予易消化、清淡饮食，多食赤小豆、冬瓜、西瓜等利水消肿类食物。限制蛋白质类食物摄入量。恢复期可进普通饮食。

(3) 服用疏风利水药物，方选越婢加术汤加减。汤药宜热服，服后盖被安卧，注意观察出汗情况，汗后切勿受凉，以防加重病情。

(4) 注意观察患者体温的变化，发热者参照 2.1 发热护理。

(5) 针刺治疗，取大杼、合谷、气海、三阴交及灸水分等穴位。

2. 湿热蕴结

临床表现

全身水肿，腹大胀满，胸闷气粗，发热口干，小便短赤，大便干结，苔黄腻，脉沉细。

护理

(1) 患者卧床休息，胸闷气粗者取半卧位。

(2) 加强皮肤护理，预防褥疮发生。

(3) 饮食同风水相搏证。

(4) 针刺治疗，取大椎、三焦俞、气海、足三里等穴位。

3. 水湿困脾

临床表现

全身浮肿，反复出现，下肢肿甚，晨起面肿甚，食后腿足较重，肢体困重，纳呆腹胀，苔白腻，脉沉缓。

护理

(1) 水肿严重者取半卧位，适当抬高下肢，减轻浮肿。

(2) 饮食宜选渗湿利水的食物，如苡仁、赤小豆、绿豆、鲤鱼、鲫鱼等。适当限制水的摄入量。

(3) 服用通阳化浊利水药物，方选五苓散合五皮饮加减。

(4) 针刺治疗，取气海、关元、阴陵泉、脾俞、足三里等穴位。

4. 脾肾阳虚

临床表现

全身水肿，日久不消，以腰腹下肢为甚，按之凹陷，不易恢复，尿少色清，食少便溏，畏寒肢冷，苔白润，脉沉细。

护理

(1) 患者卧床休息，水肿严重者取半卧位，做好皮肤护理，预防褥疮。

(2) 注意保暖，及时增加衣被，预防感冒。

(3) 多食具有渗湿利尿作用的食物，增加营养，如红枣、桂圆、蛋、豆类、水产等营养丰富的食品。

(4) 注意病情变化，若有尿闭，恶心，呕吐等症状，提示有尿毒症出现，应报告医生，采取措施。

(5) 针灸治疗，取脾俞、肾俞、三阴交等穴位。

(6) 玉米须 30 克、马鞭草 60 克，水煎代茶饮，可消水肿。

3.14　泌尿系结石

临床以腰腹钝痛，血尿、排尿困难为主症。本病属中医学砂淋、血淋、石淋范畴。

一般护理

1. 除发热患者应卧床休息外，其它应多活动，以利结石排出。

2. 鼓励患者多饮水。根据结石类型，改进饮食习惯，尿酸盐结石用低嘌呤饮食；磷酸盐结石，用高蛋白、高脂肪饮食，并多食酸性食物；草酸盐结石，少食含草酸食物，如蕃茄、土豆、菠菜等；钙盐结石，避免食牛肉。

3. 注意观察尿的颜色、量，有无结石排出。

4. 疼痛较重兼有血尿者，可服用云南白药或七厘散。

5. 针刺治疗，取肾俞、八髎、关元透中极、足三里等穴位，可加用电针。

6. "总攻"疗法，对直径在 1 cm 以内的尿路结石，无严重尿路感染，无明显肾盂积水患者均适用。早晨 6 点服排石汤 1剂，同时饮水 2000 ml，6 点 30 分口服双氢克尿塞 50 mg，7 点肌注阿托品 0.5 mg，同时电针取肾俞、膀胱俞，或在腹侧结石部位取穴，电针 15～20 分钟，然后嘱患者做跳跃运动。

辨证护理

1. 下焦湿热，蕴积成石

临床表现

腰腹绞痛，连及小腹或向阴部放射。尿频，尿急，尿痛，排尿时突有中断，尿中带血或夹有结石。苔黄腻，脉弦数。

护理

(1) 注意观察肾绞痛的情况。应向患者说明，肾绞痛发作，多属结石有排出的可能，不要紧张，并要仔细观察排石的情况。

(2) 肾绞痛发作严重时，可给予电针止痛，取肾俞、膀胱俞、三阴交、阳陵泉等穴位。亦可选用耳针止痛，取肾区、膀胱等。

(3) 服用清热利湿，通淋排石药物，方选排石汤加减。汤药宜温服，多饮水。注意排石情况。

2. 结石久停，气滞血瘀

临床表现

腰酸痛而胀，小腹胀满隐痛，尿涩痛，滴沥不尽，血尿或见血块。舌质红、苔薄，脉弦滑。

护理

(1) 注意观察患者体温的变化，预防合并泌尿系感染。

(2) 观察小便及血尿的情况，并做好记录。

(3) 服用理气导滞，化瘀通络药物，方选小蓟饮子加减。

(4) 指导患者做适度的跳跃活动，以利于结石排出。

3.15 糖尿病

糖尿病是一种常见的，有遗传倾向的，代谢内分泌疾病。其特征为血糖过高或糖尿，临床上出现多尿，多饮，多食，疲乏，消瘦等症状。常有化脓性感染，肺结核，动脉硬化及神经、肾、眼部病变等并发症。本病属中医学消渴或消瘅的范围。

一般护理

1. 症状明显有合并症时，要卧床休息，症状不明显者，可适当工作，防止过劳。

2. 节制饮食，避免过饥过饱，按医嘱给予生理需要的饮食量，严格要求患者按规定进食，饥饿明显者，可用多次煮过的菜充饥，如瘦肉、豆制品类等，忌食辛辣，厚味，甜食和戒烟酒。

3. 保持皮肤清洁，避免发生化脓性感染，一旦发生要积极治疗。

4. 对重症患者注意口腔护理，防止口腔粘膜及牙龈溃烂，给予银芩汤漱口。

5. 每周测体重 2 次，患者在控制饮食，或用药治疗的情况下体重不但不降，反而逐渐增加，示病情好转。

6. 记录 24 小时饮水量和排出尿量。及时留取尿的标本化验检查。

7. 注意观察病情，如出现头晕，心悸，出汗，软弱无力等症状时，应考虑是否引起低血糖，可立即口服糖水，如不缓解，应报告医生，给予静脉注射 50% 葡萄糖；如发现患者厌食，呕吐，腹痛，口内有苹果气味，可能为酸中毒，报告医生采取措施。

8. 使用降糖药物，应严格掌握给药时间，和进食时间。

9. 对患者加强卫生的宣传教育，使之了解自己的病情，学会检测尿糖，合理用药，及并发症的预防和一般处理措施。

辨证护理

1. 肺热津伤

临床表现

口渴多饮，咽干，舌燥，尿频，苔薄黄，脉数。

护理

(1) 患者要避免精神刺激，消除忧虑和紧张，积极配合治疗。

(2) 服用清肺润燥生津药物，方选消渴方加减，配合饮用菠菜根粥。

(3) 针刺肺俞、太渊、神门、廉泉、内庭等穴位。

2. 胃燥阴伤

临床表现

口渴多饮，多食易饥，形体消瘦，小便频数，大便秘结，苔燥，脉滑数。

护理

(1) 便秘患者可多食蔬菜，必要时可给予大黄片、番泻叶等缓泻剂。

(2) 服用清胃泻火养阴药物，方选玉女煎加减，配合饮用猪肚粥。

(3) 针刺胃俞、中脘、足三里、三阴交等穴位。

3. 肾虚精亏

临床表现

小便频数，量多，尿如脂膏，头晕，目糊，腰酸腿软，畏寒肢冷，口干，舌红，脉细数。

护理

(1) 病情严重者，应卧床休息。并告诫患者节制房事。

(2) 服用滋肾固精药物，方选六味地黄丸加减，汤药应热服。

(3) 严密观察患者病情变化，出现并发症者，及时处理。

(4) 针刺肾俞、三焦俞、关元、太溪等穴位。

3.16 类风湿性关节炎

本病以关节疼痛，局部肿胀或变形为主要症状。属于中医学痹证范畴。

一般护理

1. 病室要适当通风，保持干燥，温度适宜，空气新鲜。患者要避免受风，防止感受寒湿引起疾病的复发。

2. 发热，关节疼痛较重，肿胀明显者，应卧床休息。恢复期始可适当活动，防止过劳。

3. 一般患者给予营养丰富的普通饮食；湿寒偏盛者忌食生冷；发热者可食半流质或软饭，患者因发热耗伤津液，应多饮水，并忌食辛辣刺激性食物。

4. 患者体质虚弱，抗病能力差，出汗多，为防止外感，汗后用干毛巾擦身，及时更换汗湿衣被。夜间盗汗患者，每晚睡前用适量的五倍子粉，加水调匀，外敷肚脐。

5. 注意观察体温变化，按时测量体温，并记录，患者午后低热一般不做处理，可多喝热水，促其出汗使体温下降；体温38.5℃时，可服用解热镇痛药物，不做物理降温。

6. 观察患者发病因素，疼痛的部位、性质、时间与气候的关系。

7. 本病的发生与机体的正气，气候条件，生活环境关系密切。因此要及时根治上呼吸道感染，注意防寒、防潮，尤其季节变化时，要随时增减衣被，注意保暖，加强锻炼，增强体质。若其它部位有感染病灶，应早期治疗，以预防心脏瓣膜病的发生。

辨证护理

1. 风热偏盛

临床表现

发热多汗，关节红肿疼痛，扪之有热感，喜凉恶热，多发于手足小骨节，运动不利，苔黄腻，脉细数。

护理

(1) 注意观察发热，关节肿痛，心悸等病情变化。

(2) 观察汗出情况，出汗多者及时更换湿衣被，勿受风。

(3) 服用清热祛风，兼以解毒除湿药物，方选白虎加桂枝汤加减。

(4) 针刺曲池、外关及痛区周围穴位。

(5) 关节红肿热痛时可给予中药药膏外敷：(1) 凤仙膏：用新鲜的凤仙草适量砸烂，局部外敷，或用凤仙草膏外敷。(2) 芙蓉膏：芙蓉叶适量研粉，用蓖麻油调匀外敷。(3) 川槿皮膏：川槿皮、桃仁、羌活各等量，共研粉用蓖麻油调匀外敷。

2. 寒湿偏盛

临床表现

腰背困胀，大骨节变形，疼痛非常，重着难移，活动不便，四肢拘急，食少纳差，苔白腻，脉沉迟或沉滑。

护理

(1) 关节疼痛得热则舒，遇寒则剧，应注意局部保暖，必要时可给热水袋，坎离砂热敷或做场效应治疗等，切勿受寒或雨淋。

(2) 鼓励并协助患者进行肢体功能锻炼。

(3) 服用散寒除湿兼以祛风通络药物，方选薏苡仁汤加减，汤药应热服，可服少量黄酒为引子。

(4) 针灸风府、外关、复溜及阿是穴。

3. 痰瘀痹阻

临床表现

久痹不愈，局部关节肿疼或青紫，屈伸不利，关节变形，压之更疼，皮下结节或见瘀斑，苔厚腻，脉细涩。

护理

(1) 指导并协助患者进行肢体活动，增强关节活动能力。

(2) 配合推拿针刺、理疗或外治疗法。

(3) 脊柱变形者宜睡硬板床；关节疼痛或变形者，可加以护架，以免压迫患肢而增加痛苦；关节不利或强直者，可配合推拿、按摩、针灸等疗法，以疏通经脉，调和气血。

(4) 四肢关节疼痛肿胀者，可配合熏洗疗法，常用活血止痛散，或患者本人内服的中药渣，再煎水熏洗，每日 1~2 次，每次 30 分钟。熏洗时，注意温度适宜，防止烫伤。洗完后用干布包好，避免受风。

(5) 关节畸形者可给予牵引矫形，用力勿过大过猛，以免引起骨折。观察牵引重量，角度是否合适，以及肢体的血运情况，发现异常，及时纠正。注意皮肤护理。

4 外科常见病证及护理

4.1 疖

疖是单个毛囊及其所属皮脂腺的急性化脓性感染疾病。多发生于富有毛囊和皮脂腺的面部、颈部和背部，常见于夏、秋季节。初发为红色小硬块突起，上有黄白色脓头，数天后脓头脱出即愈。严重者可伴有发热、恶寒等全身症状。中医按其发病季节、病因、形态的不同，又分为暑疖、面疖、蝼蛄疖等。

一般护理

1. 保持皮肤清洁干燥，勤洗澡，勤换衣，勤理发，预防及减少疖病的发生。

2. 发病后疖肿周围的毛发应剃去，既便于换药，盖贴敷料，又可保持局部清洁，防止反复发作。

3. 认真观察病情，了解体温变化及局部病变的消长情况。

辨证护理

1. 肿疡期

临床表现

初起局部突起为红色小硬块，上有黄白色脓头，红肿热痛，严重者可有发热、恶寒等全身症状。

护理

(1) 伴有发热者，应卧床休息，抬高患处。局部保持清洁，外敷拔毒膏、大青膏。也可用新鲜蒲公英、马齿苋、野菊花各等量洗净捣烂外敷，或煎汤内服，以促其内消。

(2) 肿疡期切忌挤压、碰撞，面疖，尤其生于唇、鼻周围者，防止邪毒内攻脏腑，引起"走黄"（颅内感染或脓毒血症）。

(3) 针刺及放血以疏泄督脉，清除血热，常用穴位：灵台、合谷、委中等。前两穴针刺，用泻法；委中点刺放血。若伴有发热者加刺大椎、曲池等穴。

(4) 症状较轻者可内服解毒消炎丸、六神丸或万氏牛黄清心丸。另外可用六神丸加水少许研碎，涂于疖肿处。面疖多伴发热、恶寒，可服用清热解毒消肿的药物，方选五味消毒饮，煎汤宜冷服，多饮水。暑疖宜清暑化湿、清热解毒的药物，方选清暑汤。

(5) 饮食宜素普食。面疖生于唇、鼻周围及发热者，可给素流质或半流质；暑疖应多进清热消暑的食物，如西瓜、甜瓜、绿豆汁、多饮茶，或用六一散水泡代茶饮。忌食辛辣刺激之物。

2. 溃疡期

临床表现

脓肿已成，中央变软，有波动感，脓头自溃或切开，流出黄色稠厚脓液，局部肿痛随即减轻。

护理

(1) 脓肿自溃或切开，应保持引流通畅，面疖切忌早期切开。

(2) 溃后疮口用大黄油纱布换药，脓头及坏死组织不易脱落，脓液引流不畅者，可用九一丹、九黄丹以提脓祛腐。脓液多、炎症明显者先用解毒洗药煎汤温洗疮口，然后换药。脓液少、肉芽组织新生，疮口可撒少许生肌散，外盖生肌玉红膏油纱布。

(3) 换药时注意保持周围皮肤清洁，敷料整齐，毛发处固定稳妥。另外，要观察其他部位有无新的疖肿发生。

4.2 痈

痈是化脓性细菌侵入多个相邻的毛囊和皮脂腺的急性化脓性感染。初起局部红肿热痛，上有粟粒状脓头，形如蜂窝状，继之脓头间皮肤坏死，形成溃疡，逐渐生肌而愈。多伴有发热，食欲不振等全身症状。属于中医有头疽的范围。

一般护理

1. 患者多伴有轻重不同的全身症状，应卧床休息，根据痈的部位，选择舒适的体位。生于面部应少说话或咀嚼动作，以减轻疼痛。

2. 密切观察病情，注意体温、血压、舌苔、脉象的变化，如有高热者参照（2.1 高热护理）。

3. 本病多发于老年人，应根据老年人的特点，做好生活护理，对体质虚弱者应协助翻身及肢体活动，促进气血运行，防止并发症。对糖尿病患者应同时协助治疗糖尿病。

4. 颈部痈应剃去患处周围的毛发，保持患处清洁干燥，便于换药。

5. 局部病变周围的正常皮肤给予涂擦马黄酊（马钱子、黄连各 30 克，捣碎，用 75%酒精 300ml 浸泡 3～5 天，密封备用），防止病变向周围发展。

辨证护理

1. 肿疡期

临床表现

局部为红肿热痛的肿块，上有很多脓头，形如蜂窝状。实证红肿高突，根盘收束；虚证疮形平坦，化脓迟缓。伴有发热，恶寒，烦渴，便秘溲黄，舌淡或红，苔白或黄燥，脉数。

护理

(1) 局部保持清洁，红肿热痛者给予清热解毒的软膏外敷，常用大青膏、金黄膏，促其内消。

(2) 内服药：实证服用清热解毒、活血化瘀的药物，方选清热解毒饮，或兼服腥消丸，汤剂宜温服。虚证服用养阴生津、清热托毒的药物，方选竹叶黄芪汤。患者活动困难应喂服。伴有高热，烦渴，便秘，苔黄燥，脉数有力，此为里实热证，宜服清热解毒，通里攻下的药物，方选内疏黄连汤，可冷服。高热可以冷敷降温。若高热不退，可服安宫牛黄丸 1 粒或紫雪丹 0.9 克。精神萎靡或烦燥，脉数，局部红肿蔓延，属火毒内陷之征兆，应及时报告医生处理。并做好抢救准备。

(3) 饮食宜清淡易消化的素食，高热者给素流质或半流质，多食瓜类、豆类、菠菜、菠萝、香蕉等，多饮水，以助清热解毒。虚证化脓迟缓者，可给鲜发食物如：鲜鱼、虾或雄鸡头汤等，以助化脓托毒而出。糖尿病患者应严格控制饮食，可适当加食牛奶、银耳、红蕃茄、丝瓜等，以养阴清热。忌食膏粱厚味、醇酒、辛辣刺激之品，以免痰湿火毒内生加重疮疡病势。

2. 溃疡期

临床表现

脓肿形成，脓头溃破，形似蜂窝，从脓头中流出黄稠或清稀脓液，脓出毒泄，全身症状可随之减轻。

护理

(1) 脓肿自溃或切开，应保持脓液引流通畅，用解毒洗药熏洗疮口后，再外撒少许九黄丹、追毒丹，以提脓祛腐。或用药捻纳入疮底，以利于引流，及时清除坏死组织，然后用大黄油纱布换药。若脓脱肉芽组织新生，可撒珍珠生肌散，外盖生肌玉红膏油纱布，促进疮口愈合。

(2) 保持疮口周围皮肤清洁干燥，脓液多的创面，床上应铺油布，及时更换浸透的敷料，防止脓液污染被褥。

(3) 疮面较大，愈合迟缓者，可用维生素 B_1 100 毫克在双足三里穴交替注射，以促进疮口愈合。

(4) 内服药：实证服用清热解毒，托里排脓的药物，方选清热解毒汤，宜冷服。体虚邪热未退者服用补益气血，托里消毒的药物，方选托里消毒散。若热退气血两虚者，服用补益气血的药物，方选八珍汤或十全大补汤。在服药期间要认真观察证候的转化情况，及时通知医生更换方药。

(5) 饮食一般应给予营养丰富的食物。气血双虚者多为老年人，根据老年人脾胃功能的特点，给予温、热、熟、软，营养丰富、容易消化，并具有益气养血味美可口的食物，可食些肉类、蛋类、豆腐、牛奶及黄芪粥等，切忌煎、烤、炸等烹调方法。若热邪未退切忌滋补。

4.3 手部感染

手部化脓性感染，属于中医疗疮范围。多因手部轻微外伤，化脓性细菌侵入而引起发病。中医按其部位不同而有不同的名称，如甲沟炎称为沿爪疗；脓性指头炎称为蛇头疗；化脓性腱鞘炎称为蛇肚疗；掌中间隙感染称为托盘疗等。其中以沿爪疗和蛇头疗为多见。

一般护理

1. 抬高患肢，限制活动，可用三角巾或绷带悬吊前臂，以减轻肿痛。伴全身症状者应卧床休息。
2. 若手部有外伤或异物，应及早处理。
3. 认真观察病情，使局部病变得到及时恰当的处理。

辨证护理

1. 肿疡期
临床表现
局部红肿热痛，或伴有发热，头痛，口干，食欲不振，舌红，苔薄白或微黄，脉弦数。

护理

(1) 初期以消为贵，外用清热解毒，消肿止痛的药物。

①用雄黄、白矾各 10 克，蟾酥 1 克，蜈蚣 1 条，共研细末，每次 3 克，装入一个猪苦胆内（或生鸡蛋一个，打破一端装上药），搅匀套在患指上，待干后再换。

②局部敷大青膏或金黄膏，也可用鲜蒲公英、鲜马齿苋各 60 克，洗净捣烂，加适量蛋清调匀，外敷患处。

③用疔疮洗药：金银花、苦参、黄柏、地丁、蒲公英、连翘、泽兰、荆芥、防风、甘草各 10 克，煎汤趁热熏洗患处。

④用 50%芒硝溶液浸泡。

(2) 服用清热解毒，活血消肿的药物，方选五味消毒饮加味。若有发热，恶寒等全身症状者，可给蟾酥丸 3 粒吞服。

(3) 局部疼痛剧烈者，可针刺止痛（循经取穴）。或耳穴压豆，可取手、腕、交感、神门等穴。

(4) 饮食宜素食，清淡饮料，忌食辛辣燥热的食物。

2. 溃疡期

临床表现

局部红肿，剧烈跳痛，压痛显著，伴有畏寒，发热，纳差等全身症状。

护理

(1) 认真观察局部情况，脓已成者，应及时切开排脓，以防局部肿胀，气血运行障碍发生骨髓炎。切开后参照疖肿换药法处理。

(2) 有发热，寒战等全身症状者，仍可继续服用五味消毒饮加味，注意观察病情，如果并发淋巴管炎、淋巴结炎或骨髓炎应及时处理；若已发生骨髓炎有死骨形成者，待死骨松动后即应取出，疮口才易愈合。

(3) 早期进行功能锻炼，以免造成手部功能障碍。

(4) 恢复期邪退宜多进滋补生肌的食物。

4.4　急性蜂窝织炎

急性蜂窝织炎是由化脓性细菌侵入皮下、筋膜下、肌间隙或深部蜂窝组织而引起的一种急性化脓性炎症。并伴有发热，寒战，头痛等全身症状。属于中医痈、无名肿毒等范围。

一般护理

1. 全身症状较重，疼痛剧烈，应卧床休息，根据不同病变部位，选择舒适的体位。

2. 认真观察病情，头痛者可针刺百会、印堂、头维、太阳等穴，发热者参照（2.1 高热护理）。

3. 注意观察有无并发症发生，如四肢或颈部受累，常伴有相应的腋窝、腹股沟或颈部淋巴结肿大疼痛，可参照 4.1 疖肿疡期护理，颈部颌下急性蜂窝织炎，容易引起喉头水肿，严重者呼吸困难。应禁食，嘱其少说话，并做好气管切开的准备。

辨证护理

1. 肿疡期

临床表现

局部红肿热痛，发热，恶寒，舌苔黄，脉弦滑而数。

护理

(1) 早期局部用解毒洗药熏洗，然后用生大黄、大青叶各9克，山慈菇6克，共研细末，以水或蜂蜜调成膏，敷患处。

(2) 针刺：根据病变部位，循经取穴，以疏通经络，消肿止痛；发热者可加大椎、曲池、合谷。

(3) 服用清热解毒，活血化瘀的药物，方选五味消毒饮加味。

(4) 饮食宜清淡，多食具有清热解毒作用的蔬菜、水果，如各种瓜类、豆类、香蕉、菠萝等。忌食辛辣之物。

2. 溃疡期

临床表现

肿痛加重，触痛明显，按之中软而有波动感者，脓肿已成，自溃或切开疮口渐愈，如正不胜邪，肿硬不消，则脓出不畅。

护理

(1) 观察局部情况，若溃后肿硬不消，排脓不畅，此为正不胜邪，应服用扶正托里的药物，方选托里消毒散，服药后要注意病情变化，若症状不减，体温升高，发生败血症者，应报告医生，并做好抢救准备。

(2) 局部保持清洁，脓肿自溃或切开，要保持引流通畅，脓液及坏死组织多者可配合解毒洗药浸洗后，外敷大黄油纱布。坏死组织不易脱落，疮口可撒五五丹以祛腐，脓去肉芽组织新生，即可用生肌玉红膏换药，至痊愈。

(3) 饮食调养：宜营养丰富，易消化的食物。若邪去热退，气血双虚者，疮面难于生肌收口，应进高蛋白，维生素多的食物，如肉类、蛋类及新鲜蔬菜和水果，忌食辛辣、刺激性和鲜发性食物，戒烟酒。

4.5 丹毒

丹毒是溶血性链球菌引起的一种传染性急性炎症，初起局部皮肤呈红色斑片，压之退色，放手后即复原状，边缘清晰而不规则，迅速向周围蔓延，稍高出皮面，灼热疼痛，表面可出现水疱，并伴有恶寒、发热、头痛、口渴，严重者也易因邪毒内攻，发生"内陷"。中医也称丹毒，但因发病部位不同，名称也不一样。发于头面部者称为"抱头火丹"，躯干部称为"内发丹毒"，下肢丹毒称为"腿游风"。

一般护理

1. 卧床休息，发热者参照（2.1 高热护理）。

2. 观察病情，注意体温及神态的变化，若发生内陷，要积极配合医生及时进行处理，护理措施参照急性全身化脓性感染护理。

3. 饮食宜素普食或半流质，发热期间应多饮水，或饮米汁，西瓜汁，绿豆汁等。忌食辛辣、香燥性食物。

4. 皮肤、粘膜破损或有足癣者应及时处理，防止感染。

5. 处理疮口所用器械及换下的敷料，应严密消毒或烧毁，以免交叉感染。

辨证护理

1. 头部丹毒

临床表现

除局部皮肤火红、灼热、水肿外，易引起眼睑肿胀，目赤羞明，鼻翼肿大，头额胀痛，转动不便。

护理

（1）卧床时，适当抬高床头，室温不宜过高，保持湿润，光线宜暗。

（2）保持面部清洁，用黄连适量煎汤湿敷眼睑及鼻翼部，以清热泻火，减轻肿胀。

（3）头痛可针刺列缺、外关、合谷等穴，或耳穴压豆（常用王不留行或绿豆），取面、鼻、眼、交感、神门等穴。

（4）服用清热解毒，散风消肿的药物，方选普济消毒饮，服药时应多饮水。

（5）病变部位要保持清洁，外敷大青膏或金黄膏，或用双柏散以蜂蜜调后外敷，以清热解毒消肿止痛。

2. 下肢丹毒

临床表现

发于足部或胫部，有时可波及股部，下肢丹毒多为湿热下注，可反复发作，形成象皮肿。

护理

(1) 卧床时，适当抬高患肢，以减轻肿胀及疼痛。

(2) 局部用硝矾洗药（芒硝、明矾、月石各 10 克）开水冲化后熏洗，或用鲜蒲公英 90 克，白矾、青黛各 10 克，捣烂后外敷病变部位。

(3) 服用清热利湿，活血化瘀的药物，方选四妙勇安汤加味，兼服龙胆泻肝丸和活血通脉片，服药期间应注意观察药物的疗效及不良反应。

(4) 经过治疗，症状消失后，仍需要继续用药治疗 5～7 天，巩固疗效，以防止复发。

(5) 下肢复发性丹毒，易反复发作，症状逐次加重，应用白花丹参注射液 10 毫升，加在 5% 葡萄糖液 500ml 中，静脉滴注，15 天为 1 疗程；复发性丹毒形成象皮腿者，可用活血止痛散煎汤趁热熏洗，每日 1～2 次，同时患肢可用绷带加压包扎。本症一般病程较长，疗效缓慢，因此，应鼓励患者，树立信心，长期治疗，方能取得满意的效果。

4.6 急性乳腺炎

急性乳腺炎是乳腺组织的化脓性炎症。多在产后 3～4 周发病，初产妇多见，初起局部肿胀热痛或有肿块，继之跳痛，按之应指，则脓肿形成，可伴有发热，恶寒，口干等全身症状。中医称为乳痈。

一般护理

1. 伴有全身症状者，应卧床休息，环境要安静舒适，减少不良刺激。

2. 本病多因肝气郁结而发生，因此应做好精神护理，要关心体贴患者，了解思想情况，消除各种不良因素，使患者精神愉快，心境坦然，避免郁怒而加重病情。

3. 哺乳期经常用温水、肥皂擦洗乳头，乳头内陷者，洗后向外牵拉，若乳头有破裂可给芝麻油或蛋黄油外涂。

4. 宣传哺乳期卫生知识，哺乳要定时，每次哺乳应将乳汁吸空，不能吸空时，可用吸奶器或用手将乳汁挤出，以防乳汁郁积；不可让婴儿含乳头睡觉。乳母应保持心情舒畅，切忌暴怒，忧郁；饮食要有规律，以防脾胃运化失调，胃热壅滞而发病。

辨证护理

1. 初期
临床表现
患乳肿胀，触痛，有块，并伴有恶寒，发热，口渴，烦躁，厌食，便秘，舌苔黄，脉弦数。
护理。

(1) 发热者参照 2.1 高热护理。

(2) 初起乳汁积滞，可继续哺乳。行乳房按摩，术者以五指由乳房四周轻轻向乳头方向按摩，不要挤压或旋转按压，在按摩的同时用手轻提乳头数次；或用木梳向乳头方向梳理一遍，然后用手轻轻按摩肿块，自上而下顺乳头方向挤出郁积的乳汁。炎症明显时应停止哺乳，有肿块者，应用薄荷、陈皮各 30 克，煎汤热敷患处，热敷后用吸奶器吸出乳汁，再敷大青膏或金黄膏，也可用仙人掌 90 克、白矾 15 克，捣烂后外敷，促其内消。乳汁过多者，宜用芒硝外敷。

(3) 乳腺炎早期可用干棉球裹丁香粉塞鼻，左右鼻孔交替应用，每日 3～4 次，每次 1～2 小时，效果良好。

(4) 服用疏肝清胃，和营通乳，清热解毒的药物，方选括楼牛蒡汤加味，药宜温服。

（5）针刺可疏通乳道，清泻热毒，取膻中、乳根、少泽、内关等穴；或用耳穴压豆，取乳腺、神门、肾上腺、皮质下等穴。

（6）饮食宜清淡，忌食辛辣油腻、荤腥，以免助火伤阴，损及脾胃。乳汁多而稠的患者，应少喝汤。胃热重、恶心、纳差、口渴，要多饮水或用天花粉、麦冬、淡竹叶各9克水泡代茶饮，以清热益胃生津，促进食欲。

2. 溃疡期

临床表现

脓肿自溃或切开，热退痛减，但因正邪相搏的转归不同，还会出现不同的症状，如脓黄而稠，肿痛不减；排脓不畅或脓液稀，肉芽淡白，生长迟缓，疮口久不愈合。

护理

（1）患者注意休息，用乳罩或三角巾托起乳房，以减少活动时疼痛，有利于引流。

（2）乳房脓肿溃破后，脓液多，有坏死组织时，用大黄油纱布蘸少许九一丹、八二丹或化腐散塞入疮口内引流；疮口脓液少，肉芽组织新鲜时用生肌玉红膏油纱布换药；肉芽组织生长迟缓者，可应用鹿茸生肌散或珍珠生肌散换药；若形成乳房窦道者，用红升条插入窦道内，促进肉芽组织新生。

（3）密切观察病情变化，掌握病情转化表现的不同症状，配合医生辨证用药，如溃后热退，肿痛减轻，但脓液黄白而稠，身体虚弱，则为余毒未尽，宜服用补益气血，清解余毒的药物，方选四妙汤加味；若排脓不畅，疼痛不减，则为正虚毒盛，不能托毒而出，应服补益气血，托毒消肿的药物，方选托里消毒散；若脓稀，肉芽组织淡白，生长迟缓，疮口久不愈合者，为气血双虚，则应用补益气血的药物，方选八珍汤或十全大补汤，药应久煎热服。

（4）配合饮食调养。掌握疾病各个阶段的症状和用药的不同，饮食也应随症而用，以辅助药力，如脓肿溃后，毒邪已去，气血虚衰，脾阳不振，脓水清稀疮口难收者，饮食宜给予鱼、肉、禽、蛋等品，以补益气血，促进疮口愈合；若余毒未尽或正虚邪盛者，不宜滋补。

4.7 急性全身化脓性感染

化脓性细菌及其毒素侵入血液而引起严重全身性反应，称为急性全身化脓性感染。临床一般分为毒血症、败血症、脓毒血症三种类型。属于中医走黄、内陷范围。

一般护理

1. 做好精神护理，解除患者紧张情绪，积极配合治疗。
2. 严密观察病情，注意患者体温、舌苔、脉象及神态的变化，高热患者参照 2.1 高热护理。
3. 观察全身各部位的情况，如局部有感染病灶，应及时处理，早期可用金黄膏、芙蓉膏外敷，促进内消；已溃破者应认真辨证换药。若因急腹症引起者，要及时协助医生采用手术处理，清除原发病灶。
4. 患者抵抗力差，容易感染，在针刺或注射时，要做好皮肤消毒和严格无菌操作。患者常因全身无力不愿活动，因此应鼓励和协助患者翻身活动，促进气血运行，防止褥疮的发生。
5. 做好口腔护理，饭前饭后漱口，有口疮者可涂冰硼散、锡类散或柿霜，口唇干裂可以香油涂之。

辨证护理

1. 气营热盛型
临床表现
起病急剧，寒战，高热，口大渴，大汗出，小便短赤，大便秘结，舌质红，苔薄黄或黄燥，脉弦数或洪数。
护理

(1) 卧床休息，汗出过多，应及时更换汗湿之衣被，保持皮肤清洁干燥，以防受凉。

(2) 高热不退，拘急抽搐者，可以针刺大椎、曲池、合谷、太冲、三阴交等穴。也可冷敷降温，或口服羚羊粉 0.5～1.5克。

(3) 服用清气泻热，解毒清营的药物，方选白虎汤、黄连解毒汤加减，煎汤冷服。服药后注意舌苔的变化及排便情况，若舌苔由黄变薄，便通，则为病情好转。

(4) 大便秘结者，可饮用蜂蜜水，或用番泻叶 6～9 克水泡代茶饮。也可应用针刺疗法，常用穴位：大肠俞、三焦俞、阴陵泉等。

(5) 饮食宜清淡的素流质或半流质，发热易耗伤津液，应多饮水或清淡饮料，还可给双花、麦冬、天花粉各 9 克，水泡代茶饮，以清热解毒，滋阴生津；若气虚大汗淋漓者，可取黄芪、沙参或西洋参煎汤频频服之，以补气止汗。忌食辛辣、酒、炙煿之品和热性食物。

2. 热入营血型

临床表现

壮热不退，神昏躁动，发斑，衄血，舌质红绛或深绛，苔少而干，脉细数。

护理

(1) 认真观察病情，注意患者神态、呼吸、血压、脉象的变化，躁动不安者，应加床档，防止坠床。若毒邪内攻，血压下降，出现休克先兆者，要积极配合医生处理，并参照 2.3 厥证护理。

(2) 服用清热解毒，凉血清营的药物，方选犀角地黄汤、黄连解毒汤加减。药宜温服，服药时，可少量多次，频频喂服，必要时可用鼻饲给药。

(3) 神昏谵语者，可针刺人中、十宣、涌泉等穴。或喂服安宫牛黄丸或紫雪丹。

(4) 衄血者，应根据衄血情况及时处理，如鼻衄，可在额部冷敷，要静卧少动，用鲜茅根水煎代茶饮，并应注意观察出血的颜色及出血量。

(5) 病情较重者，应用支持疗法，如输液、输血和氧气吸入或给予抗菌素。

(6) 本病常由疔疮走黄或疮疡热毒内陷发展而成，因此要密切注意病情变化，若脉细数无力或脉微细欲绝，则为亡阴亡阳之征，应及时协助医生抢救，并参照 2.3 厥证护理。

4.8　胃、十二指肠溃疡穿孔

本病是胃、十二指肠溃疡的严重并发症之一，发病特点为腹痛骤然发生，刀割样剧烈，自上腹或右上腹开始迅速蔓延全腹。中医称为胃脘痛、厥心痛。

一般护理

1. 做好精神护理，消除患者的恐惧心理，鼓励其积极配合治疗。

2. 绝对卧床休息。取半卧位，若血压不稳时要采取平卧位。患者切忌蹲卧，以防发生膈下脓肿或肠间脓肿。

3. 观察病情，注意患者神态、血压、体温、舌苔、脉象的变化及治疗后的反应。

4. 做好口腔护理，用胃管后，可常用银芩汤或生理盐水漱口，口唇涂润滑油。

辨证护理

1. 第一期（中焦气血郁闭期）
临床表现
持续性剧烈腹痛，全腹压痛，反跳痛，腹肌紧张，肠鸣音减弱或消失。伴有恶心呕吐，精神紧张，烦躁不安，面白唇青，汗出肢冷，气促脉微，舌淡苔薄。

护理

（1）根据急则治其标的原则，给予针刺缓急止痛。操作前应向患者说明操作方法及疗效，取得合作。安排好体位，注意保暖。首先观察腹部情况及听诊肠鸣音，然后针刺。常取穴：中脘、梁门（双）、足三里（双）；恶心呕吐者加内关（双）；腹胀配天枢（双），留针 30～60 分钟，每 10～15 分钟行针 1 次，手法宜捻转法，也可用电疗机。每 4～6 小时针 1 次，每次针后观察腹痛、腹胀及肠鸣音的改变，以了解病情的消长。

穴位注射：用维生素 $B_1$100mg，取双足三里穴交替注射，注射时取穴要准确，针感应明显，以缓解疼痛，促进穿孔闭合。

（2）禁食，胃肠减压，吸出胃内容物，减轻中焦痞塞。应保证有效减压，并观察引流液的性质，颜色，记录引流量。

（3）中药灌肠。应用通里攻下，疏通肠道的药物，使中焦复运，气机通畅，以解郁消痛。常用大承气汤加减，煎汤 500 ml，过滤后，倒入输液瓶内，温度 39～40℃。患者取左侧卧位或平卧位，以粗导尿管插入肛门 25～27 cm，其尾端与输液瓶的玻璃接管联通，以每分钟 80～100 滴的速度，缓缓滴入结肠，滴入后观察患者的反应。如患者肠蠕动增强，有便意，排便前有暂时性腹痛加重，为正常现象，嘱患者不要紧张。

（4）患者由于长期脾胃不和，致使水谷精微吸收功能减退，正气损伤，体质虚弱，所以在禁食期间，应给予必要的支持疗法。如补液、输血等。

2. 第二期（中焦郁久化热期）

临床表现

腹胀腹痛明显减轻，腹肌紧张消失或局限在右上腹，上腹部压痛减轻，肠鸣音恢复正常，排气排便，出现发热，大便干结，小便赤黄，脉数，舌红苔黄等一派热象。

护理

(1) 急性症状缓解后为穿孔闭合的象征。此期治疗以中药为主，应用清热解毒，通里攻下的药物，方选复方大柴胡汤。用药方法：早期可经胃管注入，即将一剂中药煎后过滤，浓缩为150ml，第一次注入50ml，温度39～40℃，如有粉剂可与汤剂一起用。注药前先抽空胃内容物，然后徐徐注入，再以少量温水冲洗胃管，防止堵塞。注药后夹胃管1～2小时，此时应密切观察腹部症状及体征，若无腹痛加重等现象，肠鸣音有所恢复，即可拔出胃管，停止胃肠减压。口服中药，每次100ml，早晚各1次。如果全身症状重者，可每日两剂，分4次服。

(2) 腹腔邪热重者可配合外治疗法，常用消炎散（芙蓉叶、生大黄各300克，黄芩、黄柏、黄连、泽兰叶各250克，冰片10克，共研细粉备用）适量，用黄酒或葱、酒煎液调成糊状，敷于右上腹，以促进腹腔炎症局限或消失。

(3) 停止胃肠减压后，即可进流质饮食。初进饮食应少量多餐，不宜过饱，逐渐改为半流质或普通饭。观察进食后的反应，了解排气排便情况。

(4) 观察全身情况，注意并发症的发生。常见并发症为膈下感染及脓肿，或肠间脓肿及盆腔脓肿。脓肿形成后可出现持续发热，腹胀，脓肿部位有压痛或触及包块。如膈下脓肿形成，可出现咳嗽，吐痰等胸腔炎症，反应性症状；盆腔脓肿可出现里急后重，大便有粘液等直肠刺激症状，应协助医生辨证处理。若无并发症者，应鼓励患者适当活动。

本病经过第一、二期治疗，绝大多数患者可以治愈，但也有个别患者效果不好，需要行手术治疗，应作好手术前后的护理。

3. 第三期（恢复期）

临床表现

自觉症状基本消失，饮食体温恢复正常，大便通畅，腹肌紧张或反跳痛消失，或仅有剑突下右上腹有轻压痛。根据缓则治其本的原则，按患者不同的表现行辨证施护，临床一般分为 3 型。

(1) 虚寒型

临床表现

胃脘隐隐作痛，喜暖，喜按，面黄体瘦，食少不化，舌淡苔白。

护理

①调节饮食：宜温中健脾，进食应温、热、熟、软，营养丰富，并具有性温祛寒作用的食物，如常食些煨羊肉、猪肝汤、甲鱼、牛奶、羊奶、大枣、莲子粥、山药粥、茴香菜粥、胡萝卜粥、山楂、糖姜片等。忌食生冷、寒凉之食物。

②注意保暖：室内要温暖，局部可行热熨疗法，如麸熨、盐熨或砖熨。同时可给陈皮、姜片各 6 克，水泡代茶频饮之。

③止痛：常用针灸疗法：取中脘、足三里（双）、内关（双）穴针刺；灸中脘。

(2) 肝郁型

临床表现

胃脘胀痛，连及两胁，嗳气吞酸，胃纳不佳，口苦，善怒，脉弦。

护理

①注意精神护理，使患者心情愉快，情绪稳定，避免郁怒伤肝。肝气犯胃而加重病情。

②饮食调养：宜多食舒肝理气消食之物，如常食萝卜、菠菜、山楂、橘子或胡萝卜粥、鸡内金粥、蜜饯萝卜，用佛手 3 克水泡代茶饮。

③止痛：针刺中脘、期门（双）、太冲（双）等。或耳穴压豆，取肝、胆、脾、胃、神门、交感等穴。

(3) 血瘀型

临床表现

痛处固定，痛似针刺，眼周晦暗，大便黑粘，脉涩。

护理

①注意休息，避免剧烈活动，认真观察病情。

②做好精神护理，要患者安定情绪，有呕吐、便血者要静卧少动，避免紧张、恐惧。

③止痛：针刺中脘、足三里（双），也可给三七粉、元胡粉各1.5克，温开水送服。

④观察排便情况，如有黑便者留送标本检验，以了解出血程度，协助医生辨证用药。

⑤饮食调养：宜进营养丰富、软、烂，易消化的食物，常食具有行气，活血化瘀作用的食物，如：黑木耳、海参、海蜇、香菇、大枣、胡萝卜、芋头等。忌食油炸、煎烤以及未煮烂的食物。

4.9 急性阑尾炎

急性阑尾炎是外科急腹症中的常见病，多发生于青壮年。初起上腹部或脐周围疼痛，经数小时至1天，腹痛转移至右下腹阑尾所在部位，呈固定性疼痛，阵发性加剧，常伴有恶心呕吐，发热，便秘等全身症状。中医称为肠痈。

一般护理

1. 密切观察病情，注意腹痛的性质，有无腹膜刺激症状，以及体温、舌苔、脉象的变化，有利于辨证护理。

2. 一般应卧床休息，并发腹膜炎及阑尾脓肿的患者，应取半卧位，防止膈下或肠间脓肿的形成。

3. 中医认为，急性阑尾炎的发病原因与情志刺激有很大关系，因此，应做好精神护理，解除思想顾虑，积极配合治疗。

辨证护理

1. 瘀滞型

临床表现

体温正常或低热，脘腹胀闷，恶心，纳呆。气滞重者绕脐走窜；血瘀重者痛处固定不移。大便正常或秘结，尿清或黄。局部压痛，肌紧张不明显，或摸到局限性包块。舌苔薄白，脉弦数。属于单纯性阑尾炎。

护理

(1) 患者可适当活动，避免过劳。

(2) 针刺：取阑尾、足三里。血瘀重者加刺麦氏点；气滞重者加天枢、大横，恶心、呕吐加内关、上脘，发热者加曲池、合谷。

(3) 外治疗法：用盐熨法，即取粗盐 2 斤，放置铁锅内炒至频频发出爆裂声时，加食醋少许调匀，装入布袋内，趁热外敷右下腹压痛明显处，冷后更换，每日 1~2 次。

(4) 服用通里攻下，活血化瘀，清热解毒的药物，常用阑尾化瘀汤。气滞重者加服元胡粉。服药后应注意排便情况，一般服药后每日排便 2~3 次为宜。若次数过多应酌情减量，服药后因呕吐将药液吐出时，应追补吐出之药量，以确保药效。

(5) 认真观察病情，了解腹痛、体温及舌苔脉象的变化，若腹痛减轻，体温正常则为病情好转，若大便次数虽多，而排便不畅，症状不减，或无排便者，应及时报告医生，以便早期处理。

(6) 饮食宜清淡，容易消化的软饭或半流质，进食温度要适中，忌食辛辣及炙煿的食物。

2. 湿热型

临床表现

右下腹疼痛，压痛反跳痛，腹肌紧张或形成局限性包块。伴有发热，食欲减退，大便溏或便秘，小便短少或赤，舌红、苔黄腻，脉弦滑而数。相当于化脓性阑尾炎合并局限性腹膜炎，以及阑尾周围脓肿。

护理

（1）服用通里攻下，清热解毒的药物，常用阑尾清化汤，恶心呕吐者，可多次分服。

（2）针刺取穴同瘀滞型，若在右下腹有局限性包块者，可在包块周围施行围针，一般在周围取 3～4 点，针刺即可。

（3）外治疗法：常用芒硝外敷，即取芒硝 150～200 克，研成粉末状，然后装入纱布袋内，摊平后敷于右下腹压痛明显处。数小时后药物吸收水分而变成硬饼状，即取下，每日 2 次。

（4）认真观察病情，了解疾病的转化。如经过治疗后，腹痛减轻，压痛范围局限，体温正常，大便通畅，小便清长，舌苔薄白，脉象变缓，则为病情好转，反之则病情加重。如果病情不断恶化，应及时报告医生，并做好手术前准备。

（5）饮食宜流质或半流质，应给清淡素食，热重者口渴欲饮，应多饮水及清淡饮料；湿重者口渴不欲饮，可用双花 12 克，淡竹叶、麦冬各 9 克，水泡漱口，以促进食欲。应多食水果。需要行手术者应禁食。

3. 热毒型

临床表现

腹痛剧烈，压痛反跳痛，腹肌紧张，高热、恶寒、面红目赤，口干舌燥，恶心，大便秘结，小便赤涩，舌质红绛，舌苔黄燥，或出现黑苔，脉象洪滑数大或弦数有力。若热甚伤阴，阴伤及阳，则出现精神萎靡不振，四肢厥冷，自汗，气促，血压下降等症状。

护理

（1）此型为发热的炽盛阶段，容易发生变证。嘱患者绝对卧床休息，无休克者取半卧位。密切注意神态、体温、血压及腹部体征的变化，有高热、休克者参照 2.1 高热、2.3 厥证护理。

（2）服用清热解毒，通里攻下，行气凉血的药物。若津液亏损者，腹胀、呕吐、高热不退，苔脱，舌面干燥起刺，应及时补液，维持水、电解质平衡，以利于发挥中药的作用。

(3) 针刺疗法同瘀滞型，加刺耳穴：阑尾、大肠、神门、交感等。

(4) 外治疗法：用蒜硝黄醋糊剂，即大蒜 6～8 头，芒硝 15～30 克，大黄粉 60 克，食醋适量。将大蒜剥去皮，和芒硝共捣成泥，摊在凡士林纱布上，面积约 12×10cm，敷在右下腹相当于阑尾部位或压痛最显著点，上面再盖一层同样大小的凡士林纱布，合拢两层纱布之边缘，以防止药物外流刺激皮肤。外面覆盖一层塑料薄膜，用腹带包扎固定。一般敷 2 小时后取下，改用大黄粉加醋调成糊状敷于原处，外面覆盖一层塑料薄膜，以保持糊剂湿润。连续敷用 8～10 小时。（如用蒜硝泥直接敷于皮肤，应随时观察局部反应，防止灼伤。一般敷 15 分钟左右即可）。

(5) 经过治疗，患者腹痛减轻，体温下降，大便通畅，仍应休息，继续用药 5～7 天。若症状不能缓解，出现四肢厥逆，热深厥深等现象，应采用手术治疗。要做好手术前后的护理，手术后应协助并鼓励患者早期下床活动，以促进气血运行及肠道功能恢复。

4.10　肠梗阻

肠梗阻系指任何原因引起的肠道通畅性遭到破坏，造成一系列的症状和病理改变。临床上以腹痛、呕吐、腹胀及便闭为主要表现，同时可伴有高热，津液耗伤则大渴、唇燥、皮肤失去弹性，表情淡漠，最终导致亡阴、亡阳。中医称为关格、肠结。

一般护理

1. 做好精神护理，解除患者的紧张情绪，主动配合治疗。
2. 密切观察病情变化，如神态、体温、舌苔、脉象、血压及腹部症状，腹痛的性质、部位，呕吐的次数、性质及量，腹胀的程度，排便排气的情况，以利于辨证施护。
3. 禁食，行胃肠减压，以减轻胃肠膨胀，有利于肠壁气血运行，恢复肠蠕动及吸收功能，胃内排空，便于接受内服中药，防止呕吐。在行胃肠减压期间，应保持胃管通畅，有效减压，同时要观察引出液的颜色和量，可了解病情的转归，若抽出液由草绿色变为淡黄色乃至澄清，表示病情好转。

4. 给予补液，防止因大量呕吐，不能进食，津液耗伤，致使患者大渴、烦燥、口干唇裂、皮肤无弹性、脉细弱，头痛头晕等脱水现象。

5. 做好口腔护理，在插胃管期间经常用生理盐水擦洗口腔，用银芩汤漱口，唇干者涂润滑油，口腔有溃疡可涂锡类散或冰硼散。

辨证护理

1. 虚寒型
临床表现
腹痛较轻而腹胀较重，痛无定处，时痛时止。喜暖恶寒，腹壁压痛，无腹肌紧张。无热或低热。舌质淡或肿胖有齿痕，舌苔薄白或腻，脉象沉迟而细。

护理
(1) 环境要安静，室内应温暖，做好生活护理，保证患者充分休息。

(2) 服用温阳健脾，行气导滞的药物，方选温脾汤加减或理气宽中汤，煎汤后，经胃管注入（用法参照胃、十二指肠溃疡穿孔）。药量每次 100～200ml。注药后，要注意患者的反应。

(3) 针灸疗法：针刺上脘、关元、天枢（双）、足三里（双）以消胀止痛；灸神阙以温经散寒；穴位注射，用新斯的明0.5 毫克，取双足三里穴各注射 0.25 毫克，以促进肠蠕动。

(4) 外治疗法：采用麸熨法，即取麦麸1 斤，葱白两根（切碎）铁锅内炒热，加醋适量调匀，以布包或袋装，热熨腹部。

(5) 灌肠：用大承气汤或皂角 30 克、细辛 10 克，煎汤后灌肠（方法参照胃、十二指肠溃疡穿孔）。

（6）治疗期间认真观察病情，若腹痛腹胀逐渐减轻，肛门排气排便，可拔出胃管，口服中药。其他疗法可继续应用至好转。

（7）饮食调养：拔出胃管后，可进流质、半流质或软饭，应选用性温，营养丰富，易消化的食物，忌食油腻、刺激性食物。

2. 实热型

临床表现

腹痛剧烈，辗转不安，痛有定处，痛时可见肠型和蠕动波，肠鸣音亢进，腹部压痛，反跳痛及腹肌紧张等腹膜刺激症状。伴有发热，口渴，便秘尿少，舌质红绛，舌苔黄燥或黄腻，脉象弦数有力。

护理

（1）应用通里攻下，行气活血，攻下逐饮的药物，方选复方大承气汤或甘遂通结汤，煎汤后由胃管注入。用药期间应观察疾病的转归，若多次用药后，患者出现畏寒，口淡，呃逆，思热饮，腹痛喜按喜暖，舌质淡，苔白滑，脉虚弱而沉细，则转为里寒证，应停用泻热之剂。

（2）针刺疗法：取中脘、天枢（双）、足三里（双）、大肠俞（双）；发热者加曲池（双）、合谷（双）；穴位注射，即用阿托品0.25毫克，足三里穴注射，可预防用药呕吐及缓解剧痛。

（3）灌肠：用大承气汤。另外可用生理盐水 500ml 加阿托品 1～2ml，保留灌肠，以缓解肠痉挛，减轻患者的痛苦。

（4）因肠扭转引起的肠梗阻，可采用推拿疗法或颠簸疗法，肠套叠引起者，应用指压复位法或空气灌肠整复法。因蛔虫引起者，可采用食油疗法，即取生豆油或麻油，成人 200～250ml，儿童 80～150ml，加温后口服，或由管注入。在应用前，问患者讲明此法无任何痛苦，服后让患者静卧休息，并观察治疗效果。

（5）经治疗患者全身情况改善，能安静入睡，腹痛、呕吐腹胀症状明显减轻、肛门排便排气，示肠梗阻缓解，可进流质或半流质饮食。反之，全身症状恶化，血压下降，腹痛加重，腹胀加剧，出现腹膜刺激症状，需要行手术治疗者，应做好手术前后护理。

4.11 胆道系统感染与胆石症

胆道系统感染与胆石症是外科常见的急腹症，以右上腹部或剑突下部位隐钝痛或阵发性疼痛为主要表现。常伴有发热，寒战，恶心，呕吐，纳呆，腹胀，口苦咽干等症状。本病属于中医胁痛、黄疸等范围。

一般护理

1. 做好精神护理。慢性胆道感染可形成结石，而结石又多并发胆道感染，两者常互为因果，同时存在。胆肝相表里，同具疏泄功能，肝喜条达而恶抑郁，则常因情志不遂，肝气郁结，气血运行不畅而诱发或加重病情。因此要做好精神护理，使患者心情舒畅，从而达到行滞、消散和止痛的目的。

2. 认真观察病情，注意疼痛的性质，体温，有无黄疸，舌苔脉象的变化，以了解病邪的深浅及转化，若舌质淡红转红绛，舌苔薄白转黄燥，伴有高热，寒战，脉洪数，血压下降，则为湿热炽盛，正不胜邪，毒邪内陷，应及时报告医生并协助处理。

3. 患者有口苦咽干，影响食欲，应多漱口，或给双花、麦冬、天花粉各 9 克泡水代茶饮，以清热泻火，益胃生津，或用银芩汤漱口，多饮清淡饮料，严重者做好口腔护理。

4. 对胆石病患者用排石汤或总攻疗法时，应认真观察病情，若出现腹痛加重，发热，脉数，甚至出现黄疸，此为排石现象，排石后腹痛骤然消失，体温下降，黄疸消退，此时应注意收集大便，了解排石情况。若腹痛持续不能缓解，高热不退，寒热交作，黄疸加深时，应报告医生，并做好手术准备。

辨证护理

1. 气郁型
临床表现

右胁绞痛或窜痛，或胁脘隐痛，胀闷感，牵扯肩背，常伴有口苦，咽干，头晕，食少等，舌尖微红，舌苔薄白或微黄，脉弦紧或弦细。

护理

(1) 保持情绪稳定，心境坦然，避免抑郁。注意休息，防止剧烈活动。

(2) 饮食要有规律，常食瓜类、菠菜、茄子、萝卜粥，同时可用佛手3~6克开水泡代茶饮，以舒肝解郁，行气止痛。胆石症患者可常食金钱草粥，以利胆排石。

(3) 针刺取中脘、期门、胆囊穴；绞痛加合谷；头晕加印堂、风池；食少加足三里穴。

(4) 外治疗法：镇江膏药1贴加冰片0.25克，膏药隔火软化后，将冰片均匀撒在膏药上，然后敷于胆囊区或肩背疼痛处，每日取下膏药加温，再撒同量冰片继续敷用。具有消散行气，芳香走窜，通络止痛的功效。

(5) 服用舒肝理气，缓解止痛的药物，方选清胆行气汤。煎汤宜热服。

(6) 平日注意寒温适宜，生活规律，根据气温的变化适当增减衣被，防止气候骤冷而发病或加重病情。

2. 湿热型
临床表现

右上腹持续性胀痛，多向右肩部放射，右上腹部肌紧张，压痛，有时可触及肿大的胆囊，伴有寒热往来，口苦咽干，恶心呕吐，不思饮食，身目发黄，大便秘结，小便少而黄浊，舌质红，苔黄腻，脉弦滑或弦细。

护理

(1) 应卧床休息，待症状基本消失，可逐渐增加活动量。

(2) 服用舒肝利胆，清热利湿的药物，方选清胆利湿汤，煎后宜温服。同时可用金钱草 60～100 克，水煎频服，或用玉米须 60 克开水泡代茶饮，具有清热利湿、排石作用。

(3) 针刺：取胆囊穴、阳陵泉、中脘、太冲、胆俞；黄疸加至阴、日月穴；呕吐加内关穴。耳穴压豆，取肝、胆、十二指肠、神门、交感、胃。仍可用镇江膏加冰片外敷，缓解疼痛。

(4) 饮食宜营养丰富，易消化之素食，多食水果，少食粘食，忌食辛辣、油腻肥甘之物。核桃仁具有一定的化石作用，胆石症宜常食之。食用方法：取核桃仁 5～6 个，去皮取仁加冰糖和麻油适量，放锅内蒸熟食用，每日 1 次。

(5) 有黄疸者，皮肤瘙痒严重，患者不能休息，可用止痒剂或用苏打水、硼酸水涂擦。应经常洗浴，保持皮肤清洁。

3. 实火型

临床表现

腹痛剧烈，持续不解，范围扩大，腹肌强硬，压痛反跳痛，或有包块。高热不退，面红目赤，口干舌燥，全身深黄，大便秘结，小便黄赤。甚者神昏谵语，四肢厥冷，皮肤瘀斑，鼻衄齿衄，舌质红绛，舌苔黄燥，起芒刺，脉弦滑而数，或沉细而弱。

护理

(1) 认真观察病情，因湿热化火，热毒内陷，病情危重，应注意神志，血压，体温的变化，发热者参照 2.1 高热护理。给予必要的支持疗法，如补液、输血，或给予抗菌素。

(2) 应在准备手术的情况下，给予清热泻火、舒肝利胆的药物，方选清胆泻火汤，煎汤冷服，若呕吐严重不能口服者，可经胃管注入。仍可配合应用针刺、外治疗法。

(3) 若经上述处理，症状缓解，可继续采用上法护理。反之，需急症手术，应做好手术前后护理。

4.12　胆道蛔虫病

胆道蛔虫病是由于蛔虫钻入胆道而引起的胆道阻塞和感染，是肠道蛔虫病常见的并发症。发病特点：上腹部剑突下突发生剧烈绞痛，有钻顶之感，患者辗转不安，或伴有恶心呕吐，发冷，发热，四肢厥冷，梗阻严重者可出现黄疸。中医称为蛔厥。

一般护理

1. 密切观察病情，了解腹痛性质，协助医生及时解除患者的痛苦，解痉止痛可选用以下方法：

(1) 针刺疗法：

①体针：可选用以下几组穴位：中脘透梁门；迎香透四白；右胆俞、胆囊穴、太冲、内关均双侧。手法要强刺激，留针30分钟。

②耳针：取交感、神门、肝、胆、胰、十二指肠等穴，针刺或压豆。

③电针：取右胆俞（阴极）、中脘（阳极），进针得气后，联接电疗仪，用连续波，电流强度以患者能忍受为宜。

④穴位注射：选用阿托品或维生素 $K_3 1 ml$，取胆囊穴、胆俞、中脘、鸠尾等穴，每次注射1～2穴。

(2) 食醋疗法：取食醋100ml，加花椒少许，煮沸后，去花椒，顿服食醋。

(3) 背部叩击法：患者取坐位或左侧卧位，术者用右手掌根叩击患者之右脊肋角区，用力要均匀适度，可达止痛的目的。

(4) 拔罐疗法：在剑突下压痛区拔火罐，每次30分钟。

2. 治未病：要求患者作到饮食有节，起居有常，寒温适度。注意饮食卫生，饭前便后要洗手，切忌暴饮暴食。发现肠道蛔虫病及时治疗。按医嘱进行驱蛔，常用方法如下：

(1) 使君子仁：炒黄去皮去尖，成人每次5～10克（儿童半量），空腹嚼服。

(2) 针刺：取关元、太冲、血海、丰隆（均双侧）。

(3) 苦楝根皮 30 克，去外面粗皮，水煎服。服时可加适量红糖，以矫味。

驱蛔时要观察排便排蛔情况，以了解驱蛔效果。

辨证护理

1. 虚寒型

临床表现

脘腹绞痛，时痛时止，止则如常人，喜暖喜按，呕吐清水或吐蛔虫，四肢厥冷，面色㿠白，出冷汗，常伴有纳差，大便正常或稀薄，小便清长，舌体胖嫩，舌苔白腻，脉弦紧或沉伏。

护理

(1) 注意休息，室内温度要适宜，卧处应温暖，根据气温的变化增减衣被，防止外邪乘虚而入耗伤阳气加重病情，腹部保暖可行热熨疗法，如麸熨或盐熨等。或用灸法，灸上脘穴，以温经散寒。

(2) 注意饮食调养，以增强体质，卫护后天之本，改善机体虚弱为原则。给予温、热、营养丰富，并具有温中散寒的食物，以促进脾胃运化功能的恢复。另外根据蛔虫闻酸则静，遇辛则伏的特点，在饮食烹调时适当加些食醋、花椒等辛、酸味之品。常食山楂、山楂片（糕），多饮酸梅汤或乌梅粥。忌食生冷、油腻食物。

(3) 服用安蛔止痛，温中驱蛔的药物，方选乌梅汤，煎汤应在腹痛暂止时热服。一般服药后患者腹痛缓解，安静入睡。如果腹痛不能缓解，而呈持续性剧痛，并伴有寒热往来，应请医生处理。

2. 湿热型

临床表现

腹痛呈持续性胀痛，阵发性加剧，拒按，伴有寒热往来，口苦咽干，不思饮食，舌质红，苔黄腻，脉弦。

护理

(1) 患者卧床休息，保持环境安静舒适，发热者参照 2.1 高热护理。

(2) 服用清热利湿，理气驱蛔的药物，方选清胆利湿汤，宜温服。服药后注意排便排蛔情况。另外，要观察病情变化，若热退痛减，即为好转。如果出现高热，寒战，身目黄染，舌质红绛，舌苔黄燥，应疑为脓毒症。要密切注意患者的神态及血压变化，报告医生，并做好手术准备。

(3) 注意饮食调养。应进素流质或半流质，多食些具有清热利湿的食物，如赤小豆、蚕豆、芹菜等，多饮茶以助药力。口苦咽干，影响食欲者，应勤漱口，或用双花、麦冬、天花粉各 9 克开水泡代茶饮，以清热泻火、益胃生津。

4.13 血栓性静脉炎

血栓性静脉炎，多发生于四肢浅静脉。发病特点：局部浅静脉出现疼痛，红肿，灼热，可摸到硬结节或硬性索条状物，甚至发生静脉周围炎，可伴有发热等全身症状。属于中医脉痹范围。

一般护理

1. 做好预防工作。血栓性静脉炎多因外伤、感染、静脉输液毒邪侵入而发病。所以对局部外伤。感染应及时有效的治疗。静脉输液时，严格注意无菌操作，交替注射静脉血管，尽量少用刺激性的药物。

2. 密切观察病情变化。若肢体有间歇性、游走性反复发作的血栓性静脉炎，应协助医生检查是否有其他疾病，如血栓闭塞性脉管炎或潜在性内脏癌。

辨证护理

1. 湿热型

临床表现

局部焮红，灼热，肿痛，湿甚则肢体浮肿，沉重，可触及硬结节或硬性索条状物，压痛明显。

护理

(1) 发热者，应卧床休息，抬高患肢，治疗期间要尽量减少患肢活动。

(2) 患处可用大青膏、茅菇膏或用鲜马齿苋，捣烂外敷，也可用马黄酊涂患处。

(3) 用解毒洗药煎汤，或用硝矾洗药开水冲化后热罨患处。

(4) 针刺夹管穴（即病变静脉边缘两侧每隔 1cm 交叉排列）、膈俞、太渊穴。胸腹壁浅静脉炎加内关、阳陵泉穴；上肢浅静脉炎加合谷；下肢浅静脉炎加阴陵泉、三阴交穴。

2. 瘀结型

临床表现

局部湿热逐渐消退，转归为瘀阻经络，遗留硬性结节或硬性索条状物，局部皮肤留有色素沉着。

护理

(1) 局部用活血止痛散煎汤趁热熏洗。

(2) 可长期服用散结片或活血祛瘀片。

(3) 可多食些海带、蛤蜊、紫菜等，以助活血化瘀。

4.14 下肢深静脉血栓形成

下肢深静脉血栓形成，多发生于髂股静脉，而以左侧髂股静脉血栓形成为最常见，以下肢广泛性肿胀、疼痛为特征，属于中医脉痹、肿胀、血瘀范围。

一般护理

1. 由于发病急骤，肢体突然肿胀，疼痛，不能活动，致使患者多处于恐惧焦虑状态，故应做好思想工作，消除紧张情绪，保持心情平静，积极配合治疗。

2. 卧床休息，抬高患肢，以利于静脉血液回流，减轻患肢肿胀及疼痛。

3. 严密观察病情，髂股静脉血栓在形成后的四周内血栓容易脱落，有发生肺梗塞出现胸痛、咯血、发热等的可能。另外血栓向上发展延伸至下腔静脉至肾静脉，甚至可累及肾静脉，并发肝后型门脉高血症，出现黄疸、腹水等。因此应加强护理，随时注意病情变化，发现异常及时协助医生处理。

4. 本病的发生与患者手术后、产妇生产后长期卧床休息有关，因此医护人员对手术后患者或产妇，应劝告或协助早期下床活动，以减少此病的发生

辨证护理

1. 湿热下注型
临床表现
发病早期静脉有炎症现象，全身发热，患肢肿胀胀痛，舌苔白腻或黄腻。
护理
(1) 绝对卧床休息3～4周，抬高患肢。发热者参照2.1高热护理。
(2) 服用清热利湿，活血化瘀的药物，方选四妙勇安汤加味和活血通脉饮各1剂，交替应用，以集中药力达到消肿通络的目的。药宜温服。服药后观察患者的反应。另外可兼服活血通脉片、四虫片。
(3) 饮食宜具有清热利湿，活血化瘀作用的食物，如海带

紫菜、赤小豆汤、冬瓜汤等。忌食滋补之食品。

2. 血瘀湿重型

临床表现

深静脉炎症消退，血栓形成，下肢肿胀明显，浅静脉曲张和皮肤毛细血管扩张，舌质红绛或有瘀斑。

护理

(1) 患肢可作适当的活动，应用活血止痛散热毡患肢，以消肿，缓解疼痛，促进侧支循环的建立，改善肢体的血液循环。

(2) 服用活血化瘀，利湿通络的药物，方选丹参活血汤或活血通脉饮，兼服四虫丸、大黄䗪虫丸。

(3) 患肢肿胀，浅静脉曲张，皮肤毛细血管怒张，因此要保护患肢，防止局部皮肤损伤及感染。可应用弹力绷带缠压，以减轻瘀血及毛细血管怒张。

(4) 饮食调养：患者虽热邪退，但舌苔白腻，仍有湿邪滞留，因此，夏令时多食些西瓜、冬瓜、绿豆汤，或常食鲜菇、木耳、海参；常饮茶或以玉米须用开水泡，频饮之，以助活血化瘀，祛湿邪。

3. 脾肾阳虚型

临床表现

患肢肿胀，沉重胀痛，腰酸畏寒，朝轻暮重，倦怠无力，纳少不渴，舌质红，苔薄白。

护理

(1) 注意休息及保暖，随气候变化增减衣被，防止感冒。

(2) 保护患肢，夜间休息仍应抬高，另外可用硝矾洗药熏洗。

(3) 服用益肾健脾，利湿通络的药物，方选温肾健脾汤，煎汤宜热服。

(4) 饮食调养：应进温补健脾利水的食物，如羊肉、海参、甲鱼、木耳、莲子、大枣或用栗子、胡桃仁、山药、熟地分别加粳米煮粥常食之。胃纳差者在饮食烹调时加些姜、葱、蒜、花椒、茴香、醋等，可开胃启食；也可针刺中脘、足三里，以促进食欲。

4.15 下肢静脉曲张

下肢静脉曲张发生于大、小隐静脉，以大隐静脉为常见，多发生于中年人。发病特点：小腿沉重，胀痛，易疲劳，久站可出现小腿、足踝部浮肿，静脉曲张、隆起、弯曲，严重者扭曲成团块状，可并发血栓性浅静脉炎和下肢溃疡。中医称下肢溃疡为臁疮。

一般护理

1. 注意休息，卧床时抬高患肢，以利于静脉血液回流。

2. 避免久站及负担重物。可长期穿绵纶弹力长筒袜，或用弹力绷带，防止患肢皮肤外伤及感染。

3. 需要行手术治疗者，应做好手术前后护理。

辨证护理

1. 湿热下注型

临床表现

下肢发生血栓性浅静脉炎，或溃疡感染，红肿热痛，有湿疹样皮炎者，则局部发痒，舌苔黄腻。

护理

(1) 卧床休息，抬高患肢。溃疡面脓液多者，先用解毒洗药煎汤浸洗，然后用大黄油纱布进行换药；若脓退，肉芽组织新生，可撒少许生肌散，以促进生肌收口。

(2) 并发湿疹样皮炎，可用止痒洗药或燥湿洗药煎汤熏洗，洗后擦干，外撒黄柏散、青蛤散。应注意不要搔抓，以免发生感染。

（3）如有血栓性浅静脉炎，参照血栓性浅静脉炎护理。

2. 阴虚内热型

临床表现

局部溃疡久不愈合，肉芽淡红或微暗，脓少，肿胀，舌质红。

护理

（1）局部溃疡面可撒鹿茸生肌散或珍珠生肌散，外盖生肌玉红膏油纱布。

（2）维生素 B_1 100 毫克，穴位注射，常取足三里、阳陵泉穴交替注射，促进溃疡愈合。

（3）在服用养阴清热的药物时，多食些具有养阴清热作用的食物，如豆类、瓜类，以及鸡蛋、木耳、牛奶等，以助药力。

3. 气血两虚型

临床表现

溃疡久不愈合，肉芽组织淡红或苍白，脓液稀薄，体虚泛力，舌质淡苔薄白。

护理

（1）局部处理参照阴虚内热型，另外可采用艾条灸创面，可促进愈合。

（2）由于邪退正虚，服用补气养血，和营通络的药物，如人参养荣汤、十全大补汤加减。

（3）饮食调养：宜食些补养气血的食物，如猪肉、羊肉、牛肝、羊肝、甲鱼、海参及新鲜蔬菜和水果。

4.16 血栓闭塞性脉管炎

血栓闭塞性脉管炎，是进行缓慢的动脉、静脉节段性炎症性病变，由于全层血管炎症，血管内膜增生，血栓形成，发生管腔闭塞，导致严重肢体缺血，最后发生肢体坏疽。属于中医脱疽的范围。

一般护理

1. 做好精神护理。本病多发生于青壮年，由于病程缠绵，疼痛难忍，甚至造成患肢不同程度的残废，给患者带来极大的精神痛苦，因为长期心情忧郁，造成气血运行失调，则易导致病情加重或复发。因此，要做好精神护理，鼓励患者树立战胜疾病的信心，积极配合治疗。不仅要注意休息，还要督促养成良好的生活习惯，或指导患者练气功，通过"调心"、"调息"、"调身"的气功运动，提高机体的抗病能力。

2. 中药的应用与观察：因患者需要长期服用活血化瘀，清热解毒的药物，一般每日1剂，重症者可每日两剂。对消化道均有不同程度的影响，因此药温要适中，服药与进食时间不宜太近，以免引起恶心。同时要观察服药后的反应，如胃纳不振者，可同时服用调理脾胃的药物，或针刺中脘、足三里穴，以促进食欲。

3. 血栓闭塞性脉管炎的早期或发病过程中，均易发生游走性血栓性浅静脉炎，要经常观察患肢局部变化，如有发生应及时处理，以减轻患者的痛苦。参照血性浅静脉炎护理。

4. 吸烟不但可以引起血管功能的改变，而且会加重病情或促使复发。所以应要求血栓闭塞性脉管炎的患者，做到终生戒烟。

辨证护理

1. 阴寒型
临床表现
患肢喜暖怕冷，触之冰凉，局部皮肤苍白或潮红，舌苔薄白，舌质淡，脉象沉细或迟。
护理
(1) 患肢护理

①注意保暖。患肢穿软暖而舒适的棉鞋、棉袜、戴棉手套。冬令时不宜在室外长时间停留。卧室应温暖。

②保持患肢清洁，经常用温水和肥皂清洗，用软毛巾擦干，防止损伤皮肤。有足癣者，可用硝矾洗药熏洗，足痒时注意不要搔破。

③修剪趾（指）甲时，防止损伤，可先用温热水浸洗泡软后再修剪，有嵌甲、鸡眼不要乱用腐蚀性药膏或药粉。

④保护患肢，防止碰撞、挤压等外伤。鞋、袜要宽大柔软，避免患足受压，影响血液循环。

(2) 服用温经散寒，活血化瘀的药物，方选阳和汤加味，或兼服参桂再造丸、参茸大补丸。服药后要观察患者的反应，定时测量血压。有的患者长期服用温热药，可有口干或咽部异物感、头晕等症状，应向患者说明原因。如果血压正常，坚持继续服用，症状可自行消失。若头晕较重者，停药 3～5 天后即可好转。

(3) 患肢可用回阳止痛洗药煎汤熏洗。熏洗时，药物温度要适中，不宜过热，以避免因过热而引起疼痛。

(4) 针灸疗法具有调理气血，消除肢体动脉痉挛，促进患肢侧支循环形成等作用。上肢取曲池、合谷、内关、太渊等穴；下肢取足三里、三阴交、承山、昆仑、阴陵泉、阳陵泉，每次可针 2～3 穴；灸气海、足三里、曲池等穴。

(5) 患肢疼痛可口服通脉安片、元胡止痛片，或耳穴压豆等，以缓解疼痛，减轻患者的痛苦。切忌用麻醉药品，以防久用成瘾。

(6) 指导患者作患肢运动。即让患者平卧，患肢抬高 45度，维持 2～3 分钟，然后下垂于床沿 3～5 分钟，再平放 2～3 分钟，如此反复运动 5～10 次。每日 3 次，以促进患肢气血运行。

(7) **饮食调养：**应进营养丰富并具有性温、行气活血作用的食物，如：羊肉、鸡肉、鲤鱼、鲫鱼、草鱼、红糖、大枣、山楂、橘子、胡萝卜、韭菜等。另外可常食黄芪粥或丹参粥。忌食炙煿的食物。

(8) 注意观察患肢血液循环的变化。如皮肤颜色，温度，股，腘，足背动脉的搏动情况，了解疾病的消长，以协助医生辨证用药。

2. 血瘀型

临床表现

患肢持续性固定性疼痛，呈紫红、暗红或青紫色，皮肤有瘀点瘀斑，舌质红绛、紫绛或有瘀斑，舌苔薄白，脉象沉细而涩。

护理

(1) 患肢护理同上。另外，患肢宜平放，切忌下垂，局部皮肤有瘀点瘀斑者可涂马黄酊。

(2) 持续而剧烈疼痛，临床常采用的止痛方法如下：

①针刺止痛：一般根据疼痛部位而取穴。

②普鲁卡因穴位注射：下肢取足三里、三阴交、绝骨等穴；上肢取曲池、手三里等穴，一般每穴注射 0.5%普鲁卡因 3ml。

③股动脉周围封闭：10%普鲁卡因 20ml，加维生素 $B_1$100毫克，作患肢股动脉周围封闭或股神经干封闭。

④对疼痛剧烈，彻夜不眠或对麻醉药品已成瘾的患者，应用中药麻醉控制疼痛，效果较好。同时对扩张血管，改善肢体血液循环，有一定的作用。应用方法：中麻Ⅱ号 2~3 毫克（或中麻Ⅰ号 2.5~5 毫克）加氯丙嗪 25 毫克，用生理盐水 10ml 稀释后，静脉缓慢注入，3~5 分钟后患者即可入眠，一般可睡 6~8小时，隔日注射 1 次，连续使用 3~5 次，疼痛可缓解或消失。应用后要精心护理，认真观察体温、脉搏、呼吸、血压的变化，发现异常可对症处理。

(3) 服用疏通经络，活血化瘀的药物，方选活血通脉饮，兼服活血祛瘀片、三七片、复方丹参片。

（4）鼓励患者多进饮食，给予营养丰富易消化的食物。忌食辛辣刺激之品。

3. 湿热下注型

临床表现

患肢潮红，紫红肿胀，肢端轻度溃疡或坏疽，有炎症表现者，舌质红，舌苔黄，脉弦细而数。

护理

（1）服用清热利湿，活血化瘀的药物，方选四妙勇安汤加味，兼服四虫片、活血祛瘀片。服药后要注意观察患者的反应，个别患者可出现腹泻，这与当归、元参具有缓泻作用有关，一般无须处理，便可自行恢复，若腹泻较重，应报告医生，停药后即可恢复。

（2）局部处理：肢端干性坏疽，可用酒精棉球消毒，以消毒的干纱布包扎，保持干燥。湿性坏疽，伤口脓液多或有坏死组织，可用全竭膏外敷，以祛腐止痛，也可用解毒洗药熏洗后再换药；脓液少者应用大黄油纱布进行换药；创口脓液少肉芽组织新鲜时，用生肌玉红膏油纱布换药直至痊愈。换药时操作轻柔，细心，避免刺激增加患者的痛苦。

（3）饮食调养：宜营养丰富易消化的食物，多食些瓜类、豆类以助清热利湿。

4. 热毒炽盛型

临床表现

患肢红肿热痛，脓液多，有恶臭气味，伴有高热，恶寒，舌苔黄腻或黄燥，甚至出现黑苔，舌质红绛，脉象滑数洪大。

护理

（1）密切观察病情，注意体温、舌苔、脉象、血压的变化。如发热则为瘀血发热，属实热症，表现为壮热，面红目赤，意识模糊，烦躁不安，可用冷敷降温。应多巡视病室，床边加床档，防止坠床，并参照 2.1 高热护理。

(2) 服用清热解毒，活血化瘀的药物，方选四妙勇安汤加味、活血通脉饮各 1 剂，两剂分次交替服用，服药困难者，应少量多次频频喂服，服药后多饮水。兼服犀黄丸、牛黄清心丸。

(3) 局部处理：脓液多，有坏死组织者，应及时更换敷料，或用解毒洗药熏洗后再换药，以减轻恶臭，防止污染被褥。若坏疽继发感染扩展至踝关节或踝关节以上，持续高热，剧痛者，需要行截肢术。协助医生做好手术前准备。手术后残肢应平放，小腿以下截肢后，切忌屈曲膝关节，以免刀口直接压在床上。同时要观察全身情况，由于患者术前高烧，不能进食，术后容易出现低钾现象，应协助医生早期处理，防止低钾发生。患肢血液循环差，刀口愈合慢，应延长拆线时间。

(4) 饮食调养：给予营养丰富易消化的流质或半流质饮食，多食水果及新鲜蔬菜，多饮水或清淡饮料，或用双花、麦冬、天花粉各 9 克，开水泡代茶饮。若不能进食者，应给予补液。

5. 气血两虚型

临床表现

患者憔悴萎黄，消瘦无力，患肢皮肤干燥，脱屑，趾（指）甲干燥增厚，生长缓慢，肌肉萎缩，创口久不愈合，肉芽灰暗，脓液清稀。舌苔薄白，舌质淡，脉象沉细无力。

护理

(1) 由于久病气血耗伤，营卫不和，致使体质虚弱，因此要做好饮食调养，根据患者脾胃的运化能力，给予滋补气血的食物，如肉类、鱼类、禽蛋、海参、木耳、虾类及苹果、大枣、胡萝卜等，或以山药、当归、黄芪等分别加粳米煮粥常食之，以补气养血、健脾益胃。

(2) 患肢护理同阴寒型。另外，有创口者继续换药，若创口久不愈合，可用维生素 B_1 100 毫升，取双足三里穴，交替注射，或用艾条灸创面，促进创口愈合。

(3) 服用补气养血，调和营卫的药物，方选顾步汤加味，兼服十全大补丸或参茸大补丸。服药期间要注意观察舌苔的变化，若舌苔由薄白转黄，食欲差，则应停服。

(4) 由于局部疼痛，不能活动，久之造成关节不利，肌肉萎缩，因此在恢复期间应指导患者进行功能锻炼，促进患肢血管侧支循环的建立。常用方法：

①行局部按摩。

②应用活血止痛散行局部熏洗，熏洗后进行关节活动。

4.17 闭塞性动脉粥样硬化

闭塞性动脉粥样硬化，是全身动脉粥样硬化在肢体的局部表现，多发生于 45 岁以上的中、老年人。初发时肢体发凉怕冷，麻木，胀痛或灼热感，随着肢体缺血症状的加重，引起营养障碍，严重者可发生溃疡和坏疽。属于中医脱疽范围。

一般护理

1. 精神护理：本病多发生于中、老年人，常伴有高血压、冠心病或脑血管病变，又因患肢疼痛，坏疽，甚至可造成残废，给患者带来极大的痛苦，所以要重视精神护理。针对老年患者怕孤独，喜尊重的特点，要经常接触与其谈心，了解其心理活动。要掌握每个患者的思想情况，解除其顾虑，积极配合治疗；此外，还要做好亲属的思想工作，争取其理解与合作，特别是对截肢的患者，要指导亲属协助患者恢复自理能力。

2. 饮食调养：根据老年人脾胃功能减退的特点，饮食宜温、熟、软，营养丰富，易消化，并具有行气活血化瘀作用的食物。除主食米、面外，应多食些菠菜、胡萝卜、黑木耳、大枣、山楂等，还可常食些豆腐、鲜菇、紫菜汤、海带汤、莲子汤以及当归粥、丹参粥等。若伴有冠心病、高血压病、高血脂症等，宜清淡低盐饮食，多食豆制品及植物油。忌食辛辣及炙煿食物，另外应养成良好的生活习惯，饮食要有规律，定时定量，食勿过饱，勿因味美而贪食，不宜偏食。指导患者进食前应保持心情舒畅，做到怒后勿食，食后勿怒。食后忌卧，应适当散步。

3. 忌烟：吸烟可使患者肾上腺素和去甲肾上腺素分泌增多，使血管收缩和动脉内皮细胞损伤，并可使血液处于高凝状态，而加重病情，所以闭塞性动脉粥样硬化患者应终生戒烟。

辨证护理

1. 血瘀型

临床表现

肢体麻木，发凉，疼痛，肢端有瘀斑或呈紫红色，舌质绛有瘀点，脉弦涩。

护理

(1) 保护患肢，防止外伤，冬令时应注意保暖。局部可用活血止痛散煎汤熏洗，熏洗时，药液温度不宜过高。肢端瘀斑可涂马黄酊。

(2) 服用活血化瘀的药物，方选丹参通脉饮或活血通脉饮及活血通脉片。长期服用汤药造成胃纳减退，可加服调理脾胃的药物。

(3) 指导患者作自我推拿按摩运动。常用方法：上肢按揉肘关节周围，擦肘，捻指，搓手掌，擦手背。下肢按揉足三里，拿小腿，弹拨阳陵泉，擦涌泉，摇踝关节。按摩运动能舒筋活血，祛瘀通络，促使患肢建立侧支循环，改善肢体的营养状况，减轻疼痛。

2. 湿热下注型

临床表现

肢体坏疽感染，发红，肿胀，疼痛，舌苔黄腻。

护理

(1) 注意休息，防止过度劳累。

(2) 患肢应适当活动，防止因疼痛的关节长期不活动而失去功能。创口应辨证换药（可参照血栓闭塞性脉管炎湿热下注型换药法）。

（3）服用清热利湿，活血化瘀的药物，方选四妙勇安汤加味。

3. 热毒炽盛型

临床表现

肢体严重坏疽感染，向上扩展至踝部及小腿等，红肿热痛，溃烂脓多。伴发热，严重者意识模糊，胃纳减退。

护理

（1）卧床休息，高热者参照 2.1 高热护理。

（2）加强巡视病室，做好生活护理，协助患者翻身，防止局部长期受压，致使血瘀化热而发生褥疮。患肢疼痛参照血栓闭塞性脉管炎的止痛方法处理。

（3）服用清热解毒，活血化瘀的药物，方选四妙活血汤，兼服四虫片。

（4）注意观察病情，了解患者的神志、体温及局部变化，如果局部严重坏疽感染，可参照血栓闭塞性脉管炎热毒炽盛型换药处理。若坏疽扩展迅速，毒邪内攻，高热不退，意识模糊，需要行截肢手术者，应做好手术前后护理。

（5）给予频服清热解毒的饮料，如银花甘草汤、鲜芦根汤等，同时可给予补液，以维持水、电解质平衡。

5 妇科常见病证及护理

5.1 月经失调

凡是月经的周期、量、色、质发生异常改变，皆为月经失调。属周期改变的有月经先期，月经后期，月经先后无定期；经量改变的有月经过多，月经过少。

一般护理

1. 避免精神刺激，保持心情舒畅。

2. 观察月经周期，超前，延后及经行天数，行经的量、色、质的改变，并作好记录，向医生提供参考依据。

3. 注意观察腹痛，面色，体温，脉象，血压的变化，发现经血过多，出现血脱时，及时报告医生进行应急处理。

4. 做好经行时护理，注意保暖，经行期间忌用冷水洗浴，游泳，盆浴及房事。

5. 外阴部保持清洁，月经纸应柔软干净，以免擦伤皮肤。月经带宜勤洗勤换，并在日光下晒干，以防邪毒侵袭。

6. 经期忌食生冷瓜果和寒凉之药食，宜热饮食。

辨证护理

1. 血热型经行先期
临床表现
经行先期，量多，色紫粘稠或挟瘀块，小腹胀痛，心胸烦闷，面赤，手心灼热，舌红苔微黄而干，脉细数。
护理
(1) 加强情志护理，避免忿郁暴怒，情绪激动，保持心情舒畅。若情志不畅，造成气机紊乱，可致气血失调。

(2) 观察行经超前的时间，经量及色泽，腹痛程度等，并记录报告医生。腹痛时禁用热敷，以免血热妄行。

(3) 服用清热凉血的药物，方选用清经汤加减。汤药宜温服。

(4) 口干便燥重者，可用麦冬、玄参煎水服用，以滋阴生津。

(5) 饮食可多食黑木耳、藕汁等，以清热凉血，忌食生葱蒜、酒及辛辣温燥之食品。

2. 气虚型经行先期

临床表现

经期超前，量多，色淡清稀，倦怠乏力，纳呆，心悸气短，小腹坠感，舌质淡，苔白，脉虚大无力。

护理

(1) 行经期注意休息，避免劳累，经量过多者，应卧床休息。

(2) 服用健脾养心，益气补血的药物，方选归脾汤加减。

(3) 久病身体虚弱，出现气虚的患者，应适当增加营养，如多食牛奶、鸡蛋、豆浆、猪肝、新鲜蔬菜等食品。

3. 血寒型经行后期

临床表现

经期后延，色黯红量少，小腹疼痛，得热稍减，面色青白，肢冷畏寒、舌苔薄白，脉细数。

护理

(1) 患者平时应注意保暖，经行时注意休息，勿劳累。

(2) 服用温经散寒的药物，方选温经汤加减，汤药宜温服。

(3) 经行期，小腹疼痛者，可用热水袋热敷，或用艾条灸天枢、气海、关元等穴。

(4) 若久病阳气不足，气虚血亏的患者，喜温暖是虚寒之象，宜常服艾附暖宫丸，日服 3 次，每次 6 克，空腹温开水送下。

（5）饮食要营养丰富，行经期，忌食生冷瓜果。

4. 血虚型经期后延

临床表现

经期后延，色淡量少，小腹疼痛，面色苍白，头晕眼花，心悸，舌淡苔白，脉虚细。

护理

（1）经期注意休息，要观察记录经量、色泽变化。

（2）服用补血益气的药物，方选人参养荣汤加减。

（3）注意饮食调护，加强营养，多食猪肝、红枣、桂圆，可煎生姜大枣汤服用，以和胃消食。

5. 气郁型经期后延

临床表现

经期延后，量少，色紫红，小腹胀痛，精神郁闷，胸痞不舒，乳胀胁痛，舌苔黄薄，脉弦涩。

护理

（1）加强精神调护，对患者多进行解释、鼓励、安慰，消除思想顾虑，树立起战胜疾病的信心，积极配合调治。

（2）服用开郁行气的药物，方选七制香附丸加减。

（3）平时常用佛手、橘皮泡水代茶饮，口含金橘饼，或服逍遥丸 3 克，每日 3 次，以疏肝行气解郁。

6. 肝郁型经行先后无定期

临床表现

经期或先或后，量或多或少，小腹胀痛，胸闷不舒，胸胁乳房胀痛，时欲叹息，舌苔薄白，脉弦。

护理

（1）病房要安静、整洁、使患者静心调养，保持心情舒畅，避免精神刺激。

（2）服用舒肝解郁和血的药物，方选逍遥散加减。

（3）嘱患者常服逍遥丸，日服 2 次，每次 6 克，温开水送下，以舒肝行气开郁。

7. 肾虚型经行先后无定期

临床表现

经来先后不定期，量少，色淡质清稀，小腹坠痛，腰酸，夜尿频，舌淡苔薄白，脉沉细。

护理

（1）经期注意休息，不要参加过重的体力劳动及剧烈的体育活动，以免耗伤气血，引起行经失调。

（2）患者睡眠要充足，使精神饱满，情绪稳定，节制房事，以免损及冲任。

（3）服用补肾气，调冲任的药物，方选定期饮加减。

（4）可用益母草膏加红糖适量，每日早晚各服 20ml，以活血祛瘀。

8. 气虚型经量过多

临床表现

经量多过期不止，色淡清稀，面色苍白，心悸气短，小腹空坠，肢软无力，舌淡苔薄白，脉虚弱。

护理

（1）卧床休息，避免疲劳及房事。

（2）服用益气摄血升阳的药物，方选举元煎加减。

（3）因下血过多，身体虚弱，四肢无力，应注意饮食调摄，加强营养，给予温补脾胃的食品，如猪肝、甲鱼、红枣、桂圆、藕汁、黑木耳及新鲜蔬菜等。要忌饮酒及辛辣动火刺激食品。

（4）注意观察经量、色泽、用纸量，并记录，如经量特别多，出现血脱现象，立即报告医生，即刻针刺人中、十宣、合谷、涌泉等穴，或艾灸百会穴，给口服红参粉 3 克，以回阳固脱。

9. 血热型经量过多

临床表现

经来量多，过期不止，色红质粘稠，有紫块，腰腹胀痛，心烦口渴，面红唇干，尿黄便干，舌红苔黄，脉滑数。

护理

（1）行经期注意休息，防止劳累。经量过多者，应卧床休息。

（2）服用清热凉血的药物，方选清经四物汤加减。

10. 血虚型经量过少

临床表现

经量过少，色淡红，质清稀，头晕耳鸣，心悸怔忡，腰膝酸软，小腹空痛，面色萎黄，皮肤干燥不润，舌淡苔薄，脉虚细。

护理

（1）加强营养。因饮食失节，损伤脾胃，脾胃虚弱，气血生化来源不足，致月经量少，在经行时属虚寒者，要禁生冷苦寒收敛的食品。

（2）行经时要注意休息，防止过度劳累。要节制房事。

（3）服用补血益气健脾的药物，方选人参滋血汤加减。

11. 血瘀型经量过少

临床表现

经量过少，色紫黑有块，小腹胀痛拒按，血块排出后腹痛减轻，舌边紫黯，脉沉细。

护理

（1）要保持心情舒畅，切勿忧思过度，以免影响气机的运行，致月经量减少。

（2）腹痛拒按者，可针刺血海、少海、归来、足三里等穴，也可给耳穴压豆，取穴：子宫、交感、内分泌等穴，以促使瘀块排出减轻腹痛。

（3）服用活血行瘀的药物，方选过期饮加减。

(4) 因受寒邪外袭，引起气滞血瘀者，可用小茴香、干姜适量煎汤服用，或适当饮用红糖黄酒液，以温经祛瘀。

5.2 痛经

妇女在经期或行经前后，小腹及腰骶部疼痛，甚至剧痛难忍，伴有恶心、呕吐、头痛或出现昏厥，随着经行周期持续发作，称为痛经，亦称经行腹痛。

一般护理

1. 痛经者应注意休息，重者要卧床休息，病室要安静整洁，通风良好，温度适宜。

2. 加强精神调护，安慰病者稳定情绪，节制情欲，同时要避免各种精神刺激，保持心情舒畅。

3. 经行时，小腹部注意保暖，勿用冷水洗下肢，经前数日忌食生冷、寒凉、酸涩食物，以防寒邪侵袭。

4. 观察疼痛的时间、部位、性质、程度及经血排出情况，必要时保留标本供医生查看或送检。

5. 疼痛剧烈引起面色苍白，手足厥冷，出冷汗等症时，应立即让患者平卧，注意保暖，并报告医生，进行急救。

6. 用针灸方法，取穴：中极、气海、三阴交，或按摩下腹部、腰骶部及气海、关元、肾俞、八髎等，亦可口服延胡索片、去痛片等；寒湿痛经用热水袋热熨小腹部。

辨证护理

1. 气滞血瘀型
临床表现
经前经期小腹胀痛，行经量少或行而不畅，经色紫黑，经行有血块，腹痛拒按，块去痛减，胸胁乳房胀痛，舌质紫黯，舌边有瘀点，脉沉弦。

护理

（1）经期绝对卧床休息，避免疲劳及房事。

（2）注意情志护理，多与病人交谈，解除其忧虑情绪，使之安心调养。

（3）给予富有营养、清淡、易消化食物，忌生冷、辛辣食品。

（4）服用理气活血，化瘀止痛的药物，方选血府逐瘀汤加减，服药后让患者卧床休息。

（5）腹痛拒按，给服元胡止痛片，日服 3 次，每次 2 片，或用黑豆 15 克、红糖 30 克、红花 9 克，水煎温服。

（6）用针灸疗法，于月经前 2 天开始针灸中极、三阴交、次髎、关元、命门、足三里、气海，耳穴取内分泌、子宫、皮质下等穴，以调经止痛。

2. 寒湿凝滞型

临床表现

经前经期小腹冷痛，按之痛甚，得热痛减，经量少，色黯有块，如黑豆水样，舌青紫，苔白腻，脉沉紧。

护理

（1）嘱患者饮食要热饮，或用生姜片数片同红糖适量，煎水代茶饮，以散寒活血止痛。

（2）小腹冷痛，用艾叶、生姜适量炒热，温敷脐部，或用艾条灸，随时注意小腹部保暖。

（3）服用温经散寒止痛化瘀的药物，方选温经汤加减，汤药热服，服后卧床休息。

（4）寒湿痛经用针灸，取中极、气海、三阴交等穴，艾灸气海、三阴交，以温经止痛。

3. 气血虚弱型

临床表现

经期或月经干净后，小腹绵绵作痛，按之痛减，色淡，质清稀，面色苍白，精神倦怠，经量少，舌淡苔薄，脉细弱。

护理

(1) 经期要注意休息和保暖，切勿受凉，以防邪气乘虚侵袭。

(2) 服用益气养血的药物，方选黄芪当归通经汤加减，汤药宜热服。

(3) 气血虚者，注意增加营养，常食山药粉、猪肝、羊肉等，以补养气血。

(4) 虚寒腹痛，喜温，宜热敷，或用针灸补法，针刺艾灸命门、肾俞、关元、足三里、大赫，以调补气血，温养止痛。

4. 肝肾亏损型

临床表现

经后小腹隐痛，经色淡量少，腰部酸胀，头晕耳鸣，舌淡红，苔薄，脉沉细。

护理

(1) 要注意劳逸适度，动静结合。平时节制房事，以减少气血的耗损和伤及肝肾。

(2) 服用调补肝肾的药物，方选调肝汤加减。

(3) 腰酸腹痛可选用揉、推、点三种推拿手法，取穴：三阴交、归来、太冲，配肝俞、肾俞、足三里，以活血止痛。

5.3 闭经

发育正常的女子，一般在 14 岁左右，月经便按时来潮，若超过 18 岁，月经尚未来潮，称为原发性闭经；已有经行周期之后，又停止 3 个月以上者，除妊娠、哺乳期、更年期外，称为继发性闭经。

一般护理

1. 加强情志护理，避免各种不良的刺激，鼓励其树立治病的信心，以积极的态度配合调理。

2. 对于青春期闭经的患者，应适当增加营养，注意劳逸结合。

3. 对于身体肥胖者，鼓励进行体育活动，减轻体重。

4. 哺乳时间过长者，劝其按时给婴儿断奶。

辨证护理

1. 肝肾不足型

临床表现

月经来潮较晚，经行后又停止，面容苍老，皮肤干燥，腰膝酸软，头晕耳鸣，消瘦，手足心热，盗汗，舌质淡，苔薄黄，脉虚细而数。

护理

(1) 注意饮食调补，给予滋补肝肾的食品，如银耳、甲鱼、阿胶，以滋补肝肾。

(2) 适当调理生活起居，切勿过度疲劳，应节制房事。

(3) 服用补益肝肾，养血调经的药物，方选归肾丸加减。

(4) 用耳穴压豆法，取内分泌、卵巢、子宫等穴，调理冲任。

2. 气血虚弱型

临床表现

经量少，色淡，渐渐停止，面色苍白，萎黄，疲倦乏力，头晕目眩，心悸气短，舌质淡，脉细弱无力。

护理

(1) 要安慰患者，避免精神刺激，以增强战胜疾病的信心。

(2) 饮食勿冷饮，以防损伤脾胃，可常食红枣、桂圆、蔬菜、猪肝、鸡汤等，以补气养血。

(3) 服用益气扶脾，养血调经的药物，方选六君子汤加减。

3. 气滞血瘀型

临床表现

经停，面色青黄，精神抑郁，情绪急躁，胸闷胁痛，小腹痛拒按，舌质紫黯，边有瘀点，脉弦涩。

护理

(1) 加强情志护理，多给予精神安慰，消除患者顾虑，以配合治疗。

(2) 服用活血祛瘀，理气通经的药物，方选乌药散加减。

(3) 饮用红黄酒，即红花15克，黄酒适量，浸泡5天后服用，每天2～3次，以活血祛瘀。

4. 痰湿内阻型

临床表现

停经后身体肥胖，胸闷泛恶，痰多腹胀，不思饮食，带下量多，舌苔白腻，脉弦滑。

护理

(1) 要注意饮食护理，给予清淡，富有营养，易于消化的食品，少食脂肪、甜食，以防增加体重，助湿生痰加重病情。

(2) 患者要适当进行体育锻炼，增加抗病能力，减轻体重。

(3) 服用行气化痰，健脾燥湿的药物，方选苍附导痰丸加减。

5.4 崩漏

妇女不在行经期，阴道大量出血，或持续下血，淋漓不断，称为崩漏，亦称崩中漏下。一般以突然下血，来势急，血量多的称崩；来势缓，血量少，淋漓不断的称漏。但在发病过程中，两者易互相转化，崩和漏只是病势不同，其病因病机是一致的，所以通常崩漏并称。

一般护理

1. 做好生活起居的护理，病室要安静整洁，空气新鲜，通风良好，温度、湿度要适宜。

2. 做好精神护理，消除精神刺激，安慰患者，树立战胜疾病的信心，以积极配合调治。

3. 饮食要营养丰富，易于消化吸收，忌食辛辣、煎炸、油腻等食品。

4. 注意观察病情变化，察看阴道出血量、色、质、气味及舌苔，脉象，血压，神色的变化，并做好记录，向医生汇报。

5. 阴道出血淋漓不断或突然下血量多，挟有瘀块，可留取标本供医生察看或送检。

6. 发现面色苍白，出冷汗，血压下降，突然阴道大量下血，脉芤者，应报告医生，采取急救措施，并做好输液，输血，给氧的准备工作。

辨证护理

1. 血热型
临床表现
阴道出血量多，淋漓不止，色深红，或紫黑挟块，质粘稠，面赤口干，烦躁不安，渴欲凉饮，舌质红，苔黄，脉滑数。

护理

(1) 下血多者应注意休息，少活动，避免情志受刺激，保持心情舒畅，安心调治。

(2) 饮食选用富于营养，清淡之食物，如鸭、鱼类等，以补养气血，可多食水果、蔬菜及清热凉血之品，忌辛辣刺激，温燥助阳之物。

(3) 服用清热凉血止血的药物，方选清热固经汤加减，汤剂宜偏凉服。

(4) 腹痛者，可用推拿手法或指压三阴交、足三里、内穴等穴以止痛，不宜用热敷、艾灸，以防出血更甚。

(5) 保持大便通畅，若大便干结可用蕃泻叶 5 克泡水饮，或食香蕉、桃子、蜂蜜等，以润肠通便。

（6）下血多者可用针刺疗法，取关元、三阴交、隐白、血海、水泉等穴，以泄血中之热。

2. 血瘀型

临床表现

下血淋漓不止，或突然下血量多，挟有瘀块，小腹疼痛拒按，瘀块排出后则疼痛减轻，舌质暗红或舌尖边有瘀点，脉沉涩。

护理

（1）注意休息，避免劳累

（2）饮食宜易消化富有营养的食品，忌食生冷、酸涩刺激性食品。

（3）服用活血行瘀的药物，方选四物汤合失笑散加减。

（4）少腹疼痛拒按者，予以活血祛瘀中药研为细末，开水调敷少腹，促进瘀血排出，减轻腹痛。

（5）出血多可针刺气海、三阴交、血海、子宫等穴。

3. 脾虚型

临床表现

暴崩下血，或淋漓不净，色淡质薄，面色㿠白，身体倦怠，四肢不温，气短懒言，胸闷纳呆，大便溏薄，舌质淡，苔薄白，脉虚细无力。

护理

（1）静卧休息，避免过度思虑和劳累，体虚怕冷者，应注意保暖。

（2）加强饮食调护，增加营养，多食健脾益气的食药，如山药粉、苡米粥、黄芪、党参粥等，忌生冷硬固之食品。

（3）服用补脾摄血、养血、止血的药物，方选归脾汤加减，汤剂宜温服。

（4）暴崩下血多时，须防血脱发生，必要时急煎独参汤服之，以益气摄血固脱。

(5) 用针灸疗法，取关元、三阴交、隐白、足三里、脾俞等穴，以益气摄血；如血脱时，可灸百会、气海穴，以回阳固脱。

4. 肾虚型

临床表现

下血量少，淋漓不断，头晕耳鸣，五心烦热，失眠盗汗，腰腿酸软，舌质红苔少，脉细数无力为肾阴虚；下血量多，淋漓不断，色淡红，面色㿠白，少腹冷痛，精神萎靡，腰背酸痛，小便频数而清，大便溏薄，舌淡苔薄白，脉沉细为肾阳虚。

护理

(1) 阴虚者，衣被不宜过暖，情绪要安定。

(2) 饮食宜滋润益阴的食品，可选用鸭、甲鱼、蛋类、黑木耳、银耳及水果、蔬菜等。忌煎炸及辛辣动火之食品，以防伤阴助火。

(3) 服用滋肾固阴的药物，方选左归丸加减，汤剂宜温服。

(4) 可针刺肾俞、关元、三阴交、内关、太溪等穴，用补法以调养心肾而退虚热。

(5) 阳虚者要注意腰腹部保暖，下血减少，病情稳定后，可到室外活动。

(6) 服用温肾止血的药物，方选用右归丸加减，汤剂宜热服。

5.5 绝经前后诸证

妇女在 49 岁左右，月经开始终止，称绝经或经断　有些妇女在绝经前后，往往出现经行紊乱，头晕耳鸣，心悸失眠，烦躁易怒，易出虚汗，五心烦热，或浮肿便溏，腰酸，倦怠乏力，情志异常。以上这些症候，轻重不一的综合出现，有的可延续 2、3 年之久，名为绝经前后诸证，亦称经断前后诸证，现代医学称更年期综合症。

一般护理

1. 病室陈设舒适、安全、实用，室内阳光充足，空气流通，整洁安静，温度、湿度适宜。

2. 了解患者的病情，掌握思想状况，关心患者痛苦，做好生活起居，情志，饮食的护理。

3. 耐心解释病情，使之了解更年期的生理变化过程，消除思想顾虑，积极配合调治。

4. 注意劳逸结合，避免剧烈运动。适当参加有意义的社会活动，使生活有规律，以增强生活乐趣。

5. 应注意调节饮食，选用清淡，易消化，富于营养的食品。

6. 按时服药，认真观察服药的情况，做好服药护理，尤其在服汤药后，注意有无恶心呕吐和其它不适等变化，并及时报告医生。

辨证护理

1. 肾阴亏虚型
临床表现

阵发性面部潮红，烦躁易怒或忧郁，手足心烦热，头晕，头痛，耳鸣多汗，口唇干燥，胃纳差，腰酸骨痛，大便燥结，月经量少，色鲜红或紫红，舌质红，苔少，脉弦细略数。

护理

(1) 患者要充分休息。头晕头痛应卧床休息，闭目养神，待症状减轻后，方可下床活动。

(2) 密切注意观察患者情绪的变化，做好思想工作，积极配合调治。

(3) 头晕目眩者，应注意血压的变化，若血压增高，适当限制食盐的摄入量。多食海带、芹菜、银耳等清淡饮食，忌辛辣肥甘厚味。

(4) 服用滋阴潜阳、补益肝肾的药物,方选六味地黄汤加减。

(5) 有心肾不交表现的患者,给服补心丹,日服 3 次,每次 9 克,空腹温开水送下。或用耳穴压豆疗法,取心、肾、神门、皮质下,以宁心安神。

(6) 多参加体育锻炼,坚持打太极拳、气功疗法等,以增强体质。

2. 肾阳亏虚

临床表现

月经量多,色淡,精神不振,畏寒怕冷,腰膝酸软,神疲乏力,食少浮肿,便溏,舌淡苔薄,脉沉细无力。

护理

(1) 参照肾阴亏虚护理。

(2) 注意饮食调护,可食莲子、扁豆、薏仁、山药粉、芡实粉,进食时加肉桂、良姜,以补肾助阳。忌生冷。

(3) 服用温肾助阳的药物,方选右归汤加减,汤药以睡前温服为宜。

(4) 推拿关元、气海、脾俞、胃俞、肾俞、长强等穴,针灸命门、关元、肾俞,用补法。

5.6 带下病

妇女阴道常流出少量的无色透明的分泌物湿润阴道,通常称白带。这种分泌物在月经前期或妊娠期可能有所增加,这是正常现象。如分泌物过多,或色、质、味发生变化,并伴有全身症状者则为病态,中医称为带下病。

一般护理

1. 注意生活起居的护理,病室要清洁卫生,空气新鲜,通风良好。

2. 加强卫生教育，应经常保持外阴部清洁，每日用复方蛇床子洗药熏洗。

3. 月经期更要注意卫生，月经纸要干净、柔软，勤换内裤。在经期内，机体抵抗力较弱，不宜劳累，注意避风寒，并禁止房事。

4. 饮食宜营养丰富，清淡易消化，多食鲜菜水果，平素可食山药、芡实、扁豆、银耳等，以健脾利湿；忌生冷、辛辣、油腻煎烤之食品。

5. 观察带下的量、色、质、气味及全身症状，并记录，必要时留取样本，供医生查看或送检。

6. 外阴瘙痒者，防止抓破引起感染，应及时治疗。

辨证护理

1. 脾虚型

临床表现

带下色白或淡黄，质粘稠，无气味，绵绵不断，面色㿠白或萎黄，四肢不温，神疲乏力，纳少便溏，两足跗部浮肿，舌淡苔白或腻，脉缓。

护理

(1) 注意休息，保暖，四肢不温怕冷者，可安排在向阳温暖的病室内，室温保持在 20℃ 左右。避免过度疲劳。

(2) 做好情志护理，解除思想负担。

(3) 服用健脾益气，升阳除湿的药物，方选完带汤加减，汤剂宜睡前温服。

(4) 大便稀溏者，少食生冷、水果、宜饮热小米粥，平素多食黄芪党参粥、苡米粥、山药粉等，以健脾利湿。

(5) 每日用白果 7 枚，去壳打碎，用豆浆 1 碗煮沸冲服。

2. 肾虚型

临床表现

白带清冷，量多，质稀薄，淋漓不断，腰膝酸软，小腹冷感。小便频而清长，夜间尤甚。大便溏薄。舌质淡，苔薄白，脉沉迟。

护理

(1) 参照脾虚型护理

(2) 服用温补肾阳，除湿止带的药物，方选内补丸，每丸9克，每次2丸，日服2次，温开水送下。

(3) 服药后注意休息，节制房事。

3. 湿毒型

临床表现

带下量多，色黄绿如脓，或挟血液，或混浊如米泔水，有秽臭气，阴中瘙痒，少腹痛，小便短赤，口苦咽干，舌质红，苔黄，脉滑数。

护理

(1) 适当休息，避免劳累，安定患者情绪，保持心情舒畅。

(2) 患者应注意增加营养，多食高蛋白类食物，少食辛辣刺激厚味之食品。

(3) 服用清热解毒，除湿止带的药物，方选止带方加减。

(4) 阴中瘙痒甚者，避免盆浴及房事，可外用复方蛇床子洗药，煎熬趁热先熏后洗，或用针刺疗法，取百虫窝、蠡沟、曲骨、太冲、三阴交等穴。

5.7 阴道炎

、健康妇女阴道本身有自净作用，可形成自然防御能力，能抑制细菌生长。若防御功能被破坏，细菌侵入，便可导致阴道发炎，称为阴道炎。阴道炎症最常见的是老年性阴道炎和滴虫、霉菌性阴道炎。

一般护理

1. 督促患者注意休息，病室内经常保持整洁，安静，空气流通。

2. 做好情志护理，避免精神紧张，了解患者病情及生活起居。还要做好饮食护理，少食辛辣厚味之品。

3. 养成良好的卫生习惯，经常保持外阴清洁，勤换内裤。经期月经纸要干净柔软，月经带勤洗勤换，最好消毒后使用。若分泌物增多时应留取标本，供医生察看或送检。

4. 用外洗中药煎汤熏洗，禁止盆浴。患者单独使用瓷盆、浴巾。应节制房事。有滴虫者，禁入游泳池游泳，以防止交叉感染。

5. 痒痛甚者，切勿搔抓，防止感染，可配合针灸疗法。

辨证护理

1. 老年性阴道炎

临床表现

阴道有烧灼感，小便时外阴和阴道刺痛，其带下有时呈水样或呈血性粘液状，阴道壁及宫颈粘膜发红，轻度水肿，触痛，并有大小不等的片状出血点，舌红无苔，脉弦数。

护理

(1) 急性期宜安静休息，老年人情绪易急躁，火热伤阴，加之体质虚弱，食少，抵抗力差，需注意补充营养，给清淡易消化之品，不可过食滋补的食品。忌食辛辣、酒类和刺激性食品。

(2) 服用清热解毒，补脾益肾的药物，方选滋肾凉血解毒汤加减。

(3) 外洗中药用苦参、黄柏各 9 克，蛇床子 15 克，煎汤，趁热先熏后洗，每日 1 次。

(4) 用针灸疗法，取百虫窝、曲骨、横骨、阴阜、足三里、太溪、三阴交等，耳穴取神门、外生殖器、肺、内分泌等穴。或用地丁黄芩注射液 2 毫升穴位注射，以止痛止痒。

2. 滴虫、霉菌性阴道炎

临床表现

阴痒带下，小便短赤及外阴刺激症状。滴虫性带下为黄绿色，量多稀薄，呈泡沫状或米汤样，腥味；霉菌性带下呈乳白色块状，豆腐渣状。阴道及宫颈粘膜红肿，有散在出血点，伴有剧痒及烧灼感。

护理

(1)加强卫生教育，坚持身体锻炼，增强抵抗力。男方有滴虫或霉菌感染者，夫妇应同时治疗，治疗期间应禁止房事，以免互相传染。

(2)滴虫病患者，服用清热祛湿，杀虫解毒止痒的药物，方选三妙散加减。

(3)可用 2% 乳酸溶液冲洗阴道，擦干后放入雄蛇丸，睡时放入阴道内，晨起取出，5 天为 1 疗程，不愈者再加 1 疗程。

(4)中药外洗方：用苦参、黄柏各 9 克，蛇床子 30 克，川楝子 6 克，枸杞根、枯矾各 15 克，水煎去渣，注入阴道。并做外阴冲洗，每日 2 次。

(5)针灸疗法同 1.老年性阴道炎。

(6)霉菌病患者，服用清热化湿的药物，方选化湿汤加减。

(7)中药外洗方：用蛇床子 15 克，地骨皮、川椒、明矾各 6 克，苦参 9 克，用水煎汤熏洗患部，每日 1～2 次。

(8)冰硼散适量加甘油少许拌匀，清洗外阴后涂于阴道内，早晚各 1 次。

(9)霉菌性阴道炎剧痒者，可在无名指掌侧中节横纹血管处放血，能止痒数小时，可连续针刺数次。

5.8 妊娠恶阻

妊娠早期出现恶心呕吐，头晕厌食，或食入即吐，体倦，喜食酸咸之物等。祖国医学称为妊娠恶阻，也叫子病等。

一般护理

1. 病室内要清除一切诱发呕吐的因素，要安静，卫生，空气新鲜。一般患者要注意休息，严重者要卧床休息。

2. 注意精神护理，要给予精神安慰，解除思想顾虑，使之精神愉快，积极配合调治。

3. 饮食要给予营养丰富，易消化，清淡的半流汁；呕吐严重者，要少量多餐，给予流汁，必要时静脉补液。

4. 保持口腔卫生，每次呕吐后要用清水漱口，防止发生口腔糜烂。

5. 保持大便通畅，便秘者可食蜂蜜适量，每日 3 次，以润肠通便。

6. 注意观察病情，因剧烈呕吐可引起腰腹疼痛，阴道少量流血，胎动不安或胎漏、坠胎等现象，要及时报告医生。

7. 出现呕吐频繁，发热口渴，尿少便秘，舌红，脉滑数无力等气阴两亏的严重证候时，可能为妊娠中毒症，应及时报告医生进行抢救。

辨证护理

1. 脾胃虚弱型

临床表现

妊娠早期恶心呕吐，不思饮食，或呕吐清涎，厌闻食气，神疲思睡，舌淡苔白，脉缓或无力。

护理

(1) 呕吐剧烈，频繁者，应卧床休息。

(2) 调理情志，避免恼怒，保持心情舒畅，以配合治疗。

(3) 饮食宜清淡，富有营养，可随患者喜好选择食物，呕吐后要鼓励多饮米汤、豆浆、藕粉等，补充体液，以防脱水。

(4) 服用健脾和胃，调气降逆的药物，方选香砂六君子汤加减，服药时加姜汁数滴，以和胃止呕。服药后要静卧休息。

(5) 鼓励患者进补脾和胃的药食，多饮淡盐水，或人参、白术、陈皮煎水代茶饮，以健脾降逆；平素可咀嚼砂仁数粒，以和胃宽中止呕。

(6) 针灸疗法，根据病情，可选双侧内关，留针 20 分钟。虚寒者艾灸足三里穴，以清热止呕。

2. 脾胃不和型

临床表现

妊娠初期吐苦水，嗳气、胸闷肋胀，心烦头晕，精神抑郁，舌淡红，苔微黄，脉弦滑。

护理

(1) 病室环境要清洁，整齐,优美，舒适，定时通风换气，避免噪音干扰。

(2) 做好情志护理，多给患者精神安慰，使之心情舒畅，精神愉快，以配合治疗。

(3) 服用疏肝和胃，降逆止呕的药物，方选苏叶黄连汤加减，服药时可加姜汁数滴。

(4) 用菊花、竹茹、黄芩水煎代茶饮，以清热理气和胃。

3. 瘀滞型

临床表现

妊娠初期，呕吐痰涎，胸闷不思饮食，心悸气促，苔白腻，脉滑。

护理

(1) 参照 2.脾胃不和型护理。

(2) 服用健脾除湿，化痰止呕的药物，方选小半夏茯苓汤加减。

5.9 胎动不安（胎漏、坠胎、小产、滑胎）

妊娠后，阴道不时少量下血，时下时止，或淋漓不断，但无腰酸腹痛和小腹坠感等现象者称为胎漏；如先感胎动下坠，继则有轻微腰酸腹胀，或阴道少许出血，称胎动不安；如妊娠3个月以内，胎儿尚未成形而坠者，称为坠胎；3个月以后坠胎者则称小产。

一般护理

1. 病室要安静，，避免一切噪音和不良刺激，应绝对卧床休息，直至阴道下血停止。

2. 做好精神护理，加强情志调理，多安慰诱导，消除一切思想顾虑，使之安心治疗。

3. 饮食宜清淡，营养丰富，易于消化，多食新鲜蔬菜、水果，忌食辛辣、厚腻、煎炸之品。

4. 注意保持外阴清洁，给患者使用消毒的会阴垫，用后保留，以供医生察看。注意观察阴道下血、腹痛等症状的变化，如阴道大量下血，腹痛加剧，应及时报告医生进行处理。

5. 出现面色苍白，汗出，四肢厥冷，则是阴道流血过多所造成的血脱之象，立即报告医生，并做好急救准备，必要时输血。

辨证护理

1. 气血虚弱型

临床表现

妊娠初期，胎动下坠，阴道少量下血，腰酸腹胀，神疲肢倦，面色㿠白，心悸气短，舌质淡，苔薄白，脉细滑无力。

护理

(1) 应卧床休息,避免劳累，禁止房事，以防伤胎。

(2) 注意调和情志，鼓励患者稳定情绪，消除恐惧心理。

(3) 服用补气益血，健脾安胎的药物，方选胎元饮加减。

(4) 气血虚弱，则胎失营养，应加强饮食的护理，给予营养丰富，易于消化的食物，如老母鸡汤、鱼、肉、蛋及动物内脏，或用阿胶、黄芪、糯米煮粥，以调补气血，养胎安胎。忌食辛辣、刺激性食品。

(5) 配合针灸补法，取足三里、内庭、阳陵泉等穴，每日 1 次。

2. 肾虚型

临床表现

阴道下血，腰酸腹坠，头晕耳鸣，小便频，有滑胎史，舌淡苔白,脉沉细。

护理

(1) 参照 1.气血虚弱型护理。

(2) 有滑胎史的患者，应在停经后开始多食阿胶、核桃仁、枸杞子等补肾之品，服用到妊娠 5～6 个月。

(3) 服用固肾安胎的药物，方选寿胎丸加减，汤药宜温服。

3. 血热型

临床表现

阴道下血，色鲜红，心烦不安，手足心烦热，口干咽燥，小腹痛，潮热便干，舌红苔黄，脉滑数。

护理

(1) 病室环境宜安静、舒适，通风凉爽、有利于睡眠。要鼓励患者做到清心寡欲，保证充分睡眠。

(2) 注意饮食护理，鼓励患者多饮淡盐水，多吃新鲜蔬菜和甘酸水果，以及多营养，多蛋白饮食。忌食辛辣、炙煿之物，以免助热伤阴。

(3) 服用清热安胎的药物，方选保阴煎加减。

（4）出现口干咽燥者，常用麦冬、肉苁蓉、胖大海、竹茹泡水饮，或服用梨汁、藕汁滋阴清热凉血。

（5）针灸疗法，取神门、少海、内关、太冲、阳陵泉、足三里等穴。

4. 外伤型

临床表现

妊娠期间受伤，腹痛腹胀，胎动下坠，阴道流血，脉滑无力。

护理

（1）绝对卧床休息，稳定患者情绪，消除顾虑，保持心情舒畅，以安奠胎元。

（2）服用益气养血，固摄安胎的药物，方选圣愈汤加减。

（3）禁用活血化瘀的药物，腹部及腰部禁外用膏药，以免破血动胎，上下肢受伤，可适当进行局部按摩，以减轻疼痛。

（4）密切观察病情，对腹痛下坠，阴道流血过多，有流产先兆者，应报告医生，做好流产的准备工作。

5.10 妊娠痫证

妊娠后期，或正值分娩时，或分娩后，忽然眩晕仆倒，昏迷不知人事，四肢抽搐，牙关紧闭，目睛直视，口吐白沫，少时自睡，后又复发，或昏迷不醒，为妊娠痫证。中医称子痫或子冒。

一般护理

1. 病室环境要安静、整洁、通风良好，空气新鲜，温度、湿度适宜，避免声光刺激。

2. 加强精神护理，多劝慰开导患者，使其解除思想顾虑，消除紧张恐惧心理，安定情绪，保持心情舒畅，积极配合治疗。

3. 安排单人房间，设床档，以防坠床。应设专人守护，严密观察病情变化。注意血压及胎心音的改变，每4～6小时测量

1次。

4. 尽量避免刺激，一切诊断、检查、护理操作要轻柔，时间要集中，或在应用镇静剂后进行。不能吞咽者可鼻饲饮食，昏迷者应禁食。

5. 大小便失禁者，衣被污染后随时更换，注意保持衣被干净和皮肤清洁。皮肤水肿者，在肌注或静滴时，防止漏液，要严格局部消毒，以免引起感染。

6. 详细观察记录抽搐、神志、血压、脉象、体温，小便，浮肿等变化。备好急救药品与器械，如发现危象，立即报告医生配合抢救。

辨证护理

1. 阴虚肝旺型

临床表现

妊娠后期，头晕目眩，心悸气短，胸闷烦热，面色潮红，大便干结，小便短黄，舌质红，苔微黄而干，脉弦细滑数。

护理

(1) 绝对卧床休息，每天保证足够的睡眠，避免用脑及疲劳过度，衣被不宜过暖。

(2) 做好情志护理。由于患者常处于紧张、恐惧状态，因此在护理工作中，要用温和的语言，安慰开导患者，使之情绪稳定，增强治病的信心。

(3) 饮食可选清淡富有营养，易消化，高热量，高蛋白饮食，多食新鲜蔬菜、水果，宜食猪肝、猪心、海蜇等。禁烟酒，忌食肥甘及辛辣刺激食物。

(4) 服用育阴潜阳，平肝养血的药物，方选羚羊钩藤汤加减，必要时每日2剂，分数次服用。

(5) 患者如突发抽搐，应将头偏向一侧，用纱布包压舌板置上、下齿之间，以防咬伤舌头。针刺或指掐人中、合谷、承山、颊车、太冲、涌泉、曲池等穴。给服安宫牛黄丸1丸，水研化服或鼻饲，并及时报告医生处理。

(6) 有痰阻气道者，可针刺天突、丰隆、内关、肺俞等穴，以豁痰开窍。或用捶背法促使排痰。亦可用竹沥水60毫升加姜汁数滴，频频喂服或鼻饲，以化痰降浊。痰液排出后宜进少量热粥，以恢复胃气。

(7) 下肢水肿者，应限制食盐摄入量，多食西瓜汁、冬瓜汁，或用冬瓜皮煮水代茶饮，以利小便。大便干结者，可给蜂蜜水，润肠通便。

2. 脾虚肝旺型

临床表现

面浮肢肿，胸闷欲吐，头晕目胀，纳差便溏，苔腻，脉虚弦而滑。

护理

(1) 服用健脾利湿，平肝潜阳的药物，方选白术散加减。

(2) 其它护理同1.阴虚肝旺者。

5.11 异位妊娠

受精卵着床于子宫腔以外的组织，如输卵管、卵巢、腹腔等形成妊娠者，称为异位妊娠，亦称宫外孕。

一般护理

1. 加强情志护理，做好细致的思想工作，给予精心照顾，多安慰鼓励患者，消除思想顾虑，以积极配合治疗。

2. 绝对卧床休息，避免或减少不必要的搬动，防止体位改变和增加腹压的因素。

3. 密切观察腹痛、腹胀，阴道出血及排出物，注意神色，血压，脉象的变化，并做记录。做好阴道后穹窿穿刺术和手术前准备工作。

4. 若腹痛剧烈，面色苍白，出虚汗，肢冷，血压下降，脉微欲绝，为厥证出现，应立即报告医生，配合急救。

辨证护理

1. 休克型

临床表现

孕妇突然下腹剧痛，拒按。面色苍白，四肢厥冷，冷汗淋漓，恶心呕吐，血压下降，烦躁，脉微欲绝。

护理

(1) 设专人护理，取平卧位。

(2) 服用益气回阳救逆的药物，方选独参汤，急煎灌服，汤药可浓缩，服时加姜汁数滴，要少量多次分服，以防呕吐。

(3) 鼻饲流质、米汁等食物，以补充营养。

(4) 血压下降，大汗淋漓不止，四肢厥冷者，应注意保暖，急煎人参汤服之，或配合针刺人中、内关、足三里，涌泉等穴。耳穴取交感，升压点，肾上腺等穴，以回阳救逆。

(5) 休克症状缓解后，再给予活血化瘀的药物，方选宫外孕Ⅰ号汤内服。

2. 不稳定型

临床表现

腹痛拒按，但逐渐减轻，并有不规则的阴道流血，点滴而下，血压稳定，脉细缓。

护理

(1) 住院1～2天内卧床休息，逐渐增加活动量，妊娠试验阴性者，可下床轻度活动。

(2) 服用活血祛瘀止痛的药物，方选宫外孕汤加减.

(3) 注意观察腹痛，阴道出血量，颜色及有无血块或组织排出。若腹痛加剧，伴有汗出肢冷，血压下降,应及时报告医生，按休克型进行护理。

3. 包块型

临床表现

宫外孕流产或破裂后，形成血肿包块，下腹部有轻微的胀痛或压痛，阴道流血基本停止，舌色淡暗，脉沉弦细。

护理

(1) 服用活血化瘀，破坚散结的药物，方选宫外孕Ⅱ号方加减。

(2) 观察服药后变化，应定时检查肝功、血常规，如有改变，报告医生停药或加补气保肝的药物。

(3) 包块表浅而体弱，不宜久服中药者，可在小腹部外敷血竭散，可做理疗或外贴膏药。

(4) 胚胎已死，可适当下床活动，生活自理，逐渐增加活动量。

(5) 积极开展计划生育宣传教育，间隔受孕时间，可降低宫外孕的发病率。加强体育锻炼，增强抗病能力。

5.12 产后发热

产后发热持续或突然高热，伴有其他症状者，称产后发热。现代医学的产褥感染所致的发热也包括在本病范围内。

一般护理

1. 病室内应保持空气清新，流通，但应避免直接吹风。
2. 卧床休息，保持情志舒畅，避免精神刺激。
3. 恶露不净者，宜取半卧位，以利瘀浊流出。
4. 保持外阴清洁，每日定时擦洗，使用消毒的会阴垫，有伤口者每日应清洁换药一次。
5. 注意口腔及皮肤护理，嘱患者勤漱口，防止细菌生长，出汗多的用干毛巾擦身，勤换内衣。
6. 热邪亢盛者，根据病情适当采用温水擦身，嘱患者多饮开水，必要时静脉补充液体。

7. 肠燥便结者，应多饮果汁，多食蔬菜、麻油、蜂蜜、黑芝麻、胡桃仁等润肠通便。

8. 注意观察并记录热象，脉象，舌象，神志，面色，腹痛，二便，恶露等变化，若出现神昏谵语，面白肢冷，脉微而数等热厥之象，应报告医生，采取治疗措施。

辨证护理

1. 血虚型
临床表现
产后下血过多，身有微热自汗，不恶寒，面赤头晕目眩，耳鸣心悸，口燥不欲饮，大便干结，舌淡红，苔薄，脉细弱无力。

护理

(1) 注意休息，衣被不宜过暖，观察体温变化，嘱患者不要直接吹风，以防受凉。

(2) 饮食要根据病情选择，鼓励患者多食营养丰富，易消化的食品，如鸡汤、鱼汤、银耳、牛奶等。要忌食生冷辛辣动火刺激性食物。

(3) 服用补血益气，养阴清热的药物，方选八珍汤加减。

(4) 忌用物理降温及各种以发汗为主的退热法，防止汗出过多。

2. 外感型
临床表现
产后发热恶寒，头痛无汗，肢体酸楚，或有咳嗽流涕，苔薄白，脉浮。

护理

(1) 卧床休息，注意避风。

(2) 服用养血祛风的药物，方选荆防四物汤加减，汤药趁热服。服药后以微微汗出为佳，若无汗出者，可喝热粥或生姜红糖汤，以助发汗。

(3) 注意患者服药后汗出的情况，发汗不宜过多，汗出后及时揩干身体，更换汗湿内衣，关好门窗，以防受凉。

3. 邪毒型

临床表现

发热恶寒，或有寒战，烦燥口干，小腹作痛，恶露量多腥臭，小便短赤，大便燥结，舌红苔黄，脉数有力。

护理

(1) 病室要空气新鲜，经常通风换气，衣被不宜过暖。

(2) 高热期给予足够的饮料，饮食宜清淡富有营养，可多饮新鲜果汁，西瓜汁等以补充体液。

(3) 服用清热凉血解毒的药物，方选凉血解毒汤加减。

(4) 高热不退者，可用 75%酒精浸泡桂枝、细辛、肉桂、生姜、红花等加温擦浴，可起到温经活络降温的作用。

(5) 配合针刺合谷、曲池、风池、列缺等穴，用泻法。

(6) 严密观察病情变化，如突然出现面色苍白，四肢不温，大汗不止，脉转微细无力时，是阳气衰微的表现，应立即报告医生，急煎参附汤频服，或服安宫牛黄丸 1 丸，以回阳救逆。

4. 血瘀型

临床表现

产后数日，寒热时作，恶露不畅，小腹疼痛，舌紫黯有瘀点，脉沉弦。

护理

1. 注意观察恶露的情况，包括量、色、质的变化。恶露不畅，血色紫黯伴有瘀块者，应给益母草膏 20 毫升，每日 3 次，温开水冲服。

(2) 服用活血祛瘀的药物，方选生化汤加减。

(3) 腹痛者，可热敷或艾灸少腹部。

5.13 恶露不绝

妇女分娩后 2～3 周内，有少量暗红色的血性液体从阴道排出，称为恶露。一般在产后 20 天左右，恶露便应排尽，如超过 3 周以上，恶露仍淋漓不断或继续流血，称恶露不绝，或叫恶露不止。

一般护理

1. 病室要空气新鲜，经常通风换气，以祛除秽浊之气。

2. 卧床休息，注意保暖，出汗后及时更换内衣，防止受凉。

3. 观察恶露量的多少、色泽，有无血块，腹痛，热象等情况，并做好记录。恶露量多时，取半卧位，以利恶露排出。

4. 若恶露多，色红有块，腹痛，面色苍白，头晕出汗，心慌气短，应考虑是残留胎盘，应报告医生，采取治疗措施。

5. 保持外阴清洁，会阴垫要消毒，勤换，禁房事、盆浴，防止邪毒入侵。

辨证护理

1. 气虚型

临床表现

产后恶露过期不止，淋漓不断，量多，色淡红，质稀薄，小腹下坠，精神倦怠，面色㿠白，舌淡，脉缓弱。

护理

(1) 调理情志，保持心情舒畅，精神愉快，积极配合治疗。

(2) 注意避风保暖，防止外邪乘虚侵袭，耗伤正气。

(3) 加强饮食营养，多食鳖肉、鸡汤、桂圆汤等。忌食生冷瓜果、辛辣及不易消化的食品。

(4) 小腹下坠可艾灸天枢、气海、归来等穴。

（5）服用补血摄血的药物，方选补中益气汤加减。

2. 血瘀型

临床表现

恶露淋漓不止，量少，色紫黯有块，小腹疼痛拒按，舌质紫黯或边有紫点，脉沉弦。

护理

（1）加强精神护理，保持心情舒畅，使气机条达，以利恶露下行通畅。

（2）服用活血化瘀的药物，方选生化汤加减。

（3）小腹疼痛拒按，可给予热敷或艾灸天枢、气海、归来、三阴交等穴，以促血块下行，减轻腹痛。

（4）益母草膏20毫升，每日3次，温开水冲服。

3. 血热型

临床表现

恶露过期不止，量多，色鲜红或深红，质稠而臭，面色潮红，口干舌燥，舌红苔黄，脉细数。

护理

（1）注意观察恶露量、色、气味及全身情况的变化。

（2）避免情志受刺激，使患者保持乐观情绪，以增强治疗信心。

（3）服用清热凉血，养阴止血的药物，方选保阴汤加减。

（4）口干舌燥，给金银花、麦冬泡水代茶饮，以养阴清热。

5.14 盆腔炎

妇女盆腔器官发生的炎性病变，包括子宫内膜炎、输卵管炎，卵巢炎，盆腔腹膜炎及盆腔结缔组织炎等。根据临床表现属于祖国医学的热入营血、带下病、症瘕等范围。

一般护理

(1) 注意休息，嘱患者生活起居要有规律，急性期应卧床休息。

(2) 做好精神护理，鼓励患者树立战胜疾病的信心，积极配合治疗。

(3) 加强饮食营养，要给予富有营养、易消化的食品。高热期多饮水，多食新鲜水果。

(4) 保持外阴清洁，月经期禁盆浴、房事，以防感染。

(5) 采用穴位注射，用丹参、苦参、野菊花注射液，取足三里、三阴交等穴，交替注射。每日 1 次，每穴 1ml。

辨证护理

1. 实热型

临床表现

多见于急性盆腔炎，发热恶寒，口干欲饮下腹疼痛拒按，腰部酸坠，带下增多而臭，质稀色黄，小便短赤，舌质红，苔黄或腻，脉洪数或滑数。

护理

(1) 发热伤阴，应给清淡易消化的食品，多饮淡盐水、梨汁、果汁、西瓜汁，以养阴清热。忌食煎烤、油腻、辛辣甜粘之品。

(2) 服用清热解毒，活血化瘀利湿的药物，方选清热解毒化瘀汤加减，每日 2 剂，每 6 小时服 1 次。

(3) 高热者，可参照 2.1 高热护理。

(4) 中药保留灌肠。红藤 60 克，水煎 100ml，温度 38℃，缓缓灌入。嘱患者灌肠后卧床休息半小时。每日 1 次，5～10 次为 1 疗程。经期前后禁用。

(5) 肌肉注射穿心莲、双花注射液 2ml，隔日 1 次。

2. 气滞血瘀型

临床表现

小腹胀痛，经前经后为甚，乳房胀痛，月经后期量少有块，白带多，清稀，舌质淡，苔白腻，脉细弦。

护理

(1) 服用行气活血，破瘀止痛，清热利湿的药物，方选清热化瘀汤加减。

(2) 加强营养，多食肉、蛋等营养之品，忌食生冷，辛辣刺激性食品。

(3) 注意外阴清洁，每日清洗 1 次，月经期避免受凉，勿冒雨涉水，以免加重病情。

3. 寒湿凝滞型

临床表现

胸闷胁痛，经期或经后小腹胀痛，大便溏薄，小便清长，舌质暗，苔薄，脉沉迟或沉数。

护理

(1) 服用温经行气活血的药物，方选温经汤加减。

(2) 小腹胀痛，可用炒盐或坎离砂加醋调热敷。

(3) 经期应注意保暖，避免受寒。

5.15 阴挺

子宫体位置下移,甚至脱出阴道口外，称为阴挺，或称阴脱，现代医学称子宫脱垂。

一般护理

1. 病室要整洁，安静，保证患者充分休息，避免活动和劳累。

2. 饮食应营养丰富，易于消化，多食调补脾肾的食物，忌食生冷、辛辣之品。

3. 保持大便通畅，便秘时可给缓泻剂，切勿努责。

4. 注意观察子宫脱出的程度，表面有无红肿，出血，糜烂，如出现糜烂，流黄水时，应将局部擦洗干净，用青黛散外敷局部。

5. 保持外阴清洁，内裤应柔软干净，每日换洗一次。

6. 搞好计划生育，避免生育过多过密。产后勿过早负重。

7. 配合功能锻炼，多做膝胸卧位或提肛运动，增强盆腔肌肉的功能。

辨证护理

1. 气虚型

临床表现

子宫脱出阴道，劳则加重，伴有小腹下坠，四肢乏力，少气懒言，面色少华，带下量多，质稀色白，小便频数，舌淡苔薄白，脉细虚。

护理

(1) 注意饮食调护，增加营养，多食蛋类、鱼类、瘦肉、甲鱼、可食黄芪或党参粥等，以调补脾肾。忌食生冷、辛辣刺激性食品。

(2) 服用补气升提的药物，方选补中益气汤加减。

(3) 针灸疗法取百会、气海、大赫、子宫、三阴交、太冲、照海等穴，用补法以提升固脱。

(4) 子宫脱出后摩擦损伤而红肿溃烂，流黄水的感染者，可用枳壳 60 克、乌梅 60 克、蛇床子 30 克煎水熏洗坐浴，洗后外涂，用黄柏粉、煅蛤粉、乌贼骨粉、炉甘石粉各适量加青黛或冰片少许，用香油调成膏，外涂患处，每日 1 次。

2. 肾虚型

临床表现

子宫脱出阴道，伴有腰酸腿软，小腹下坠，头晕耳鸣，小便频数等症状。舌淡红，脉沉细。

护理

(1) 参照 1.气虚型护理

(2) 服用补肾养血，温阳益气的药物，方选大补元煎加减。

(3) 用附子 9 克、肉桂 6 克、炮姜 6 克煎水服，或隔姜片灸百会穴，每日 2 次。

6 儿科常见病证及护理

6.1 儿科护理特点

小儿在生理、病理上独具特点。生理方面，脏腑娇嫩，形气未充；生机蓬勃，发育迅速。病理方面，发病容易、变化迅速，易寒易热，易虚易实。总之，小儿具有长而未全，气血未充，卫外不固，病情多变的特点。加之不能完整、准确地表达病情，生活起居不能自理，因此，儿科的护理工作有其独特的内容。

1. 要求护理人员有高度的责任心。对患儿的生活起居、治疗及护理等方面，切实做到耐心细致，和蔼可亲，与患儿建立感情，消除对医护人员的恐惧心理、进行各项操作要轻柔、稳准，取得在治疗、护理上的合作。

2. 病室要保持清洁，空气新鲜、流通，温、湿度适宜。室温一般为 18～20℃、夏天以 26℃ 左右为宜，相对湿度为 55%～65%。每天开窗通风换气时，勿直接吹向患儿，防止受凉。整理病室卫生宜用湿式法扫床、擦地。患儿的排泄物应及时清除。环境要安静，勿大声喧哗，以免使患儿受惊。

3. 做好消毒隔离工作，防止交叉感染。病室按病种要求定期进行物品消毒及空气消毒。每天做晨护时，床及床头桌等用消毒液擦抹。按病种分别安排房间，严格控制探视，尽量减少探视人数，以防交叉感染。患儿的奶瓶、食具每次用后宜洗净消毒；玩具、脸盆要保持清洁，定期消毒。应教育和帮助患儿饭前、便后洗手，培养成良好的卫生习惯。

4. 衣着护理。衣着要舒适，应以轻软宽松为原则，不宜穿的过多，否则出汗后常易感冒，并应根据具体病情和气候而增减。夜间盖被厚薄要适度。小儿尿布以质软，吸水性强的棉布为宜，要用水洗净并用热水浸泡。尿布要在日光中曝晒，个别情况按需要分别进行消毒处理。

5. 精神方面的护理。小儿情感丰富，真挚而外向，对平日接触较多的物和所喜爱的人，如果偶然离开，会引起他的留恋，思念和不乐，甚至出现病态表现如胃纳呆滞，情绪异常，不利于疾病的恢复。所以小儿的精神护理，要注意掌握其心理动态。对年龄较大儿童要鼓励其树立战胜疾病的信心，可通过适当的文化娱乐教育，消除顾虑和恐惧心理。

保证足够的睡眠时间。患儿药后出汗或病重初愈，往往疲倦、嗜睡，尤其是恢复期的患儿更需要充分的休息和睡眠。只要患儿睡中面色、呼吸正常，不要随意唤醒。

6. 病情的护理。小儿病情变化主要依靠医护人员详细观察而获知，因此，要求观察病情要及时，并要做到耐心细致，全面、准确、根据病情变化，施以不同的护理方法.

7. 服药方面的护理。小儿苦于服药，药量宜少煎，汁宜浓，小量多次喂服。喂药方法：将患儿抱起，用小匙将药液慢慢自口角送到舌根部，使之自然吞下；或用滴管，每2～3滴，慢慢喂下。切勿捏鼻，以防呛入气管。可以加适量调味品。婴幼儿服用丸剂、片剂、必须研成细末或用温水化开，用乳汁、米汤或蜂蜜调服。鼓励大龄儿童自己服药，护理人员要协助患儿将药服下，然后离开。严格遵守服药要求及禁忌，不能将药发给患儿，以免遗忘或隐瞒不服。注意观察服药后有无不良反应。此外，要掌握小儿服药剂量。有些也可采用贴敷、雾化吸入、激光针刺等方法，

8. 饮食调护。根据患儿年龄和病情的不同，一般提供食物的原则是：先稀后干，先素后荤，先少后多，多蛋白，少脂肪，糖适量，多食蔬菜、水果。饮食要定时，定量,定质。注意饮食卫生，饭前要洗手，不要在进食时嬉戏，以免食物误入气管。在疾病恢复期或病愈后。要掌握进食量，不可进食过多，以防食

复。

9. 安全的护理。由于小儿年幼无知，好奇心强，常可发生坠床，中毒，触电，烧伤，气管异物，外伤等意外事件，护理人员必须格外小心，加强安全教育，认真保护。凡带有尖刃的金属玩具及玻璃制品，禁止给患儿玩。热水袋温度不得超过 60℃，袋口要拧紧，外加布套，以防烫伤。特别注意防止患儿坠床。

6.2 麻疹

麻疹是以发热、咳嗽，口腔出现粘膜斑，全身出现红色皮疹为特点的急性呼吸道传染病，好发于冬春季节，病后获终生免疫力。属中医学温病范畴。

一般护理

1. 参照 6.1 儿科护理特点。

2. 执行呼吸道隔离至出疹后 5 天，有并发症者延长到出疹后 10 天。

3. 环境要安静。冬季病室温湿度宜稍偏高（室温 20～22℃，相对湿度 60%）以利诱疹透发。病室内要空气新鲜流畅，注意空气消毒，预防交叉感染。室内挂有色窗帘和遮盖灯光，使光线柔和，以免刺激眼睛。

4. 卧床休息，体温基本正常后可下地活动。疹退后方可到室外活动。

5. 保持口、鼻腔清洁。口腔可用双花水或生理盐水擦洗或漱口。口唇干裂可涂油剂。发生口疮者。可涂冰硼散、锡类散、珠黄散等。鼻腔干燥有痂时，先用石蜡油润泽后，再清除鼻痂，防止患儿用手抠鼻损伤鼻粘膜或引起出血。

6. 接触麻疹的易感儿，应检疫观察 17 天，并采取预防措施。

辨证护理

1. 初热期（前驱期）　　　一般 3～4 天。

临床表现

发热恶风寒，咳嗽流涕，目赤畏光，或伴呕吐、泄泻。发热 2～3 天，口腔粘膜上出现麻疹粘膜斑。此为麻疹早期诊断的依据。舌苔薄黄，脉浮数。

护理

(1) 此期护理同感冒。自发热的第二天起要每日两次检查口腔，观察是否出现麻疹粘膜斑，一旦发现，应进行有利透疹及保疹的护理。也有少数病例只有腮粘膜充血粗糙而无典型粘膜斑，特别近期接受免疫注射者，症状可不典型，麻疹粘膜斑可不出现。但不应忽视调护。

(2) 麻疹为发疹性疾病，疹透毒出，疹净毒净。疹前期，诱疹透发是护理麻疹的关键。发热者一般常用鲜芦根 60 克，或鲜茅根 60 克，水煎代茶饮；也可用香菜 60 克，煎汤频服。使其微微汗出，以利透疹。要注意保暖，切忌受凉，免使肌表腠理闭塞，疹出不利而发生逆证。

(3) 服辛凉透表药物，方选银翘散加减。若发热无汗，舌苔薄白者，服辛温透表药物，方选荆防败毒散加减。服药后应覆被安卧，使微汗出为宜，以利透疹。切忌大汗淋漓，耗伤阴液。

(4) 加强眼睛护理。眼眵多或有干痂者，用温开水擦洗，或涂红霉素眼药膏，待润软后再擦除。目赤流泪，眼睑红肿者，可用银花、菊花各 9 克，黄连 3 克，煎水薰洗。睡前用黄连水湿敷双眼，或涂以抗菌素软膏。

(5) 饮食宜清淡，给予富有营养、易于消化的流质或半流质食物，可食芫荽粥，有助透疹。并应供给充足的水分。

2. 出疹期　　　一般 3～5 天。

临床表现

高热气粗，心烦不安，咳嗽，目赤加重。皮疹开始由耳后颈部出现，继之扩散至前额、面颊部，尔后到胸、背、四肢，至手、足心见疹为出齐。疹色鲜红。舌质红，苔黄，脉洪数。

护理

(1) 此期为麻疹透发阶段，宜服清热解毒透疹药物，方选清解透表汤加减。服药后，注意观察出疹的顺序，颜色，疹出密度及透发是否彻底，若发现异常及时报告医生。

(2) 发热的护理。麻疹发热是自身排毒的一种手段。因此，在麻疹未出齐前，患儿虽高热而神志安宁，皮肤有汗，一般体温在 38℃ 左右，不急于退热。如体温升至 39℃ 以上，要适当降温。可用微温的湿毛巾敷前额，或用温热水洗脸、颈及手脚，使其腠理开微汗出，疹毒易于外达。另外可用西河柳 120 克、芫荽 30 克，水煎加黄酒适量，温擦皮肤，用以帮助透疹。高热惊厥者，可针刺神门、十宣、丰隆穴。

(3) 咳嗽的护理。咳嗽与出麻疹的轻重成正比。可服止咳、镇咳药；或以止咳化痰的药物煎汤，行雾化吸入，每日可进行数次，以缓解呼吸道因干燥而引起的刺激性咳嗽。

(4) 保持皮肤清洁。搔痒时，可用湿芫荽水、荆芥、苏叶水擦洗局部，即可止痒又助透疹。剪去患儿指甲，以免抓破皮肤继发感染。

(5) 观察病情。重点观察出疹后的顺证和逆证。顺证为疹色鲜红，出疹匀称，按时出，按时退，愈后良好。逆证常见壮热，疹点稠密紫暗；或精神不振，出疹迟缓，色淡而稀少；或皮疹尚未出齐而突然隐没；或出现喘促、紫绀、烦躁、惊厥、昏迷等。此期易发生变证及并发症，如肺炎、喉炎、心衰、脑病等，应密切观察病情变化。

(6) 加强眼、鼻、口腔的护理。

(7) 注意饮食调护，仍以清淡素食为宜。

3. 恢复期　　一般 5～7 天。

临床表现

皮疹出齐后，按出疹的顺序由上向下依次隐退。与此同时，发热，目赤，咳嗽诸证也随之消失，精神和食欲恢复正常。疹退后皮面留下脱皮及棕色斑痕。斑痕经 2～3 周自行消失。舌质红，苔淡，脉细稍弱。

护理

(1) 服养阴益气和胃的药物，方选沙参麦冬汤加减，以扶阴虚气弱之体。

(2) 恢复期脾胃功能逐渐好转后，可适当增加营养。给予奶类、蛋类、瘦肉和各种鲜菜、水果，亦可食莲子粥、山药粥等。可用红皮白萝卜或荸荠煎汤代茶饮，以清余毒。忌食油腻、坚硬和刺激性的食品。饮食要避免过量，以防损伤脾胃。注意饮食卫生，观察大便形态变化，防止发生疹后泻、疹后痢。

(3) 加强皮肤护理。疹退脱屑，皮肤瘙痒，可用炉甘石洗剂擦洗局部，防止抓破发生感染。

(4) 避风寒，防止交叉感染，注意劳逸有度，慎防他邪乘虚而入，引起后期并发症。

6.3 水痘

水痘是由水痘病毒引起的急性发疹性传染病。临床以发热，皮肤、粘膜分批出现斑丘疹、疱疹及结痂的痘疹为特征。一般于起病发热 24 小时内开始出现红色斑丘疹，数小时内发展成疱疹，经 1～2 日疱疹自中心干瘪结痂，数日后变为干痂，脱落后，留下短期色素沉着。水痘皮疹的特点为向心性分布，头面躯干多于四肢。在 3～5 日内分批陆续出现，因此皮肤上同时可见到各期形态及大小不一的皮疹。好发于冬春季节，散见于四季。1～6 岁的儿童发病率最高。患病后获终生免疫。属中医学温病范畴。

一般护理

1. 参照 6.1 儿科护理特点。

2. 水痘传染性极强，严格执行呼吸道及接触隔离，至痘疹完全干燥结痂为止。工作人员接触患儿时应带口罩，穿隔离衣，事后双手用 0.1%过氧乙酸浸泡。患儿的玩具、餐具等应消毒处理。病室空气要流通，注意空气消毒。

3. 饮食宜清淡，给予富有营养，易于消化的食物。忌食海腥发物和辛辣刺激性食品。

4. 床铺保持清洁干燥，衣服、被褥应松软舒适，勤换内衣，以防擦破痘皮。注意皮肤清洁，但不宜淋浴和接触冷水，防止痘疹溃破继发感染。

5. 保持患儿双手清洁，剪短指甲，防止抓破痘疹，使皮肤感染。皮肤瘙痒时，可用炉甘石洗剂或 5%碳酸氢钠溶液外涂止痒。已抓破者涂以 1%龙胆紫保持干燥。已发生感染者，用茶青散或青黛散外涂。

6. 发热时应卧床休息。多饮水，给予果汁或绿豆汤代饮料，以助清热解毒。适当降温。

7. 注意口腔、眼及外阴部的护理。眼内生有痘疮者，涂红霉素眼药膏或滴氯霉素眼药水，以保护眼睛。口腔及外阴粘膜溃疡者，用冰硼散、锡类散涂敷，每日 2～3 次。

8. 接触过水痘患儿的易感儿，应检疫观察 21 天。可肌肉注射丙种球蛋白预防。

9. 禁用激素，以免病毒扩散加重病情。

辨证护理

1. 卫气证（轻型）

临床表现

轻度发热，流涕，微咳嗽。痘疹稀疏，疱浆稀薄、清亮、瘙痒。精神食欲如常。舌苔薄白或浮黄，脉浮数。

护理

(1) 水痘透发期。应卧床休息，注意保暖，勿受风寒。汗出用软毛巾蘸干。并注意观察体温，痘出稀密，形态，色泽，分布情况及全身症状，做好记录。

(2) 服疏风解表，清热祛湿药物，方选银翘散加减。汤药不宜久煎。

(3) 轻微发热者，勿须降温，多饮水，可饮梨汁、橘子汁等。

(4) 轻症可不服汤药，用芦根 60 克、野菊花 10 克、或银花 12 克、甘草 3 克，水煎代茶饮.

2. 气营证（重型）

临床表现

壮热，烦躁或嗜睡，痘疹密布全身，散及手足。疱大，疱浆浑浊，疹周红晕，色深或呈紫红出血性。舌苔黄腻，脉洪数。

护理

(1) 服清气凉营药物，方选清瘟败毒饮加减。汤药宜冷服。

(2) 高热者，绝对卧床休息，多饮水。可用竹叶 15 克、芦根 30 克，煎水代茶饮。口服小儿退热药。注意观察体温变化及透疹情况。如壮热不退，痘出稠密，疱色红赤、紫暗、疱浆浑浊，为毒热内蕴血分证。可加犀角、羚羊角。有惊厥者，参照 2.1 高热护理。

(3) 加强对痘疹的护理，以防继发感染，加重病情。尤其是眼及外阴部有痘疹或溃疡者，要对局部进行处理。外用药，参照一般护理。

6.4 流行性腮腺炎

流行性腮腺炎是以发热，耳下腮部漫肿，疼痛为主要特点的一种急性呼吸道传染病。患儿先有发热，咽痛等外感症状，1～2 天后一侧或两侧耳下腮部肿起。部分病人发热与腮肿几乎同时出现。腮部呈漫肿形式，有触痛但不红，边缘不清楚。有时颌下腺及舌下腺也先后肿起，颊内腮腺管口红肿。病程约 1～2 周。中医学称痄腮、蛤蟆瘟。属温病范畴。长年皆可发生，但以冬春季节为多，是学龄前及学龄期儿童的常见病，病后获终生免疫力。

一般护理

1. 参照 6.1 儿科护理特点。

2. 严格执行呼吸道隔离，至腮腺完全消肿为止。食具应煮沸消毒。

3. 患儿卧床休息至腮肿消退。轻症可在室内适当活动，注意并发症的发生。

4. 给予富有营养和清淡的食物。忌食酸辣，以免刺激腮腺管口，引起疼痛。腮腺高度肿胀，张口、咀嚼困难者，勿进固体食物。

5. 注意口腔护理。肿胀期颊内腮腺管口红肿，应保持口腔清洁，防止细菌进入腮腺内引起化脓性炎症。用板蓝根水、淡盐水漱口，婴儿可擦洗口腔。

6. 注意腮腺肿胀疼痛程度及体温、脉象、神志、睾丸等变化，以识别轻重及有无并发症。若出现高热，神志恍惚，呕吐，项强等症状，为并发脑膜脑炎的征象；若出现上腹痛，呕吐，高热者，为并发胰腺炎的征象。青春后期的儿童，可见并发睾丸炎及卵巢炎。观察时间要持续到病后 3～4 周。

7. 外治法：腮腺肿胀处，可用药外敷，消肿止痛。敷药范围要超过红肿范围，每日换药 1～2 次。注意腮部清洁。外敷药及用法如下：

(1) 大青膏、金黄膏、芙蓉膏外敷。

(2) 如意金黄散、用温水调匀后外敷。

(3) 紫金锭或青黛散，用醋调研后外敷。

(4) 芒硝、青黛各等分，用醋调糊状后外敷。

（5）万应消核膏，将局部温水洗净后外贴。

（6）鲜马齿苋、鲜蒲公英、鲜仙人掌、任选一种，捣烂成泥，每次加冰片 0.5 克，调匀后外敷患侧。

（7）吴茱萸 12 克，研为细末，加面粉 30 克，用醋（醋用砂锅烧开）调糊状，临睡前贴敷双脚心，以引火下行。

患侧肿胀明显时，局部可拔火罐，每日 1 次。1～2 次即愈。

8. 有接触史的易感儿，可用板蓝根 15～30 克，水煎服；或服板蓝根冲剂，连服 3～5 天.

辨证护理

1. 热郁卫分证（轻型）

临床表现

低热，咽痛，恶心呕吐，腮腺肿起，咀嚼时有酸胀感。精神及食欲如常。持续 3～5 天后，逐渐消肿而痊愈。舌苔薄白，脉浮数。

护理

（1）服疏风清热，消肿散结药物，方选银翘散加减。

（2）用单方验方配合治疗。如全蝎 7 条，香油炸后顿服，日 1 次，连服 3 天。婴幼儿可研成细粉冲服。

（3）给予半流质或软食为宜。如鸡蛋羹、粥、面条等。

（4）低热者，多饮水；或用菊花 6 克，夏枯草 10 克，泡水代茶饮。

2. 热郁营卫证（重型）

临床表现

壮热，头痛，嗜睡或烦躁，时有恶心呕吐，腮部漫肿，疼痛拒按，张口、咀嚼困难，颌下亦可肿胀。大便干燥，小便短赤。或见并发症。舌苔薄黄或黄腻，脉滑数。

护理

（1）本证为热毒蕴结，故服清热解毒，消肿散结药物，方选普济消毒饮加减。汤药宜冷服。

（2）外治法，见一般护理 7，单方验方同 1 热郁卫分证。

（3）饮食给予流质为宜，如奶类、蛋花汤、豆浆、藕粉等。

（4）高热口渴烦躁者，因热邪入里，毒热亢盛，耗损津液所致。应多饮水或清凉饮料，如菊花露、板蓝根液、绿豆汤等；亦可用针刺降温，取大椎、曲池、合谷穴。如高热持续不退，可服羚羊粉或安宫牛黄丸。

（5）呕吐频繁者，给玉枢丹冲服，并加强口腔护理。

（6）大便干结者，可用番泻叶泡水代茶饮，多吃香蕉，必要时可用甘油灌肠。

（7）睾丸肿大局部坠痛，可用丁字带托起，以减轻坠痛。用中药马齿苋、蒲公英煎水薰洗阴囊；也可针刺三阴交、血海穴，日 1 次。或用中药外敷（见一般护理 7 外治法）

6.5 流行性乙型脑炎

流行性乙型脑炎是以起病急骤，头痛，高热，昏迷，抽风为特点的急性传染病。由疫蚊为媒介传染，好发于夏秋季节的 7～9 月份。3～6 岁的儿童最易感染，属中医温病学的暑厥、暑风范畴。轻症一般 7～10 天即可恢复，重症需要 2～3 周.在急性期可伴发内闭外脱证而危及生命。病后 6 个月尚未消退的症状，称后遗症。

一般护理

1. 参照 6.1 儿科护理特点。

2. 隔离患儿于有防蚊设备的病室内，直到体温正常为止。重症患儿安放在抢救室。室温维持在 24℃～26℃之间，保持衡定的适宜湿度。

3. 给予高热量、高蛋白饮食及充分的水分，特别是持续高热，惊厥多汗的患儿，更要及时补给，以固正气。饮食可给牛奶、浓豆浆、绿豆粉粥、赤小豆粉粥，加适量白糖调服。水分供应除静脉补给外，可给西瓜汁、百合绿豆汤等。对神志不清不能进食者，应鼻饲。恢复期神志清晰者，进半流质和软食，如羹类食品。

4. 保持口腔清洁。高热患儿每日用藿香水（藿香 30 克，水煎 200ml）清拭口腔，尔后涂以冰硼油（冰硼散 5 克、香油 10ml），保持口腔粘膜润泽，防止口腔感染。高热伴昏迷者，鼻唇部需涂油剂并覆盖湿纱布，以保持口唇和呼吸道湿润。

5. 保持呼吸道通畅。惊厥昏迷的患儿，由于咳嗽、吞咽功能障碍，唾液及痰涎潴留，易引起呼吸道堵塞，甚则发生窒息。应及时吸出痰涎，使呼吸道通畅。取侧卧位，经常翻身拍背，以促进排痰和改善肺部血液循环。素有蛔虫的患儿，可因蛔虫逆行于食道、口腔、气管，引起恶心、呕吐、呛咳或窒息，一旦发生，要及时将蛔虫取出。呼吸困难时，给予氧气吸入。

6. 病情严重或昏迷、瘫痪的患儿，易发生褥疮。故床铺应保持平软、整洁、干燥，皮肤保持清洁，以预防褥疮发生。对瘫痪的肢体，应定时进行按摩，以促使气血流畅及功能恢复。

7. 对昏迷伴大小便失禁者，应勤换尿布，保持臀部清洁，干燥；对小便潴留，膀胱膨胀者，先按摩阴包、箕门穴 2～3 分钟，继摩膀胱，由患儿右侧向左运行。

8. 观察病情。急性期病情发展迅速，应随时注意患儿精神，意识，体温，呼吸，脉象，血压及瞳孔的变化，以做到早期发现呼吸衰竭，心力衰竭，惊厥，出血，窒息及其他并发症。

辨证护理

1. 急性期

（1）卫气同病证

临床表现

突然发热，无汗或微汗出。面红目赤，头痛呕吐，嗜睡，项强，小便短赤。舌苔薄白或微黄而腻，脉浮数。

护理

①服解表清热降暑药物，方选银翘散合白虎汤，加减。汤药宜轻煎。

②卧床休息，多饮水，前额施以冷敷。若出现惊惕不安，神志朦胧时，加用回春丹3～5粒，1次冲服，或牛黄镇惊丸1丸，化服，用以清热镇惊化痰开窍。

③频繁呕吐者，取侧卧位，头偏向一侧，以防呕吐物呛入气管发生窒息。可加服玉枢丹，以化浊止呕；或在汤药内加姜汁少许止呕；也可针刺止吐，取中脘、内关、足三里、公孙穴或揉合谷。

(2) 气营两燔证

临床表现

病情逐渐加重，3～4天后体温增至40℃以上，证见壮热，多汗口渴，烦躁谵语，神志不清，颈项强直，兼反复惊厥。舌苔黄厚或黄糙，舌质红绛，脉洪数或弦数。

护理

①此期是乙脑的极期，高热，惊厥，昏迷为热邪内闭，热、痰、风交炽的三大主要症状。病情危重，易于变化，故应有专人守护，注意病情转变，以配合医生处理。

②服清气凉血，益阴清热，镇惊熄风药物，方选白虎汤和清营汤加减。汤药宜冷，徐徐喂服。

③高热的护理参照2.1高热护理。体温高达40℃以上，应积极采取降温措施，以减少惊厥及脑水肿的发生。降低室温，调节室温降至26℃以下；以温水或用30%的温酒精擦浴降温，头部及大血管处放置冰袋。必要时用冷盐水灌肠；针刺降温，可取大椎、曲池、合谷、风府穴，有汗加复溜穴。

④惊厥的护理。惊厥时解开衣服扣带，避免呼吸运动受限。

用压舌板裹纱布，垫于上、下齿之间，以防止咬伤舌头。床边加床挡，以防坠床。同时针刺人中、合谷、太冲、内关、安眠、涌泉等穴。配用成药紫雪丹1～2克；安宫牛黄丸1/2～1丸；至宝丹1/2～1丸化服，日2次。或用醒脑静6～10ml静脉注射，每日2次，以清热开闭，止惊醒神。

⑤昏迷的护理（参照2.2昏迷护理）。喉中痰声漉漉，可加鲜竹沥10～50ml顿服，以减少喉部分泌物，或给猴枣粉0.3克冲服，以化痰开窍，疏利气机。昏迷而眼睛不能闭合者，用生理盐水棉球擦拭后，涂眼药膏，或用盐水湿纱布覆盖眼部，以防角膜干燥。若有吞咽功能障碍，可鼻饲给药。

⑥严密观察病情变化，注意防止发生脱证。

（3）热入营血证

临床表现

壮热不退，身热灼手，深度昏迷，反复惊厥，或手足震颤，躯体强直拘急，皮肤发斑，或见呕血、便血。唇干舌躁少苔，脉细数。

护理

①营血证是乙脑极期的危重阶段，是关系到能否留有后遗症的关键阶段。应采取综合医疗和护理措施，以救危急。

②服凉血解毒，清心开窍，镇静熄风药物，方选神犀丹加减。汤药宜冷服。

③继续施行气营两燔证的各项护理措施。对持续高热，抽风，昏迷者，酌情增添以下措施：

持续高热者，加羚羊粉、犀角粉2克冲服，同时十宣点刺放血，或穴位注射降温药物。

反复或持续惊厥者，可加镇惊散1.5～2克冲服，或蝎尾粉0.5～1克冲服，日2次。惊厥发作时间较长者，宜给高浓度吸氧，以减轻脑缺氧。

深度昏迷者，加雄黄1克，冰片、皂荚子粉各0.3克，共研细末，每次 0.3～0.6 克，用鲜石菖蒲汁调服，日 2 次，以化痰开窍醒神。

④出血的处理。注意观察出血的部位，如鼻衄，用堵塞法止血。选用黑山栀或百部霜、马勃、云南白药等粉末，撒于纱布卷内填压出血区；如出血部位较深，可用凡士林纱布条填塞止血。同时前额用冷毛巾湿敷。吐血、便血者，服云南白药 0.5～1.5 克,日 3～4 次，或用大黄粉、白及粉、乌贼骨粉各 1 克，三七粉 0.5 克，水化服，日 3 次.注意观察止血效果。

⑤出现脱证者，采取中西医结合医、护方法抢救。

2. 恢复期

临床表现

此期临床表现个体差异很大。常见症状有低热，头痛，狂躁或少语少动，呆滞木僵，言语不利，肢体强硬或拘紧，手足震颤，时发癫痫等。

护理

(1) 恢复期的护理，是以促进症状好转，防止各种并发症的发生为重点。除口服药外，需配合针灸、推拿、捏脊、理疗、药物穴位注射，以及进行主、被动的功能锻炼等，综合治疗与护理，以帮助患儿语言、运动及生活能力的恢复。

(2) 加强营养，补充急性期的消耗。在饮食中最好调配海参、鸡、鱼类等做汤、羹食之，以加快补肾益精，扶正固本。训练进食困难患儿的健全进食能力。不能吞咽者，仍需鼻饲，但要耐心训练，以便早日恢复吞咽功能。

(3) 对瘫痪强直的患儿，除进行功能锻炼外，还应加强皮肤护理，预防褥疮。并注意保暖，按气候的变化增减衣服，避免外感。

(4) 对有言语、运动功能障碍，生活能力差及有癫、狂后遗症的患儿，要时刻注意保护，防止发生意外事故。

6.6 猩红热

猩红热是以发热，咽喉肿痛或伴有溃烂，全身出现弥漫性猩红色（鲜红色）皮疹，及皮疹退后，出现大片状脱皮为特点的一种急性发疹性传染病。起病急，多数在 1～2 天内出现皮疹。皮疹自颈、胸、背部迅速遍及全身，同时出现环口苍白、杨梅舌等特征。皮疹消退后，出现片状脱屑，以手足为明显。中医学称烂喉痧、丹痧、疫喉.属温病范畴。多在冬春季节发病。2～8 岁儿童易感染。

一般护理

1. 参照 6.1 儿科护理特点。

2. 严格执行呼吸道隔离。隔离期限，自发病起至症状消失，一般为 6～7 天。患儿的衣被、食具、玩具、杂物等注意消毒。

3. 病室温度适宜，空气流通。发疹期应卧床休息，注意心脏的并发症。恢复期活动要适度。起病 1～2 周后，开始定期做小便检查，观察有无肾炎发生。

4. 保持口腔清洁。饭前、饭后和睡前，用双花水、温盐水擦拭口腔，较大患儿可多次含漱，以利咽部解毒及帮助清除鼻咽分泌物。

5. 注意皮肤清洁。出疹期皮肤瘙痒，可用防风、白藓皮、蛇床子煎水湿敷皮肤止痒。皮肤干燥涂搽油剂，禁用肥皂水擦洗。脱屑期，可用炉甘石洗剂涂搽,或用上述中药煎汤做洗浴，以减轻痒感。如有大片状脱皮，可用消毒的剪刀修剪，切勿用手撕剥。要经常为患儿修剪指甲，以免抓痒时划破皮肤而发生感染。注意床铺被褥清洁。

6. 饮食给予富有营养的流质、半流质和软食，食味宜淡，勿过咸、过甜。咽部炎症明显时，患儿不要食酸，避免刺激咽喉部加重疼痛。忌食辛辣食品。供给充足的水分。

辨证护理

1. 邪在肺胃证（轻型）

临床表现

突然发热畏寒，咽喉疼痛红肿或溃烂，皮疹色猩红，出疹较稀少。舌苔白或白腻，舌边尖红，脉浮数。

护理

（1）服清热利咽喉药物，方选银翘马勃射干汤加减。服药后不可大发汗。

（2）咽喉肿痛，口服喉症丸；可用青黛散、朱黄散吹喉，日3～4次；也可用清咽雾化液，做雾化吸入，日1～2次。

（3）选易于吞咽的食物。如稀粥、面食、蛋羹、牛奶等，多饮果汁，或用鲜芦根煎水代茶饮。

2. 气营两燔证（重型）

临床表现

壮热，面颊绯红，咽部肿烂疼痛，疹色猩红，弥漫全身,胸背部常融为一片，瘙痒。口渴，便干。舌红绛，起刺（杨梅舌），脉洪数。

护理

（1）服解毒化斑剂，方选清瘟败毒饮加减。汤药宜冷服。

（2）咽喉局部处理同前邪在肺胃证。

（3）注意观察体温变化，出疹期大都持续高热（39～40℃），皮疹出满全身后体温才逐渐下降。注意心率，心律的变化，和惊厥，昏迷等症状的出现。

（4）给予流质饮食。高热伤津要及时补充水分，可给甘寒生津的饮料，如梨汁、荸荠汁、藕汁或鲜芦根煎水代茶饮。

6.7 百日咳

百日咳，临床以阵发痉挛性咳嗽，伴吸气喉鸣为特点。本病四季都可发生，冬春季节尤多。好发于 5 岁以下的儿童，新生儿也可发病，年龄愈小病情愈重。并易见多种并发症。起病可呈流行，也可散发。中医学称顿咳、疫咳、肾咳。

一般护理

1. 参照 6.1 儿科护理特点。

2. 严格执行呼吸道隔离。隔离时间从发病开始至 40 天，或从痉咳起至 30 天。患儿的衣被、用具等应在阳光下曝晒，或紫外线照射，或煮沸消毒后方可使用。衣被要勤洗晒，保持清洁。

3. 病室应空气流通、安静，避免混杂烟雾、灰尘及各种刺激性气味，以免诱发痉挛性咳嗽。

4. 注意休息，保证充足睡眠。若夜间咳甚，影响入睡时，可在睡前给枣仁粉冲服，或取耳穴神门穴压豆，有助安睡。必要时可给少量镇静剂。

5. 给予热量充足，营养丰富，易于消化的流质、半流质饮食。食物不宜过甜，过咸，过冷，过热。进食时不可过急，以免诱发咳嗽。忌食辛辣、异味和刺激性食品。

6. 注意精神护理。患儿因受痉咳折磨的痛苦，造成情绪紧张。护理人员要态度和蔼可亲，精心照料，安慰患儿，尽量勿使哭闹或大笑；对较大患儿组织做活动量不大的游戏，讲故事，看图画等，使之安静并分散注意力，减少痉咳发作。

7. 要特别注意口腔护理。由于患儿长期痉咳、呕吐，影响B 族维生素的吸收，可致口腔粘膜及舌体，尤其是舌系带发生糜烂或溃疡，故应注意口腔清洁（参照 6.2 麻疹一般护理）。

8. 患儿痉咳发作时，取侧卧位或坐位，以防呕吐物呛入气管；轻拍患儿背部，变换体位，以利呼吸和减轻咳嗽。痰粘稠者，可用小儿清肺雾化剂做雾化吸入，使痰液稀释，易于咳出。痉咳严重时，可服祛痰药，但忌用收敛、镇咳之药，以免影响肺气宣达。腹部可加束带，以防二便失禁，脱肛，疝气等发生。

9. 观察咳嗽阵发持续的时间，轻重程度，痰的色、质、量及呼吸，面色，神志，出汗和有无呕吐，衄血，皮肤出血点，抽搐等情况。

10. 可配用拔火罐和推拿疗法，辅以治疗，以清肺降气，镇咳化痰。

(1) 拔火罐：取肺俞、大椎穴，每日 1 次，两穴交替应用。注意拔罐时间，每次不超过 5～15 分钟，否则皮肤出现水泡。

(2) 常用推拿法：清肺经，掐揉小天心，按揉天突，分推膻中，摩肋，按揉肺俞、膈俞。

11. 易感儿童与患儿密切接触后，应检疫观察 23 天，可肌注丙种球蛋白进行预防。凡出生 2 个月的婴儿，应接种百白破三联菌苗，全程注射 3 次，以后定期加强，才能获得免疫效果。

辨证护理

1. 初咳期

临床表现

自起病至出现痉挛性咳嗽为初咳期，一般 7～10 天。初起咳嗽、流涕或伴轻度发热，1～2 天后，发热和外感症状减轻。咳嗽日渐加重。舌苔薄白或薄黄，脉浮数。

护理

(1) 此期传染性最强，应注意隔离，严格控制探视，以防交叉感染。加强病室空气消毒。未确诊前，劝患儿带口罩，少出门，少接触儿童。

(2) 服宣肺解表化痰止咳药物，方选桑菊饮加减。

2. 痉咳期

临床表现

从出现痉咳开始至逐渐减轻，一般 2~6 周或 2 个月左右。证见咳嗽阵作，咳声急迫频发，涕泪同出，伴吸气喉鸣及呕吐，日轻夜重，可见面目浮肿，目、鼻出血，面部皮肤尤以眼窝部分出现出血点。舌苔白或黄，脉有力。

护理

(1) 服祛痰止咳药物，方选苏葶滚痰丸加减。尚可配服蜈蚣、甘草各等份，研末，蜜水调服，每次 1~2 克，每日 3 次；或用鲜鸡苦胆 1 个，加糖适量，1~2 岁每日 1 个，分 2 次服下，2 岁以上每次 1 个，每日 1~2 次。应加强服药护理

(2) 患儿应卧床休息，避免一切不必要的刺激。各种检查、治疗与护理要集中进行，以免诱发痉咳。

(3) 加强进食的护理。患儿有时因惧怕进食引起咳嗽呕吐而拒食，护理人员应劝解患儿自觉进食，或耐心、细心地喂食。咳嗽时暂停进食，以免呛入气管引起窒息。若食后即呕吐，应再补充，以保证营养。可给萝卜汁、梨汁、荸荠汁作饮料，以化痰润肺，生津止咳。

(4) 婴幼儿痉咳频繁发作时，应有专人守护，以防呕吐物吸入气管发生窒息。小婴儿由于痰粘无力咳出，阻塞气道，常出现憋气，甚至窒息或抽搐，应立即给予吸痰、吸氧，并做人工呼吸，配合医生进行抢救。

(5) 密切观察病情变化，注意发生合并症。若出现高热、气喘、鼻翼煽动，或高热神昏，甚则抽风。提示热闭肺、脑，并发肺炎或脑炎，应速采取急救措施，并报告医生。

3. 恢复期

临床表现

恢复期约 2~3 周，阵发痉挛性咳嗽逐渐减轻，至咳嗽消失，并见少神乏力，纳呆多汗。舌苔薄白，脉细无力。

护理

(1) 痉咳后期由于邪衰正虚，损伤肺脾，可服补气养阴，润

肺健脾药物，方选人参五味子汤加减。

（2）加强饮食调护，逐渐增添营养，调补肺脾。可给牛奶、蛋类、鸡汤、瘦肉等食物，多吃新鲜蔬菜、水果和清凉饮料。可用人参、黄芪、百合、沙参煮粥，也可食银耳、赤小豆粥，以滋补脾胃，生津润肺。饮食宜清淡，勿进油腻，以免生痰。食品饭菜要多样化，以增进食欲。

（3）患儿体弱多汗，容易感冒，感冒后可重新出现痉挛性咳嗽。故出汗时要及时用毛巾擦干，避免受凉受寒。可适当活动，多晒太阳，增强体质.

6.8 小儿肺炎

肺炎是以发热、咳嗽、喘促为主要症状的一种呼吸道感染性疾病。四季皆可发生，冬春季节多见。年龄越小发病率越高，病情越严重。肺炎可为原发病，也可续发于其他疾病，如感冒、麻疹、百日咳，或某些重病久病的过程中。属中医学咳嗽、喘证及温病的范畴。

一般护理

1. 参照 6.1 儿科护理特点。

2. 做好呼吸道隔离。工作人员、探视者与患儿接触时应带口罩，防止交叉感染。

3. 病室要空气流通，湿润，温度适宜。注意空气消毒，每日可用紫外线照射 1 次。

4. 卧床休息，保持安静状态，以减少机体耗氧量和防止心力衰竭发生。避免过多的检查，治疗与护理要集中进行，以免影响患儿休息和睡眠。定时更换体位，轻拍背部，以减轻肺部瘀血及痰液阻塞气道。

5. 饮食宜清淡，给予富有营养易于消化的流质、半流质，多饮水。忌食油腻、辛辣刺激性食物。

6. 注意口腔护理，经常用厚朴煎汤或淡盐水清洁口腔。

7. 保持呼吸道通畅。鼻腔、口腔分泌物较多者，要及时清除鼻痂、鼻涕及口腔积物。痰多者，鼓励儿童咳嗽排痰；经常翻身拍背，以助排痰。必要时用吸痰器吸出。痰粘稠不易咳出者，可用小儿清肺雾化剂，做超声雾化吸入，使痰液稀释便于排出，改善通气功能。注意检查插管给氧的鼻导管是否通畅。

8. 密切观察患儿面色，体温，呼吸，脉象和心率，在短时间内肝脏大小的变化，咳嗽、痰喘的轻重，神志的改变及有无抽搐等，以便早期发现心衰、脑炎等并发症。

辨证护理

1. 风邪犯肺证。肺炎的初期，根据受邪的不同，可分风寒闭肺和风热闭肺。

(1) 风寒闭肺证

临床表现

发热无汗，咳嗽气促，痰白稀，口不渴。舌苔薄白，舌质正常，脉浮紧。此证多见于寒冷季节。

护理

①注意保暖，随气温的变化及时增减衣服和调节室内温度。

②服辛温宣肺药物，方选华盖散加减。汤药趁热服。服药后继进热饮或热粥，并稍加盖衣被，使全身微微汗出。注意观察出汗情况。

③高热时，可针刺大椎、曲池、合谷等穴。慎用物理降温，以免影响病邪由表外达。

④可用艾条温灸肺俞、大椎穴，以温肺散寒。

⑤忌食生冷瓜果等凉性食物。

(2) 风热闭肺证

临床表现

发热有汗，口渴，咳嗽吐黄稠痰，气促鼻煽，面赤唇红，大便干结或伴有粘液。舌苔黄，舌质红，脉浮数。

护理

①室内应适当通风，衣被适中，不宜过暖。

②服辛凉解表，宣肺化痰药物，方选麻杏石甘汤加减。服药后宜微汗出。

③高热、口渴者，可多饮梨汁、荸荠汁，配合针刺降温（取穴同（1）风寒闭肺证）。

④咳嗽，痰黄稠，可配用竹叶、鲜芦根煎水代茶饮，或用去皮梨1个，川贝粉6克，蜂蜜适量拌匀蒸熟取汁频服。

⑤大便秘结者，用大黄片，或番泻叶开水冲泡代茶饮。

2. 痰热闭肺证

临床表现

壮热烦躁，咳嗽，痰黄粘，不易咳出，面赤口渴。气促，鼻翼煽动，甚则抬肩撷肚而喘，口周紫绀。大便干结或稀臭，小便甚少。舌苔黄，质红，脉洪数。易伴发心衰、脑病等兼证。为肺炎极期。

护理

(1) 服清热泻肺平喘止咳药物，方选清肺饮加减。汤药宜冷服。

(2) 饮食给予清淡的流质、半流质，不宜食过甜的食物和饮料，以免助湿生痰。可多吃橘子、枇杷、梨、西瓜等水果或果汁，以助清肺热养阴化痰。

(3) 体温超过39℃以上者，应绝对卧床休息。多饮水。用温水或30%温酒精擦浴，前额冷敷；或用针刺降温（取穴同(1) 风寒闭肺证）。若伴惊惕给五粒回春丹3～5粒，1次化服，或服紫雪丹0.5～2克，1次冲服.

(4) 患儿咳喘，口周微青，可间断吸氧，或用冷空气疗法。若见气喘急剧，鼻煽，面色紫绀，呼吸严重困难时，应持续吸氧，取半卧位或给予高枕静卧，以利呼吸，减轻喘憋现象。

（5）肺热咳嗽痰喘，或痰黄粘咳出不利者，应加强祛痰措施。可服鲜竹沥水、喘咳散，或用喘咳散加醋外敷涌泉、肠俞穴。亦可用青萝卜切丝，煮水加蜂蜜适量频饮。

（6）腹胀者，多属肠腑气机不利，可用大黄粉加蜂蜜调匀外敷腹部，或用松节油涂腹，肛管排气，减轻腹胀，有利调整呼吸。

（7）对危重患儿要随时巡视，加强观察。特别注意心阳虚，内闭外脱，邪陷心包等危症的发生。若患儿呼吸困难突然加重，烦躁不安，或精神不振，面色苍白或紫绀，汗出肢凉，脉微细数，心率加快达 160～200 次／分以上，肝脏增大，是伴发心阳虚衰。应立即配合医生处理。急服参附龙牡救逆汤或生脉散，注意保暖，艾条灸气海、关元、神阙穴，以温补心阳，救逆固脱，或用生脉注射液 10～20ml，枳实注射液 5～10ml，加 5～10% 葡萄糖注射液稀释后静推或静滴。宜早期应用强心剂。

3. 正虚邪恋证

临床表现

咳嗽痰喘迁延日久不清，时因外感而加重。精神不振，面色发黄，食欲低下。咳嗽多痰，低热多汗。舌苔白,舌质偏红，脉细数。多见于肺炎恢复期。

护理

（1）恢复期患儿饮食应增加营养，饭菜多样化，以诱导食欲。可多食水果、蔬菜，添加奶类、蛋类、鱼类、瘦肉等，以健脾益精，阴不足，宜食百合红枣汤。多给荔枝,枇杷、梨子、橘子等，以养肺生津止咳。

（2）服益气养阴清肺化痰药物，方选补中益气汤合沙参麦冬汤加减。

（3）患儿可适当进行活动,以调整气血循环，有利排痰，健脾，增强体质。但活动时间要适度。气候适宜时，可做户外活动，多晒太阳。注意预防感冒及交叉感染。

(4) 慢性、迁延性肺炎，肺部湿罗音经久不消或肺部拍片病灶久不吸收者，可用物理疗法，如拔火罐、芥末泥敷胸、超短波、紫外线照射等，促进病变吸收。

6.9 支气管哮喘

支气管哮喘是以反复发作性呼吸困难，呼气延长，伴哮鸣音为特点的一种呼吸道疾病。婴幼儿期即可发病，一般多见于4～5岁以上的儿童。属中医学哮证范畴。

一般护理

1. 参照6.1儿科护理特点。

2. 保持病室安静，温、湿度适宜而稳定。环境力求简单，禁止吸烟及摆放有刺激气味的花草、药物等。

3. 注意保暖，防止感冒。在气温转冷时，及时增减衣服。尤须注意颈项部如天突、百劳、肺俞等处的保暖。

4. 饮食宜清淡，进食不宜过饱。发作期，勿食过甜过咸及生冷之品；缓解期，给予富有营养，容易消化吸收的食物，避免给诱发哮喘发作的食物，如奶、蛋、鱼、虾等。忌食油腻、辛辣刺激性食物。

5. 哮喘发作时卧床，取半卧位或给予高枕，保持体位舒适。要安慰患儿，消除恐惧心理，避免哭闹加重病情。缓解期可适当活动。

6. 患儿呼吸困难时，可间断吸氧或用洋金花液雾化吸入，以缓解支气管痉挛。要保持呼吸道通畅，注意口腔卫生。

7. 若发作严重，喘甚欲脱，出现喘促出汗，面色、唇、甲紫绀征、肢冷、脉细等，应立即吸氧，可急服参附汤以回阳固脱。报告医生并做好抢救的准备。

8. 观察病情

(1) 一般观察哮喘发作时间，轻重程度，咳痰难易及痰液性质，面色，出汗等变化。

(2) 观察发作前先兆，如患儿感到胸部发紧，呼吸不畅，喉部发痒，干咳等，做到早期发现及时处理，可减轻或控制发作。如哮喘有规律，可在发作前1～2小时服药，有利减轻或缓解症状。

(3) 观察诱发因素，如情志抑郁，气候骤变，或吸入粉尘，接触花粉、绒毛、煤气、油漆等，寻找过敏源，以避免诱发哮喘，或缓图根治。

9. 哮喘菌苗：国内自制三联哮喘菌苗，一般每周用1次，或用长效剂型，每3～4周1次，直至不再发作。

辨证护理

1. 发作期

部分病人发作时，先突然出现鼻塞、喷嚏、喉痒、胸闷等先兆症状，继而哮喘发作。部分病人无先兆症状，骤然咳嗽喘促，呼吸困难，不得平卧，随呼气喉间发出哮鸣声。有寒哮、热哮的区分。

(1) 寒哮证 (冷哮)

临床表现

突然哮喘，伴面色灰黄，咳嗽气促，喉间哮鸣，鼻塞，语声重浊，痰白稀多沫，口不渴或喜热饮，无汗。舌苔白滑，脉浮紧。

护理

①寒哮多在春秋季节发病，邪为风寒，遇冷加重。注意保暖，切勿受凉。室温宜偏高。通风换气时，勿吹向患儿。

②服宣肺、散寒止咳平喘药物，方选小青龙汤加减。汤药宜热服。可同时口服地龙粉，每次1～3克，每日3次，饭前吞服，以镇静，平喘。

③忌食生冷。

④哮喘发作期，可配合针灸、耳穴压豆、拔火罐等疗法，以控制症状。发作时，针刺定喘、解喘、天突、大椎等穴位，每日1次。哮喘严重者，可用艾条灸肺俞、大椎穴，并配合拔火罐。拔火罐：取平喘穴，先针刺后拔罐，双侧交替治疗，日1次，每次10分钟。注意拔罐时间勿长，以免皮肤起泡。耳穴压豆：选用喘点、内分泌、平喘穴。可治疗各型哮喘。

以上方法可任选一种，或交替使用。

⑤哮喘发作后，咳嗽吐痰清稀，色白多沫者，可服用冷哮丸，温肺化痰，缓图根治。

(2) 热哮证（痰热哮）

临床表现

突然哮喘，伴面色红晦，咳嗽喘促，喉间痰鸣，胸高气粗，烦闷不安，痰稠色黄，或质粘咳出不利。口渴喜饮，出汗。舌苔黄腻，脉滑数。

护理

①室温宜偏低。患儿出汗时应随时擦干，及时更换汗湿的衣服，以防受凉。

②服清热化痰止咳平喘药物，方选定喘汤加减。同时可加服白果10克，水煎服，日3次，以养肺益肾纳气。

③痰黄稠咳出不利者，可轻拍其背部，并服蛇胆川贝液或鲜竹沥水等中成药，化痰止咳。

④发作期，可用冰片3克，调凡士林50克，敷贴膻中穴。针灸、耳穴压豆、拔火罐等疗法同 (1) 寒哮证。

2. 缓解期

反复发作的哮喘症状消失，即进入缓解期。此期的长短，与个体的正气虚实，肺、脾、肾三脏功能的平衡与协调，以及气候的转变有直接关系。

临床表现

多见身体瘦弱，咳嗽痰多，动则短气喘促，食少，乏力或畏寒，大便稀软，或手足心热，夜间盗汗。舌质淡，苔少，脉沉细。

护理

(1) 服益肾健脾补肺药物，方选金匮肾气丸合玉屏风散加减。手、足心热，夜间盗汗阴虚者，服六味地黄丸合玉屏风散加减，兼服紫合车丸。

(2) 敷贴法：用白芥子 3 克，细辛 0.6 克，胡椒 1 克，白附子 1 克，共研细末，用生姜汁调匀敷于肺俞穴，每晚睡前敷上，次日晨取下。如局部反应重时，亦可敷 1～2 小时取下。1～2 日进行 1 次，7 次为 1 疗程。

(3) 注意寒暖适宜，劳逸结合，适当进行户外锻炼活动，多接触新鲜空气及阳光，增强体质，以减少发作。

6.10 口腔炎

口腔炎是以口腔粘膜、舌及齿龈发生充血，疱疹，糜烂，溃疡，坏死或滋生痂膜等病变为特点的口腔疾病。可为原发性疾病，也可呈继发性存在。中医学有口疮、口疳、走马疳之分，一般统称为口疮。

一般护理

1. 注意口腔清洁。一般常用淡盐水漱、洗口腔，日 3～4 次。口腔粘膜糜烂、溃疡者，用苏叶、厚扑煎汤清洗口腔。

2. 防止交叉感染，口腔护理用具必须消毒，每人一套。做护理前后要洗净双手，患儿的奶瓶、奶头、餐具等，每用一次必须洗净消毒。指导乳母注意哺乳卫生，喂奶前先洗手，后用酒精棉球洗擦乳头，再进行哺乳。多次喂水，以代清洗口腔。

3. 饮食宜清淡，避免过酸，过咸及刺激性食品，以减少进食痛苦。母乳喂养者，母亲忌食辛辣、酒类等刺激性食物。患儿常因口腔疼痛而拒食，护理人员应耐心地喂饭。

辨证护理

1. 心脾郁热

临床表现

口舌红赤，溃烂成疮，口臭疼痛，流涎拒食，哭闹不安。大便干结，小便短赤。舌质红，舌苔黄腻而厚，脉滑数。

护理

(1) 服清热泻火药物，方选清热泻脾散加减。汤药宜冷服。

(2) 外治法：口舌红赤溃烂成疮者，轻症用冰硼散、蜂蜜调成糊状搽口腔患处，重症用锡类散、珠黄散、青黛散涂口腔。可配用吴茱萸15克，研为细末，醋调敷足心，12小时除去。涂药时要看清病变部位，注意观察原有疮面有无好转和是否有新的病变发生。口腔涂药后半小时内勿进水和食物等。

(3) 大便干结者，可多饮淡盐水，亦可多吃香蕉和蜂蜜，以润肠通便。

2. 虚火上炎

临床表现

口舌生疮，疮面充血，疼痛及口臭皆轻微，但经久不愈，或反复发作长久不息。心烦口干，颧红盗汗，手足心热。舌红苔少，脉细数。

护理

(1) 服养阴清热，活血生肌敛口药物，方选知柏地黄汤加减。

(2) 外治法，同心脾郁热。配用生附子粉3～5克，用醋调匀，贴于一侧足心，以引火归元。

(3) 对急性热病，久病，久泻的患儿加强护理，经常检查口腔。若出现破损应及时涂搽凉心散。积极防治全身疾病，增强小儿体质。

3. 鹅口疮

临床表现

口腔粘膜及舌上满布如凝乳块状的白屑，可互相融合，不易拭去，重拭可见潮红粗糙的粘膜面，不痛，白屑周围绕以红晕，其他症状表现较少。

护理

基本同 6.10 口腔炎的护理

(1) 外用药可选用硼砂水洗口腔后涂芒硝、川扑粉，日 3～4 次。

(2) 本证也可延至食道、气管，影响吞咽及呼吸，延及肠道可引起腹泻。注意观察患儿呼吸、吮乳及大便情况。

(3) 本病多起伏迁延，经久不愈，故应加强食具、用具消毒处理。

6.11 小儿腹泻

小儿腹泻是以大便次数增多，便质稀薄为主要症状的消化道疾病，四季皆有，但以夏秋季多见，中医称泄泻。小儿脾胃功能较成人薄弱，所以泄泻的发病率高于成人。年龄越小发病率越高，病情转变也越快，易出现伤阴伤阳的变证。

一般护理

1. 参照 6.1 儿科护理特点。

2. 注意饮食调养，以控制饮食为主。对轻症宜适当减少食量，或延长喂奶时间。对重症及兼有频吐者，初起即需禁食 8～12 小时，禁食期间可少量多次喂水或淡米汤。解除禁食后，可给少量乳汁或浓米汤等易于消化的食物。饮食应从少量渐加到多量，由流质到半流质，随着病情好转，采取先稀后干，先少后多，先素后荤的供食原则来调摄饮食。忌食油腻、生冷及不易消化的食物。各型泄泻皆应多饮水、米汤、山楂汤、乌梅汤或口服补液盐水（配方：氯化钠 3.5 克、碳酸氢钠 2.5 克、氯化钾 1.5

克、葡萄糖 20 克，溶于 1000ml 米汤中或用水代汤），以补阴液。

3. 做好床边隔离。护理患儿后要洗手，食具、尿布等要消毒处理。

4. 保持口腔清洁湿润，防止并发口疮、鹅口疮。可用金银花水或淡盐水清洗口腔，涂以消毒的植物油或冰硼油。伤阴脱水及张口睡眠的小儿，口、鼻覆盖双层湿纱布，时时更换，以保持口、鼻腔粘膜湿润。

5. 保持臀部清洁，干燥，勤换尿布。便后用温水洗臀，以软布轻轻擦干，涂上油脂保护皮肤。若已发生臀红，用解毒敛口燥湿的药物，如黄连水局部洗浴，拭干后，轻者扑松花粉、炉甘石粉，重者用紫草油、蛋黄油外涂，或曝晒臀部，或用红外线烘烤局部湿疹面，促使干燥，生肌敛口。

6. 有呕吐的患儿，取侧卧位或半卧位，防止呕吐物吸入气管引起窒息。频吐者，口服玉枢丹、姜汁，可针灸或推拿内关、合谷穴止吐。

7. 腹痛阵作者，可用针灸疗法，取足三里、中脘、天枢穴，灸长强。婴幼儿可行推拿、捏脊疗法，贴胃安膏，或腹部放热痛灵，要注意局部皮肤的反应，勿起烫伤。

8. 观察病情：注意观察呕吐和腹泻的次数、量、气味及性质，观察腹胀、腹痛及进食情况，有无伤阴、伤阳证。

辨证护理

1. 湿热泻
临床表现
泄泻便次频繁，便色黄或黄褐，便质如糊状或蛋花汤样，每次便量较多，便味臭浊。便后肛门热痛，肛周皮肤红晕，尿短赤。多伴有呕吐，兼有腹胀，腹痛，口渴喜饮,或伴发热。舌苔黄腻，脉滑数。

护理

(1) 服清热利湿理气和胃药物，方选葛根芩连汤加减。药汁浓煎，少量多次喂服，防止呕吐。

(2) 饮食调养按一般护理。

(3) 湿热泻，易致肛周皮肤红晕，要做好臀部护理。

(4) 重症泄泻腹胀者（中毒性肠麻痹），可用皮硝30克，或大黄粉加蜂蜜外敷脐部。注意补钾。

(5) 婴幼儿可兼用葎草30～60克，煎水泡足，日2～3次，每次15～20分钟。

(6) 推拿：清脾胃、清大肠、清小肠、退六腑、揉天枢、揉龟尾，以清热利湿，调中止泻。

2. 寒湿泻

临床表现

便色淡黄或淡褐，大便清稀多泡沫，臭味较轻。腹胀腹痛明显。口渴不欲饮，或兼有发热恶寒的表现。

护理

(1) 服温中散寒，理气止痛药物，方选和气饮加减。汤药宜热服。服药后安卧，并加盖衣被。

(2) 兼有发热恶寒，咳嗽，流涕等外感表证者，要卧床休息，注意保暖。可用艾条灸大椎、神阙穴，加用散寒解表药。

(3) 腹胀痛者，应温经散寒，理气止痛。可用外治法：给予腹部热熨，可用盐熨法（参照4.8急性阑尾炎护理），或用葱姜泥敷脐；也可顺时针按摩神阙穴；或用艾条灸足三里、中脘、气海、三阴交穴；用食盐填脐中，隔姜灸。灸时防止烫伤。

(4) 饮食调养除按一般护理要求外，宜食辛温及温热食品，以助温中散寒。如温饮生姜红糖水、稀藕粉等。

(5) 推拿：补脾经、推三关、补大肠、揉外劳、揉脐、推上七节骨、揉龟尾、按揉足三里。

3. 伤食泻

临床表现

便色黄或褐，便质粗糙杂有未消化的食物，味酸臭，嗳气及呕吐物亦酸馊腐臭。腹痛阵作，腹胀欲呕，吐泻之后腹痛随减。厌食，有伤食史。舌苔黄腻垢浊，脉滑数。

护理

(1) 节食和胃是护理要点。服消食和胃的保和丸，以消积食而止泻。积不除泻不止，故积食未除尽者，禁用固涩止泻药，积在胃者，可用压舌板探吐。

(2) 发病后禁食 4~8 小时，尔后给予稀软易于消化的流质，忌食油腻及生冷食品。宜食山楂汁，麦芽、谷芽汤和焦米稀饭汤，以助消化。

(3) 用吴茱萸 30 克、丁香 2 克、胡椒 30 粒，研末，每次用药 1.5 克，用陈醋调成糊状，敷脐部。

(4) 推拿：补脾经、清大肠、揉板门、运内八卦、揉中脘、摩腹、揉天枢、揉龟尾。或用捏脊法，以调理脾胃功能。

4. 脾虚泻

临床表现

泄泻日久不愈，或反复发作不止。便色黄或绿，便质稀薄或粗糙不成形。面色萎黄，肢冷，肌肤松弛，睡时目闭露睛。或进餐后即便，便质粗糙。舌质淡，苔薄白，脉沉少力。

护理

(1) 饮食除按一般护理要求调理外，应注意补脾益气。可给予莲子、山药、苡仁、红枣、扁豆粥。进食要有规律，定时定量勿过饱，不宜吃甜食及冷食。

(2) 服温中健脾益气止泻药物，方选参苓白术散加减。

(3) 久泻身冷肢凉为阳气不足，要注意保暖，特别是下肢保暖，可加用盐附子捣烂，合肉桂末，或吴茱萸粉加面粉调匀，敷手足心，以温阳止泻。

(4) 推拿：补脾经、补大肠、推三关、摩腹、揉脐、推上七节骨，揉龟尾、捏脊。

5. 伤阴伤阳。泄泻皆能伤阴伤阳。暴泻以伤阴为主，久泻以伤阳为主。但阴阳互根，相依并存，伤阴者必伤阳，伤阳者亦必伤阴，故症状往往交互并存而又有所偏重。

(1) 伤阴证

临床表现

眼窝及前囟凹陷,皮肤干涩，弹性减退，心烦，口渴，尿少。重者啼哭无泪，无尿，口唇樱红色，呼吸深快，或呈叹息样呼吸。兼有抽风。舌苔干燥，脉沉细数。

(2) 伤阳证

临床表现

精神萎靡，面色苍白或㿠白，目闭露睛，四肢软弱无力，是腹泻伤气伤阳的早期表现。出现表情淡漠，四肢不温，皮肤发花，呼吸表浅发凉，为阳脱证。脉微弱。

临床上多见伤阴、伤阳证同时并存，所不同者仅是各自呈现的程度有差异。

护理

①以伤阴为主者，在原证所用方剂中加乌梅、石斛、天冬、麦冬、五味子、人参。以伤阳为主者，在原证所用方剂中加人参、附子、五味子、麦冬。呈现阴竭阳脱者，采用中西医结合方法，救阴固脱。

②抽风者，应熄风镇惊。针刺人中、十宣、涌泉穴。能吞咽者口服蝎尾粉镇痉。

③体温不升者，保温，并隔姜灸气海。

6.12 营养不良症

营养不良症是以面黄肌瘦，毛发枯稀，饮食异常，精神疲惫为主要症状的一种脾胃虚损证。属中医学疳症范畴。

一般护理

1. 参照 6.1 儿科护理特点。

2. 加强生活护理，按时令气温及时增减衣服及调节室温，以免感受六淫时邪。预防交叉感染。

3. 根据患儿年龄、病情选择食物品种，合理喂养。乳儿的母乳不足或无母乳，可给牛奶、羊奶、豆奶或豆浆及代乳品。喂养要定质、定量、定时。增加辅食，要掌握先稀后干，先少后多的原则。随患儿消化能力的提高，应相应增加食量和进餐次数。纠正小儿偏食、挑食的不良饮食习惯。对无食欲的患儿，要耐心喂养，并及时寻找和纠正其厌食的原因。增加适当的活动量，以改善食欲。

4. 寻求导致营养不良症的病因，针对病因可进行推拿或捏脊疗法。有营养素不足症表现者，给予针对性的补充。

5. 每周测体重两次，并做记录，比较体重增长情况，以便分析病情。

6. 掌握患儿心理活动，解除精神因素对食欲的不良影响。

7. 做好口腔、眼睛护理，每日用淡盐水或紫苏叶水清洁口腔，防止发生口腔炎。如已发生齿龈出血，溃烂，口舌生疮者，可涂锡类散或珠黄散。每日用生理盐水棉球清拭眼睛。注意预防眼睛的并发症，及维生素缺乏症。

8. 适当进行户外活动，多晒太阳，增强体质。经常进行四肢按摩，或用温淡硫磺水擦浴。

9. 注意观察并发症。在营养不良的基础上，常伴随一种或多种营养素的缺乏症，或因抵抗力低下，时常受外邪干扰，因此要经常检查患儿，及时发现及时纠正。

10. 要向家长宣传合理的喂养方法及添加辅助食品的知识，指导家长培养儿童良好的饮食习惯。

辨证护理

1. 脾气虚弱型

临床表现

面色萎黄，毛发稀疏，形体消瘦。厌食纳呆，脘腹胀满，手足心热，烦躁不宁，舌苔薄白,脉沉滑。

护理

(1) 服健脾益气，消积和胃药物，方选参苓白术散加减。

(2) 饮食调养，应多进益气健脾消食的食物，如山药粥、黄芪粥、莲子粥等。另外给予足够的蛋白质、碳水化合物及维生素。蛋白质以奶、蛋、禽、鱼类为好；碳水化合物以谷类为佳。

(3) 脘腹胀满，用揉腹、捏脊法调整胃肠功能，以消积理气，宽肠行大便。

2. 气血两虚型

临床表现

面色萎黄，肌肤消瘦，毛发焦稀，头大颈细，腹凹如舟，懒言少语，表情呆滞。发育迟缓或停滞。舌质淡，舌苔薄腻，脉沉细。

护理

(1) 加强饮食调理，除按脾气虚弱型调理饮食外，可给浓缩的鸡汤、鱼汤、甲鱼汤、人参粥、燕窝粥等以补其精。此型患儿病情复杂，常表现顽固的食欲不振，故要耐心喂养。因其消化力弱，所以喂养时采用少量多餐法为宜。注意观察大便，以了解消化功能。

(2) 本型病情较重，气血皆虚，故服补气养血健脾和胃药物，方选人参养荣汤加减。辅以小儿升血灵。

(3) 做各种操作时，动作要轻柔，尤其是重症营养不良患儿，以防引起突然的心衰暴脱。

6.13 肾病综合征

肾病综合征，临床以全身浮肿，大量蛋白尿，低蛋白血症，血胆固醇增高为特点。多见于 3～8 岁儿童。属中医学水肿的阴水范畴。

一般护理

1. 参照 6.1 儿科护理特点。

2. 浮肿期患儿应卧床休息，浮肿严重者应绝对卧床。如有胸水、腹水而致胸闷、气促者，可取半卧位。浮肿减轻后可适当活动，但不宜活动过度，以免劳复。

3. 饮食原则：给予高蛋白、高热量、低脂肪及维生素丰富，易于消化的清淡食物。水肿期应限制钠盐和水的摄入。对水肿兼尿少的患儿，给予无盐饮食。小便增多，水肿消退后，给低盐饮食。但不宜长期忌盐。长期忌盐不仅可减低食欲，又可因低钠血症加重水肿及影响患儿的生长发育。可酌情增加瘦肉、蛋类、乳品等，以补充由尿丢失的蛋白。也可用莲子、茯苓、山药煮粥，以助补益之力。也可用鲤鱼 1 条约 250 克，赤小豆 50克，砂仁 10 克，煮熟食用，对利水消蛋白有一定的作用。

4. 防止感染及复发。由于患儿精微外泄——大量蛋白由尿中排出，气血两虚，身体抵抗外邪的能力减低，易发生上呼吸道、皮肤感染和传染病等。此类感染性疾病，大多数又可导致本病的加重或复发。故应做好预防及必要的隔离工作，彻底治疗感染病灶。

5. 注意皮肤护理。每日用荆芥煎水或用 30%酒精擦拭皮肤，以保持皮肤清洁及气血流畅，促进散瘀消肿；衣服应轻软、宽松；被褥、床辅要清洁、干燥、松软。尽量避免肌肉注射，因严重水肿可使药物滞留或吸收不佳。久病卧床者，每日要多翻身，防止发生积坠性水肿及褥疮。

6. 保持口腔清洁。用厚朴水擦拭或漱口。注意消除咽喉、牙、龈等处的感染病灶。

7. 记出入量。浮肿及利尿期每天记录出入量，并留尿送常规化验。每周测量体重、腹围及血压2～3次。

辨证护理

1. 湿热型

临床表现

发热，咽喉肿痛或皮肤生疮疡。全身浮肿，口渴但不欲饮，尿少色黄。舌苔黄厚，脉滑数。

护理

(1) 服清热解毒利湿药物，方选五味消毒饮加减，水肿明显者加用鲜玉米须60～120克，水煎服，或多吃西瓜、冬瓜，以祛湿，利水，消肿。

(2) 卧床休息或减少活动，以减轻肾脏负担是首要事项。血压偏高者，应注意降压。并观察体温、血压、小便的变化。

(3) 消除病灶是早期治疗护理的重要环节。咽喉肿痛者，局部用锡类散、珠黄散吹喉，或用清咽雾化液，做雾化吸入，以消肿散结止痛；也可用开水泡双花、桔梗、麦冬代茶饮，以利咽喉。皮肤疮疡者参照外科4.1疖治疗、护理。

2. 脾肾两虚型

临床表现

面色苍白，全身浮肿以下肢较重，呈凹陷性，倦怠少力，脘腹胀闷，大便溏薄。舌苔白，脉沉细。

护理

(1) 服温阳行水药物，方选实脾饮加减。配服五苓散，增强利尿作用。

(2) 高度浮肿者绝对卧床。可用赤小豆30克，黑豆30克，加水煮后全食之，以助利尿；浮肿以下肢较重者，可将小腿适当抬高，以利消肿；严重浮肿者，两腿、臀部用软枕垫高，阴囊用三角巾吊起，可避免磨损皮肤和下肢性水肿加重。血浆蛋白低者，静脉输血浆或血浆蛋白，饮食选鸡汤、甲鱼汤、牛奶等优质蛋白食品，增加血浆蛋白。

(3) 脘腹胀闷者，饮食宜少量多次摄入。腹部可做热敷，取半卧位。

3. 肝肾阴虚型

临床表现

浮肿尿少，头痛、头晕，心烦少寐，腰膝酸软。舌苔少或薄白，脉弦细。

护理

(1) 服滋阴潜阳药物，方选杞菊地黄汤加减。

(2) 饮食可选择一些淡渗、利湿之品，以增进治疗。如食用黄芪加苡米煮粥，可加强渗湿利尿作用。可食黑木耳、甲鱼、肝类，以补阴虚。

(3) 心烦少眠者，可针刺安眠、神门穴，或晚上睡前食牛奶适量，有助眠作用。

(4) 注意观察血压变化。若血压升高或持续高压，每日测血压两次。头晕者服脑立清。多吃芹菜、山楂等，以助降压，进低盐饮食。同时配合耳穴压豆，取神门、交感穴。

6.14 遗尿

遗尿是指 3 岁以上的儿童，经常反复发生睡中遗尿，醒后方知的一种疾病，也称尿床。轻者数夜遗尿 1 次，重者一夜数次，或入睡即遗，午睡也可发生。3 岁以下小儿，脏腑功能发育尚属不足，言语、动作的表达能力及自控能力发育不全，虽有遗尿，不属病态。

一般护理

1. 睡眠时侧卧位为宜，可使腹壁肌肉松弛，以减轻对膀胱的压力。床铺被褥薄厚适宜，脚不宜过暖或受压过重。

2. 对较大儿童，给予精神护理，耐心教育和诱导，消除患儿紧张、羞怯的心理状态，建立战胜疾病的信心。

3. 尿床后及时更换衣被，保持皮肤清洁干燥及温暖。

4. 汤药在白天服完。晚餐宜给干食为主，饭后控制饮水量。睡前让患儿排空小便。

5. 观察小儿排尿时间，掌握规律，按时唤醒，敦促排尿。

6. 平时生活应有规律，白天不宜过度玩耍，精神不宜过度兴奋或紧张，以免因疲劳贪睡或自控力失衡而遗尿。要培养晚间自行排尿的习惯。

7. 用氦-氖激光仪刺激肾俞、中极及夜尿穴（手针）。耳穴压豆取肾俞、膀胱、皮质下。

8. 注意全身情况，排除神经系、内分泌系、泌尿系疾病，分清为原发性或继发性（症状）遗尿。

辨证护理

1. 下元虚寒证
临床表现
遗尿发作较频，病程较长，多甜睡不易唤醒，手足偏凉，怕冷，喜静少动，小便清长。舌苔薄白，脉沉迟。
护理
(1) 服温肾固涩药物，方选巩堤丸加减。汤药宜热服。
(2) 平时给红枣、莲子、芡实煮粥食，或用狗肉250克、黑豆100克共煮，肉汤顿服，以温补肾气。
(3) 针灸：针刺百会、中极、三阴交穴，灸关元。
(4) 验方：用鸡肠一具（烧存性）、牡蛎、茯苓、桑螵蛸各

16 克，肉桂、龙骨各 8 克，共为细末，每服 3～4 克，日 2～3 次，以滋补肾气，收涩固摄；硫磺粉 10 克，葱根适量，共捣烂成泥状，加少许植物油，调匀敷脐部，3～5 日换药 1 次。

2. 脾肺虚寒证

临床表现

遗尿，面色苍黄，短气自汗，食欲不振，大便溏薄或食后即便，部分患儿易患感冒或昼间尿频。舌苔薄白，脉沉弱。

护理

(1) 服健脾益气固涩药物，方选补中益气汤加减。汤药宜热服。

(2) 平时常食用山楂、红枣、山药粥。或以猪膀胱一只，黄芪 60 克，同煨煮烂，分次吃完，以增强膀胱固摄功能。

(3) 大便溏薄，用炮姜加红糖煎服，以温脾去寒。

(4) 贴敷法：用五倍子、何首乌各 3 克，研末，用醋调敷于脐部，以纱布覆盖，每晚 1 次，连用 3～5 次。注意皮肤刺激反应。

(5) 遗尿频者，可针刺夜尿穴（在掌面小指、二指关节横纹处），或取阴陵泉、三阴交、关元、中极、肾俞穴。体虚者加灸。

(6) 平时加强体格锻炼，预防感冒，但勿过度疲劳。

3. 肝肾郁热证

临床表现

遗尿每夜多次，每次量少或滴沥而出，断断续续。情绪急躁，有夜游症。手足心热或兼盗汗。舌苔薄白或薄黄，脉细数。

护理

(1) 服滋阴泻火药物，方选知柏地黄丸加减。

(2) 每日晚睡前，洗涤外阴，擦干后涂以爽身粉，以减少外阴的刺激，防止手淫摩擦。勤换衬裤。

(3) 尿频量少，滴沥而出者，可针刺中极、横骨、三阴交、太冲穴。

(4) 可用桑螵蛸、益知仁、金樱子、补骨脂各 15 克，水煎服，以固肾涩尿。

(5) 中药穴位贴敷：麝香 3 克、蟾酥 2 克、桂枝、麻黄、雄黄、没药、乳香各 5 克，共研细末，贮瓶备用。同时，将药物加入适量酒精，调成糊状，贴敷在气海、中极、三阴交穴位上。3～4 日换药 1 次。

THE ENGLISH-CHINESE ENCYCLOPEDIA OF PRACTICAL TCM

(Booklist)

英汉实用中医药大全

(书目)

VOLUME	TITLE	书名
1	ESSENTIALS OF TRADITIONAL CHINESE MEDICINE	中医学基础
2	THE CHINESE MATERIA MEDICA	中药学
3	PHARMACOLOGY OF TRADITIONAL CHINESE MEDICAL FORMULAE	方剂学
4	SIMPLE AND PROVEN PRESCRIPTION	单验方
5	COMMONLY USED CHINESE PATENTMEDICINES	常用中成药
6	THERAPY OF ACUPUNCTURE AND MOXIBUSTION	针灸疗法
7	*TUINA* THERAPY	推拿疗法
8	MEDICAL *QIGONG*	医学气功
9	MAINTAINING YOUR HEALTH	自我保健
10	INTERNAL MEDICINE	内科学